T0329088

NEGATIVE AFFECTIVE STATES AND COGNITIVE IMPAIRMENTS IN NICOTINE DEPENDENCE

NEGATIVE AFFECTIVE STATES AND COGNITIVE IMPAIRMENTS IN NICOTINE DEPENDENCE

Edited by

F. SCOTT HALL

JARED W. YOUNG

ANDRE DER-AVAKIAN

AMSTERDAM • BOSTON • HEIDELBERG • LONDON
NEW YORK • OXFORD • PARIS • SAN DIEGO
SAN FRANCISCO • SINGAPORE • SYDNEY • TOKYO

Academic Press is an imprint of Elsevier

Academic Press is an imprint of Elsevier
125 London Wall, London EC2Y 5AS, United Kingdom
525 B Street, Suite 1800, San Diego, CA 92101-4495, United States
50 Hampshire Street, 5th Floor, Cambridge, MA 02139, United States
The Boulevard, Langford Lane, Kidlington, Oxford OX5 1GB, United Kingdom

Library of Congress Cataloging-in-Publication Data
A catalog record for this book is available from the Library of Congress

British Library Cataloguing-in-Publication Data
A catalogue record for this book is available from the British Library

ISBN: 978-0-12-802574-1

For information on all Academic Press publications
visit our website at https://www.elsevier.com/

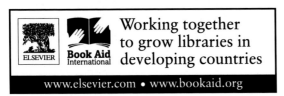

Working together
to grow libraries in
developing countries

www.elsevier.com • www.bookaid.org

Publisher: Mara Conner
Acquisition Editor: April Farr
Editorial Project Manager: Timothy Bennett
Production Project Manager: Karen East and Kirsty Halterman
Designer: Matthew Limbert

Typeset by TNQ Books and Journals

To Athina Markou,
a courageous leader, mentor, colleague, and friend,
whose tireless contributions to the field of nicotine research
paved the way for much of what is written in this book.

~ FSH, JWY, AD ~

Contents

14. Nicotine and Tobacco Smoking and Withdrawal in Schizophrenia
K. KOZAK AND T.P. GEORGE

15. Emergent Cognitive Impairment During Early Nicotine Withdrawal
R.M. SCHUSTER AND A.E. EVINS

16. Nicotine and Posttraumatic Stress Disorder
D.T. ACHESON AND D.E. GLENN

17. Nicotine Withdrawal and Depression: Clinical Studies—A Four-Factor Model for More Accurate Characterization
D.G. GILBERT AND M.L. PERGADIA

18. Neuroimaging Insights Into the Multifaceted Nature of the Nicotine Withdrawal Syndrome

M.T. SUTHERLAND, J.A. YANES AND E.A. STEIN

List of Contributors

D.T. Acheson University of California San Diego, La Jolla, CA, United States; VA San Diego Center for Excellence in Stress and Mental Health, San Diego, CA, United States

A.N. Anderson University of Houston-Clear Lake, Houston, TX, United States

Y. Arime Dokkyo Medical University School of Medicine, Mibu, Japan

A.W. Bruijnzeel University of Florida, Gainesville, FL, United States

D. Bruijnzeel University of Florida, Gainesville, FL, United States

A.R. Burns Yeshiva University, Bronx, NY, United States

L.M. Carcoba The University of Texas at El Paso, El Paso, TX, United States

H. Esan Yeshiva University, Bronx, NY, United States

A.E. Evins Massachusetts General Hospital, Boston, MA, United States

S.G. Ferguson University of Tasmania, Hobart, TAS, Australia

C.D. Fowler University of California Irvine, Irvine, CA, United States

M. Frandsen University of Tasmania, Hobart, TAS, Australia

O. George The Scripps Research Institute, La Jolla, CA, United States

T.P. George University of Toronto, Toronto, ON, Canada

D.G. Gilbert Southern Illinois University–Carbondale, Carbondale, IL, United States

D.E. Glenn University of California San Diego, La Jolla, CA, United States; VA San Diego Center for Excellence in Stress and Mental Health, San Diego, CA, United States

T.J. Gould Temple University, Philadelphia, PA, United States

P. Goyarzu University of Houston-Clear Lake, Houston, TX, United States

F.S. Hall University of Toledo, Toledo, OH, United States

E. Holliday Temple University, Philadelphia, PA, United States

G.F. Koob The Scripps Research Institute, La Jolla, CA, United States; National Institute on Drug Abuse, Baltimore, MD, United States; National Institute on Alcohol Abuse and Alcoholism, Rockville, MD, United States

K. Kozak University of Toronto, Toronto, ON, Canada

M.G. Kutlu Temple University, Philadelphia, PA, United States

D.H. Malin University of Houston-Clear Lake, Houston, TX, United States

M.E. McIlwain University of Auckland, Auckland, New Zealand; University of California San Diego, La Jolla, CA, United States

A. Minassian   University of California San Diego, La Jolla, CA, United States

L.E. O'Dell   The University of Texas at El Paso, El Paso, TX, United States

T. Ontiveros   The University of Texas at El Paso, El Paso, TX, United States

M.L. Pergadia   Florida Atlantic University, Boca Raton, FL, United States

W. Perry   University of California San Diego, La Jolla, CA, United States

J.A. Pipkin   The University of Texas at El Paso, El Paso, TX, United States

X. Qi   University of Florida, Gainesville, FL, United States

Y. Saber   University of Toledo, Toledo, OH, United States

T. Schneider   University of Central Lancashire, Preston, United Kingdom

R.M. Schuster   Massachusetts General Hospital, Boston, MA, United States

K.S. Segal   Yeshiva University, Bronx, NY, United States

S. Shiffman   University of Pittsburgh, Pittsburgh, PA, United States

M. Shoaib   Newcastle University, Newcastle, United Kingdom

I. Sora   Kobe University Graduate School of Medicine, Chuo-ku, Kobe, Japan

E.A. Stein   National Institute on Drug Abuse/NIH, Baltimore, MD, United States

M.T. Sutherland   Florida International University, Miami, FL, United States

M. Thorpe   University of Tasmania, Hobart, TAS, Australia

J. van Enkhuizen   Utrecht University, Utrecht, The Netherlands

A.H. Weinberger   Yeshiva University, Bronx, NY, United States

J.A. Yanes   Florida International University, Miami, FL, United States

J.W. Young   University of California San Diego, La Jolla, CA, United States; VA San Diego Healthcare System, San Diego, CA, United States

Preface

Addiction researchers have long struggled with the problem of notoriously low quit success rates for smokers (and those dependent on other drugs), associated with high rates of relapse. Despite increasing knowledge about the mechanisms underlying the positive reinforcing effects of nicotine over the past several decades, the effectiveness of treatments has improved only marginally.

In concordance with modest improvements in quit rates, there has been a paradigm shift within the field of addiction recognizing that different processes are involved in the initial phases of drug dependence than those in later phases. Many researchers have contributed to these ideas, but they are perhaps most associated with Dr. George Koob, whose chapter provides an introduction to these ideas and the framework for this book. Briefly, although initial drug taking may be driven by positive reinforcement and the initial desirable effects of nicotine, subsequent drug taking is driven more by negative reinforcement. The primary reasons for this shift are the neuroadaptations produced by extensive nicotine exposure resulting in nicotine tolerance and nicotine withdrawal. Affective and cognitive deficits are associated with nicotine withdrawal, which are then alleviated by subsequent drug taking, resulting in negative reinforcement. Hence, subsequent drug taking is driven more by negative reinforcement than positive reinforcement.

This type of drug taking can be described as self-medication for the negative consequences associated with nicotine withdrawal, as described in particular by Dr. Athina Markou and colleagues. This conception of nicotine self-medication in the face of affective and cognitive impairments suggests two rather important things about nicotine dependence: (1) if individuals have preexisting affective or cognitive impairments, even initial experiences with nicotine may produce negative reinforcement; and (2) there may be substantial heterogeneity of the primary reasons for smoking in the first place, eg, to alleviate different types of affective and cognitive impairments. A few years ago, the task of writing a review on animal models of nicotine dependence fell largely to one of us (FSH, along with co-authors Hall, Markou, Levin, and Uhl (2012)). In writing that review, he was struck by an odd feeling about the consequences of nicotine use: nicotine relieved anxiety and stress, and it improved mood; it had analgesic properties; it improved cognition, attention, and memory; it was a wonder drug! Of course, this had to be taken in the context of smoking being a leading cause of preventable death worldwide and massive health costs associated with nicotine dependence, but all of these positive effects of nicotine certainly spoke to the *reasons* why people smoked in the first place. Indeed, the *reasons* for smoking were often left out of considerations in nicotine research for why people began smoking, why people continued to smoke despite obvious health concerns, and why people relapsed to smoking when they attempted to quit.

Of course, as we have mentioned, many clinical and preclinical researchers have long been interested in the relationship between the affective and cognitive effects of nicotine, affective and cognitive symptoms of nicotine withdrawal, and affective and cognitive effects of nicotine use to alleviate withdrawal-induced impairments. What has grown out of these studies is an appreciation of the diverse effects of nicotine that may drive nicotine use in different individuals that may be more prone to certain effects, either based on premorbid impairments, impairments that emerge during withdrawal, or both. Moreover, quite different neural mechanisms (at biochemical, molecular, genetic, and anatomical levels) are involved in the diverse affective and cognitive effects of nicotine. This diversity may imply that quite different approaches may be necessary for effective treatment of nicotine dependence depending on the underlying causes, and that to develop these effective treatments, different experimental approaches will be necessary that address the various affective and cognitive domains involved.

In this book, we attempted to collect a representation of this work from among the leading researchers in the field of nicotine dependence, from both preclinical and clinical perspectives. It should be noted that these perspectives were initially developed as part of a symposium presented at the 2014 annual meeting of the International Behavioral Neuroscience Society and published initially as a summary review in a special issue of *Neuroscience and Biobehavioral Reviews* (Hall et al., 2015). Based on those initial ideas, we brought together the most representative group of leading researchers possible to summarize their work and the state of nicotine dependence research, going far beyond what was considered in that initial review, although the main idea and impetus remained the same. Indeed, overviews of this perspective are provided for preclinical studies by George Koob and Olivier George (Chapter 1), and for clinical studies by Mai Frandsen, Saul Shiffman and colleagues (Chapter 12) in this book, from whom many of these ideas originated. Consideration of preclinical models and findings in relation to different aspects of cognition are provided by Jared Young, Mohammed Shoaib, Thomas Gould, and their colleagues (Chapters 2–4). Consideration of different aspects of affective models and findings are considered by Adriaan Bruijnzeel, Christie Fowler, and colleagues (Chapters 10 and 11), as well interactions with other neurotransmitter systems that may affect multiple aspects of nicotine withdrawal and nicotine actions by Meghan McIlwain, David Malin, and colleagues (Chapters 8 and 9). Of particular interest in recent years has been that nicotine exposure early in life may affect the brain differently than nicotine later in life, and these issues are considered by Tomasz Schneider, Laura O'Dell, and colleagues (Chapters 5 and 6). Special attention to the genetic underpinnings and resulting genetic models of drug dependence is given by F. Scott Hall and colleagues (Chapter 7). The clinical counterpart of many of the preclinical affective and cognitive models discussed in earlier chapters involve different psychiatric comorbidities. These issues are considered specifically for schizophrenia, posttraumatic stress disorder, depression, and other conditions by Tony George, Karolina Kozak, Dean Acheson, David Gilbert, Michele Pergadia, Andrea Weinberger, and colleagues (Chapters 13, 14, 16, and 17). A broader perspective on cognitive impairments associated with nicotine withdrawal is given by Randi Schuster and Eden Evins (Chapter 15) and of imaging studies in nicotine dependence by Matthew Sutherland, Eliot Stein, and Julio Yanes (Chapter 18).

This work, covering such a range of preclinical and clinical research in nicotine dependence, naturally contains a broad perspective on this topic, with each of the authors certainly having their own unique perspectives. However, we (the editors) hope that part of what emerges from the collected work discussed in this book is that there are multiple causative factors that contribute to nicotine dependence and multiple reasons for people to initiate and maintain smoking behavior. Collectively, these issues will require different experimental approaches in preclinical models to facilitate research efforts and will require different therapeutic interventions to effectively treat nicotine dependence. We believe that the field is now sufficiently advanced to explicitly consider what the nature of these preclinical models should be and how these new therapies for nicotine dependence may be developed. Finally, given the substantial comorbidity of nicotine dependence with other psychiatric conditions, it is quite likely that this work will also have the additional benefit of contributing to our understanding and effective treatment of those conditions.

F. Scott Hall, Ph.D.
Jared W. Young, Ph.D.
Andre Der-Avakian, Ph.D.

References

Hall, F. S., Der-Avakian, A., Gould, T. J., Markou, A., Shoaib, M., & Young, J. W. (2015). Negative affective states and cognitive impairments in nicotine dependence. *Neurosci Biobehavr, 58,* 168–185.

Hall, F. S., Markou, A., Levin, E. D., & Uhl, G. R. (2012). Mouse models for studying genetic influences on factors determining smoking cessation success in humans. *Annals of the New York Academy of Sciences, 1248,* 39–70.

Acknowledgments

The editors would first like to thank the contributors to this book, without whom this book would not have been possible. We would also like to acknowledge the contributions of the editorial staff at Elsevier, especially Tim Bennett, and express our appreciation for their patience through the long process of producing this book. Additionally, we would like to thank our mentors, both past and present, who have contributed to our academic development, resulting in the opportunity to bring this work together. These mentors include Athina Markou, Mark Geyer, Hugh Marston, Ros Brett, Steven Maier, James Stellar, Ann Kelley, Trevor Robbins, Markku Linnoila, and George Uhl. Our thoughts and ideas that lead to the initial concepts behind this book are the direct result of the scientific and intellectual heritage that was passed to us by these great scientists, to whom we owe a great debt, one that can only be paid in full by passing on that heritage to our own students in turn. We would also like to acknowledge the International Behavioral Neuroscience Society (IBNS), without whom we would not have met on this topic, nor we would have discussed its production with Elsevier. The initial ideas that lead to the development of this book were presented as a symposium at the 2014 annual meeting of IBNS. Finally, we hope that future researchers will be inspired by this work to develop the novel personalized therapeutics required for the successful treatment of nicotine dependence in all individuals.

1

Overview of Nicotine Withdrawal and Negative Reinforcement (Preclinical)

O. George[1], G.F. Koob[1,2,3]

[1]The Scripps Research Institute, La Jolla, CA, United States; [2]National Institute on Drug Abuse, Baltimore, MD, United States; [3]National Institute on Alcohol Abuse and Alcoholism, Rockville, MD, United States

INTRODUCTION

Studies on the neurobiological substrates of tobacco addiction largely depend on the availability of suitable animal models. In this review, we first describe the features of tobacco smoking and nicotine abuse and dependence in humans and animal models. We then discuss the roles of positive and negative reinforcement in nicotine use and dependence. Lastly, we provide an overview of the possible neurobiological mechanisms of nicotine that underlie positive and negative reinforcement.

TOBACCO DEPENDENCE AND NICOTINE

Tobacco smoking is the leading avoidable cause of disease and premature death in the United States, and it is responsible for over 480 000 deaths annually (Agaku, King, & Dube, 2014) and USD$289 billion in direct healthcare costs and productivity losses each year. Smoking is implicated in ~70% of deaths from lung cancer, ~80% of deaths from chronic obstructive pulmonary disease, and ~50% of deaths from respiratory disease (Agaku et al., 2014). Much evidence indicates that individuals use tobacco primarily to experience the psychopharmacological properties of nicotine and that a large proportion of smokers eventually become dependent on

1

Negative Affective States and Cognitive Impairments in Nicotine Dependence
http://dx.doi.org/10.1016/B978-0-12-802574-1.00001-6

nicotine, significantly contributing to the motivation to smoke (Balfour, 1984; Stolerman, 1991). An estimated 13.7% of the US population age 18 and over smoked every day in the past month (Agaku et al., 2014). Electronic cigarette use has rapidly grown in the general population, further emphasizing the key role of nicotine in tobacco dependence (Palazzolo, 2013). According to the latest report from Bloomberg Industries, the combined sales of electronic cigarettes have doubled every year for the past 5 years, generating over USD$1 billion in revenue in the United States in 2014. The sale of electronic cigarettes is predicted to pass that of traditional cigarettes by 2047. Moreover, electronic cigarettes are marketed and viewed by the general public as safe because they do not produce compounds other than nicotine. However, considering the high level of nicotine in electronic cigarette vapor (~500–750 mg/m^3; Goniewicz, Hajek, & McRobbie, 2014), such nicotine intake likely has profound effects on the brain that can facilitate the transition to tobacco dependence, particularly in adolescents. Indeed, preliminary reports demonstrated that high levels of nicotine vapor exposure alone can lead to increased dependence and motivation to take nicotine in rodent models (George, Grieder, Cole, & Koob, 2010; Gilpin et al., 2014). The pervasiveness of tobacco use and the rapid growth of electronic cigarettes associated with the extensive costs to smokers and society provide a compelling basis for elucidating the actions of nicotine within the central nervous system that lead to potential neuroadaptations in the motivational systems that mediate the development of dependence and withdrawal symptoms.

THEORETICAL FRAMEWORK

Nicotine addiction can be defined as a chronic, relapsing disorder that has been characterized by a compulsion to seek and take nicotine, loss of control over nicotine intake, and emergence of a negative emotional state (eg, dysphoria, anxiety, and/or irritability) that defines a motivational withdrawal syndrome when access to nicotine is prevented (Koob & Le Moal, 2008). Addiction has been conceptualized as a three-stage cycle—binge/intoxication, withdrawal/negative affect, and preoccupation/anticipation—that worsens over time and involves allostatic changes in the brain reward and stress systems. Two primary sources of reinforcement, positive and negative reinforcement, have been hypothesized to play a role in this allostatic process (Fig. 1.1A). The term *reinforce* means "to strengthen" and refers to any stimulus (reinforcer) that increases the probability of a specific response that follows. Positive reinforcement is defined as the process by which the presentation of a stimulus increases the probability of a response. Negative reinforcement is defined as the process by which removal of an aversive stimulus (or aversive state of withdrawal

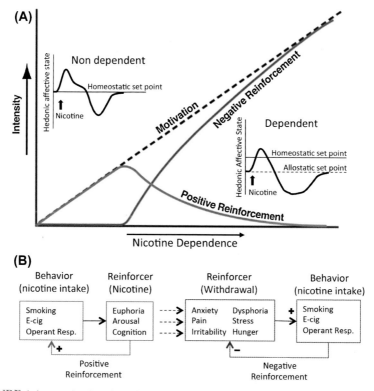

FIGURE 1.1 **Motivational mechanisms in nicotine dependence.** (A) Change in the relative contribution of positive and negative reinforcement constructs and associated changes in homeostatic and allostatic set points during the development of nicotine dependence. (B) Constructs associated with positive and negative reinforcement.

in the case of addiction) increases the probability of a response. In the case of nicotine use and dependence, nicotine is the positive reinforcer, and the negative affective state of nicotine withdrawal is the negative reinforcer (Fig. 1.1B).

Nicotine acts as a positive reinforcer in only a very narrow dose range in both humans and rodents. Moderate to high doses of nicotine can be aversive, particularly in nondependent subjects, producing conditioned place aversion and leading to decreases in nicotine self-administration (Fowler & Kenny, 2014). From an experimental psychology perspective, at a high dose, nicotine can be considered an aversive stimulus that produces punishing effects that lead to a decrease in the probability of nicotine self-administration (Goldberg & Spealman, 1983; Koffarnus & Winger, 2015). The roles of positive reinforcement, negative reinforcement, and punishment are key to understanding nicotine use and the development of nicotine addiction. This review mainly focuses on positive and negative reinforcement, but emerging work on the punishing effects of nicotine has recently suggested that it may be an important factor in excessive nicotine intake in dependent subjects (Fowler, Lu, Johnson, Marks, & Kenny, 2011).

POSITIVE REINFORCEMENT ASSOCIATED WITH NICOTINE USE

Although many components in cigarette smoke may contribute to smoking, much evidence indicates that individuals use tobacco primarily to experience the psychopharmacological properties of nicotine. A large proportion of smokers eventually become dependent on nicotine (Balfour, 1984; Stolerman, 1991). Nicotine acts as a positive reinforcer and will support intravenous self-administration in various species, including humans, nonhuman primates, and rodents (Fig. 1.2), even at doses and regimens that do not lead to a withdrawal syndrome (Corrigall & Coen, 1989; Donny, Caggiula, Knopf, & Brown, 1995; Goldberg & Henningfield, 1988; Goldberg & Spealman, 1982;

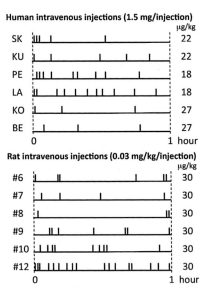

FIGURE 1.2 **Pattern of nicotine self-administration in humans and rats.** Vertical lines indicate a single nicotine self-administration. Notice the similarity in the pattern of nicotine self-administration in humans and rats. The unit dose for each subject is indicated on the right side of each record. Letters and numbers on the left axis are the initials (humans) or number of subjects (rats). *Human data are reproduced from Henningfield, J. E., Miyasato, K., Jasinski, D. R. (1983). Cigarette smokers self-administer intravenous nicotine.* Pharmacology, Biochemistry, and Behavior, 19, 887–890. *Rat data are from George et al. (unpublished results).*

Goldberg, Spealman, & Goldberg, 1981; Goldberg, Spealman, Risner, & Henningfield, 1983; Goodwin, Hiranita, & Paule, 2015; Watkins, Epping-Jordan, Koob, & Markou, 1999). For example, nicotine-containing cigarettes support higher breakpoints on a progressive-ratio schedule of reinforcement than denicotinized cigarettes in humans (Rusted, Mackee, Williams, & Willner, 1998; Shahan, Bickel, Badger, & Giordano, 2001; Shahan, Bickel, Madden, & Badger, 1999). The positive reinforcing effects of nicotine are generally attributed to its acute effects on mood and cognition. In humans, nicotine acutely produces positive rewarding effects, including mild euphoria (Pomerleau & Pomerleau, 1992), increased energy, and heightened arousal (Benowitz, 1996; Stolerman & Jarvis, 1995). Smoking cigarettes produces arousal, particularly with the first cigarette of the day, and relaxation when under stress (Benowitz, 1988). In animals, intravenous nicotine self-administration has been reliably demonstrated in numerous strains of rodents and different laboratories (Corrigall, 1999; Donny et al., 1995; Rose & Corrigall, 1997; Watkins et al., 1999). Systemic injections of the competitive nicotinic receptor antagonist dihydro-β-erythroidine and noncompetitive antagonist mecamylamine decrease intravenous nicotine self-administration in rats with limited access to nicotine (1 h/day; Corrigall & Coen, 1989; Watkins et al., 1999). Moreover, nicotine increases attentional processes (Kaye et al., 2014; Young et al., 2004; Young, Meves, & Geyer, 2013), lowers brain reward thresholds (Epping-Jordan, Watkins, Koob, & Markou, 1998), increases wakefulness (Salin-Pascual, Moro-Lopez, Gonzalez-Sanchez, & Blanco-Centurion, 1999), and increases learning and memory (Davis, Kenney, & Gould, 2007; Gould & Leach, 2014) in rodents and humans. The similar effects of nicotine on mood and cognition reported in humans and rodents provide a behavioral mechanism of action for the positive reinforcing effects of nicotine. However, preclinical studies have found that nicotine is a weak reinforcer. The reinforcing effectiveness of nicotine is approximately 10 times lower than that of cocaine in a progressive-ratio schedule of reinforcement (Risner & Goldberg, 1983). Although the acute positive reinforcing effects of nicotine are important in establishing self-administration behavior and may be sufficient to maintain nicotine self-administration in nondependent subjects, they do not appear to be sufficient to explain the intense craving for nicotine that is observed in dependent subjects and the escalation of nicotine intake during the transition from initial nicotine use to nicotine dependence and after relapse (Cohen, Koob, & George, 2012). Our hypothesis is that during the transition from nicotine use to nicotine dependence, there is a switch in the neurobiological mechanisms that underlie the motivation for nicotine self-administration that reflects a transition from positive to negative reinforcement mechanisms (Fig. 1.1).

NEGATIVE REINFORCEMENT ASSOCIATED WITH NICOTINE USE

A nicotine withdrawal or abstinence syndrome after chronic nicotine exposure has been characterized in both humans (Hughes, Gust, Skoog, Keenan, & Fenwick, 1991; Shiffman & Jarvik, 1976) and animals (Epping-Jordan et al., 1998; Hildebrand, Nomikos, Bondjers, Nisell, & Svensson, 1997; Malin et al., 1994, 1992; Malin, Lake, Carter, Cunningham, & Wilson, 1993; Watkins, Koob, & Markou, 2000) and has both somatic and affective components. In humans, acute nicotine withdrawal is characterized by affective symptoms, including depressed mood, dysphoria, irritability, anxiety, frustration, increased reactivity to environmental stimuli, and difficulty concentrating, as well as somatic symptoms, such as bradycardia, gastrointestinal discomfort, and increased appetite that leads to weight gain (American Psychiatric Association, 2000; Hughes et al., 1991). The enduring symptoms of nicotine withdrawal (protracted abstinence) include continued affective changes, such as depressed mood, irritability, sleep disturbances, and stress responsivity (Hughes et al., 1991), with abstinent smokers often reporting powerful cravings for tobacco (Hughes et al., 1984). Although the somatic symptoms of withdrawal from drugs of abuse are unpleasant and annoying, it has been hypothesized that avoidance of the affective components of drug withdrawal, including those associated with nicotine withdrawal (negative reinforcement), play a more important role in the maintenance of nicotine dependence than the somatic symptoms of withdrawal (Koob, Markou, Weiss, & Schulteis, 1993; Markou, Kosten, & Koob, 1998).

Abrupt abstinence from chronic nicotine administration also leads to a withdrawal syndrome in rodents (Malin et al., 1992) that has somatic and motivational components. Both spontaneous and antagonist-precipitated nicotine withdrawal produce various somatic signs (eg, eye blinks, body shakes, chewing, gasping, writhing, ptosis, and teeth chattering) and motivational effects (eg, elevated reward thresholds, anxiety-like responses, and conditioned place aversion; Epping-Jordan et al., 1998; Ghozland, Zorrilla, Parsons, & Koob, 2004; Stinus, Cador, Zorrilla, & Koob, 2005; Watkins, Stinus, Koob, & Markou, 2000). Several groups have established that rats will self-administer nicotine when given chronic extended access to the drug (Fu, Matta, Kane, & Sharp, 2003; LeSage, Keyler, Collins, & Pentel, 2003; O'Dell et al., 2007; Paterson & Markou, 2004; Valentine, Hokanson, Matta, & Sharp, 1997). Passive nicotine administration decreases nicotine self-administration in chronic self-administration paradigms (LeSage et al., 2003), and mecamylamine increases nicotine self-administration (O'Dell et al., 2007). Rats that are dependent on nicotine show anxiogenic-like effects during spontaneous withdrawal (Pandey, Roy, Xu, & Mittal, 2001; Slawecki, Thorsell, Khoury, Mathe, & Ehlers, 2005) and mecamylamine-precipitated anxiety-like responses in the elevated plus maze (George et al., 2007). Rats that self-administer nicotine when given limited access to it (1 h/day, 5 days/week) show very limited, if any, signs of somatic or motivational withdrawal (Paterson & Markou, 2004) and do not exhibit the escalation of nicotine intake after abstinence (Cohen et al., 2012, 2015; George et al., 2007), suggesting that nicotine self-administration is mostly driven by positive reinforcement mechanisms in this model. However, rats that are given extended access to nicotine self-administration with days of deprivation between each session (23/day, every 24–48 h) show the escalation of nicotine intake (Fig. 1.3C) and emergence of somatic and motivational signs of withdrawal, including anxiety-like behavior and hyperalgesia (Fig. 1.3D and E; Cohen et al., 2012, 2015) that predict the magnitude of nicotine intake after abstinence, suggesting that nicotine self-administration in this model is mainly driven by negative reinforcement.

One hypothesis to explain the increased self-administration of nicotine during 23 h access, particularly after periods of deprivation, is that nicotine self-administration becomes more heavily motivated by negative reinforcement mechanisms that are driven by recruitment of brain systems that are involved in anxiety-like symptoms and dysphoria (Koob & Le Moal, 2005, 2006). Recent work has confirmed this hypothesis by demonstrating that 2 days of nicotine abstinence was sufficient to increase nicotine self-administration when access to nicotine resumed (Cohen et al., 2012). Moreover, this nicotine deprivation effect was observed even after 6 weeks of abstinence (Fig. 1.3B) and was only observed in dependent rats with extended access to nicotine and not limited access (George et al., 2007). The reinforcing effects of nicotine can also be measured by using a progressive-ratio schedule of reinforcement, in which the responses that are required to obtain a discrete dose of nicotine increase after each trial until the animal stops responding (breakpoint). Both increasing doses of nicotine and nicotine withdrawal increase breakpoints under a progressive-ratio schedule (Cohen et al., 2012, 2015), demonstrating that the reinforcing effects of nicotine are dose- and withdrawal-dependent. Moreover, repeated periods of 2–3 days of abstinence lead to the escalation of nicotine self-administration with increased responding under a progressive-ratio schedule (Cohen et al., 2012). Again, only dependent rats with extended access to nicotine self-administration were sensitive to the effect of abstinence and showed the escalation of intake. We also recently showed that abstinence-induced anxiety-like behavior and hyperalgesia predicted subsequent nicotine self-administration when access to nicotine resumed (Fig. 1.3D and E; Cohen et al., 2015), suggesting that the removal of an aversive state that is characterized by increased anxiety-like behavior and pain is a key driving force behind excessive nicotine intake in dependent subjects (Fig. 1.1).

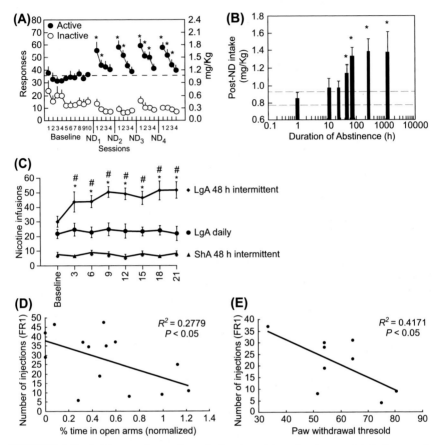

FIGURE 1.3 **Evidence of negative reinforcement in rats given extended access to nicotine self-administration.** (A) 72 h of nicotine deprivation (ND1-4) produces a robust increase in nicotine intake in rats with access to nicotine self-administration for 23 h/day. (B) Abstinence-induced increase in nicotine intake is observed after acute (24 h) and protracted (6 weeks) abstinence. (C) Repeated periods of abstinence (48 h) between each session produce a robust and sustained escalation of nicotine intake only in rats with long access (LgA) but not short access (ShA). (D) Abstinence-induced anxiety-like behavior (low percentage time on open arms) predicts high nicotine intake when access to nicotine resumes. (E) Abstinence-induced hyperalgesia (low withdrawal threshold) predicts high nicotine intake when access to nicotine resumes. *Reproduced from (A and B) George, O., Ghozland, S., Azar, M. R., Cottone, P., Zorrilla, E. P., Parsons L. H., et al. (2007). CRF-CRF¹ system activation mediates withdrawal-induced increases in nicotine self-administration in nicotine-dependent rats.* Proceedings of the National Academy of Sciences of the USA, 104, 17198–17203; (C) Cohen, A., Koob, G. F., George, O. (2012). *Robust escalation of nicotine intake with extended access to nicotine self-administration and intermittent periods of abstinence.* Neuropsychopharmacology, 37, 2153–2160; (D and E) Cohen, A., Treweek, J., Edwards, S., Leão, R. M., Schulteis, G., Koob, G. F., et al. (2015). *Extended access to nicotine leads to a CRF¹ receptor dependent increase in anxiety-like behavior and hyperalgesia in rats.* Addiction Biology, 20, 56–68.

There is significant face validity of the deprivation model to the human condition. The nicotine deprivation effect in rats is similar to the human condition, in which one observes an increase in smoking after abstinence (ie, an increase in the number and duration of puffs) followed by a titration period of nicotine intake (Benowitz & Jacob, 1984; Isaac & Rand, 1972; Madden & Bickel, 1999; Nil, Woodson, & Battig, 1987; Rusted et al., 1998). A critical point is that rats with 23 h access (without an abstinence period) show, as in humans, stable nicotine intake for months, and the nicotine deprivation effect is a short-lasting phenomenon that allows one to unveil and investigate the neural basis of the motivation to take nicotine under a negative reinforcement framework. Additionally, the similarity in blood nicotine levels in dependent humans and rats in a chronic access/deprivation model supports the relevance of this model to human addiction. Blood nicotine levels range between 10 and 25 ng/ml over the course of 24 h in humans who smoke at least one pack of cigarettes per day and reach 15 ng/ml after one cigarette (Benowitz & Jacob, 1984; Benowitz, Porchet, Sheiner, & Jacob, 1988). In previous studies, we measured blood nicotine levels in rats (O'Dell et al., 2006) and found that 1.0 mg/kg/day of nicotine via a minipump produced blood levels of 22 ng/ml. The rats in our self-administration studies self-administer 0.8–1.2 mg/kg/day using a unit dose of 0.03 mg/kg (Cohen et al., 2012; George et al., 2007; O'Dell et al., 2007). In actual measurements after an infusion of nicotine at the dose used for self-administration, nicotine levels ranged from 10 to 30 ng/ml (see Guillem et al., 2005, from our laboratory, and LeSage et al., 2002). These results suggest that under certain conditions, intravenous nicotine self-administration in rodents reaches levels well beyond those that are required to produce dependence as defined by the manifestation of a withdrawal syndrome during abstinence.

Altogether, these results suggest that extended access to nicotine itself can lead to the escalation of intake and dependence (as measured by withdrawal when nicotine is removed or nicotinic receptors are blocked). Dependence appears to be manifested by a negative emotional state, and negative reinforcement processes drive escalation. Thus, the transition from nicotine use to nicotine dependence is hypothesized to involve neuroadaptations within brain reward and stress circuitries and neuroadaptations (Koob & Le Moal, 2005) that contribute to negative emotional states that drive negative reinforcement (Koob & Bloom, 1988).

NEUROBIOLOGICAL MECHANISMS OF POSITIVE REINFORCEMENT

The neurobiological mechanisms that are involved in the acute reinforcing effects of nicotine have largely focused on the mesocorticolimbic dopamine system, a system that is heavily implicated in the reinforcing effects of indirect sympathomimetics, such as cocaine and amphetamine (Koob, Sanna, & Bloom, 1998). Nicotine is an agonist at nicotinic acetylcholine receptors (Lindstrom, 1997), and nicotinic acetylcholine receptors have been shown to be localized on cell bodies and dendrites of dopamine neurons in the ventral tegmental area and terminal fields of the mesocorticolimbic dopamine system, such as the nucleus accumbens (Clarke & Pert, 1985; Swanson, Simmons, Whiting, & Lindstrom, 1987). Systemic nicotine administration also increases extracellular dopamine levels in the shell of the nucleus accumbens, an effect that is observed with other major drugs of abuse (Nisell, Marcus, Nomikos, & Svensson, 1997; Pontieri, Passarelli, Calo, & Caronti, 1998; Pontieri, Tanda, Orzi, & Di Chiara, 1996). Neurochemical in vivo microdialysis studies have shown that nicotine can release dopamine via actions at both sites, with more evidence for the actions of nicotine at the level of the ventral tegmental area (Corrigall & Coen, 1991; Corrigall, Coen, & Adamson, 1994; Corrigall, Franklin, Coen, & Clarke, 1992; Enrico et al., 2013; Nisell, Nomikos, & Svensson, 1994; Panin, Lintas, & Diana, 2014). The recruitment of dopamine and γ-aminobutyric acid (GABA) neurons in the ventral tegmental area through the activation of α4β2*, α6β2*, and α5* but not α7* subunit-containing receptors appears to be critical for the positive reinforcing effects of nicotine (Maskos et al., 2005; Morel et al., 2014; Orejarena et al., 2012; Pons et al., 2008; Tolu et al., 2013). Other neuropharmacological systems that are implicated in the positive reinforcing effects of nicotine include cholinergic (Azam, Winzer-Serhan, Chen, & Leslie, 2002; Oakman, Faris, Kerr, Cozzari, & Hartman, 1995; Tago, McGeer, McGeer, Akiyama, & Hersh, 1989), serotonergic (Carboni, Acquas, Leone, & Di Chiara, 1989), glutamatergic (McGehee, Heath, Gelber, Devay, & Role, 1995; Schilstrom, Nomikos, Nisell, Hertel, & Svensson, 1998), GABAergic (Corrigall, Coen, Adamson, Chow, & Zhang, 2000; Corrigall, Coen, Zhang, & Adamson, 2001; Dewey et al., 1999), and opioidergic (Houdi, Pierzchala, Marson, Palkovits, & Van Loon, 1991; Pomerleau & Pomerleau, 1984) systems.

NEUROBIOLOGICAL MECHANISMS OF NEGATIVE REINFORCEMENT

The neurobiological substrates for the dependence-inducing effects of nicotine are beginning to be elucidated. Neurotransmitter systems that are implicated in nicotine withdrawal include decreases in dopamine and opioid peptide system activity, increases in corticotropin-releasing factor (CRF), dynorphin, and norepinephrine activity, and changes in serotonin activity (Cohen & George, 2013; Tejeda, Natividad, Orfila, Torres, & O'Dell, 2012; Watkins, Koob, et al., 2000). Decreases in the extracellular levels of dopamine in the nucleus accumbens and central nucleus of the amygdala, but not the prefrontal cortex, have been observed during nicotine withdrawal (Hildebrand, Nomikos, Hertel, Schilstrom, & Svensson, 1998; Panagis, Hildebrand, Svensson, & Nomikos, 2000), with decreased tonic activity of ventral tegmental area dopamine neurons (Grieder et al., 2012). Decreases in serotonin synthesis have also been observed during chronic nicotine exposure (Benwell & Balfour, 1979). Increases in CRF have been observed in the central nucleus of the amygdala during withdrawal (George et al., 2007). The somatic and affective/aversive signs of nicotine withdrawal have also been precipitated by the opioid receptor antagonist naloxone and nicotinic receptor antagonist mecamylamine, and opioid and nicotinic receptor agonists can reverse the somatic signs of nicotine withdrawal (Hildebrand et al., 1997; Malin et al., 1993). Moreover, nicotinic receptor blockade in the ventral tegmental area and interpeduncular nucleus produces somatic and motivational withdrawal (anxiety-like behavior) in nicotine-dependent rats (Hildebrand, Panagis, Svensson, & Nomikos, 1999; Zhao-Shea et al., 2015), possibly through the blockade of α7 nicotinic receptors (Nomikos, Hildebrand, Panagis, & Svensson, 1999).

Acute nicotine administration has also been shown to activate hormonal and neurotransmitter stress responses (Faraday, Blakeman, & Grunberg, 2005; Matta, Beyer, McAllen, & Sharp, 1987; Okada, Shimizu, & Yokotani, 2003; Sharp & Matta, 1993), and such activation is dose dependent (Mendelson, Sholar, Goletiani, Siegel, & Mello, 2005). Nicotine not only acutely activates the hypothalamic-pituitary-adrenal (HPA) axis (Matta et al., 1987) but also activates CRF neurons extrahypothalamically (Matta, Valentine, & Sharp, 1997). Withdrawal from chronic nicotine elevates CRF in the basal forebrain (Slawecki et al., 2005), and a CRF receptor antagonist that was injected intracerebroventricularly blocked the anxiogenic-like effects of withdrawal from bolus injections of nicotine (Tucci, Cheeta, Seth, & File, 2003). The hypothesis that CRF is activated during nicotine withdrawal (Bruijnzeel & Gold, 2005) is based on the observation that acute withdrawal from nicotine can increase circulating corticosterone, and extracellular CRF has been shown to be increased in the central nucleus of the amygdala during withdrawal from chronic nicotine (George et al., 2007) as well as during withdrawal from chronic administration of other major drugs of abuse (Koob et al., 1998). The anxiogenic-like effects of precipitated nicotine withdrawal were blocked by a CRF_1 receptor antagonist, and local infusion of CRF in the central nucleus of the amygdala produced anxiety-like behavior (George et al., 2007). Nicotine also enhanced norepinephrine release in the paraventricular nucleus of the hypothalamus (Sharp & Matta, 1993). However, activation of the HPA axis showed a subsensitive response during withdrawal from chronic nicotine administration (Matta, Fu, Valentine, & Sharp, 1998; Mendelson et al., 2005; Semba, Wakuta, Maeda, & Suhara, 2004). Chronic self-administration increases norepinephrine release in the paraventricular nucleus of the hypothalamus (Fu, Matta, Brower, & Sharp, 2001) and amygdala (Fu et al., 2003). The blockade of noradrenergic α1 receptors can decrease nicotine self-administration and nicotine reinstatement (Forget et al., 2010). Given that norepinephrine, CRF, and glucocorticoids interact in the basal forebrain in a feedforward system, in which each system enhances the release of the other neurotransmitters (Koob, 1999; Vendruscolo et al., 2012), these results would be consistent with the hypothesis that chronic nicotine activates extrahypothalamic CRF systems during the development of dependence. From a developmental perspective, increased CRF-like immunoreactivity was observed in adult rats that were exposed to nicotine during adolescence and has been linked to an anxiety-like phenotype (Slawecki et al., 2005).

Animal models that incorporate aspects of negative reinforcement in nicotine dependence have unveiled the existence of a novel CRF–CRF$_1$ system in the ventral tegmental area–interpeduncular nucleus pathway. Indeed, chronic nicotine exposure and withdrawal from nicotine recruit a population of dopamine–CRF neurons in the ventral tegmental area, and the activation of such dopamine–CRF neurons produces anxiety-like behavior and the escalation of nicotine intake (Grieder et al., 2014; Zhao-Shea et al., 2015). Moreover, the recruitment of CRF neurons in the ventral tegmental area during withdrawal is paralleled by a decrease in the tonic activity of ventral tegmental area dopamine neurons (Grieder et al., 2012), suggesting that the decrease in dopaminergic tone that is observed in human smokers may be caused by the recruitment of CRF neurons. Altogether, these reports suggest that downregulation of the dopamine system in the ventral tegmental area, nucleus accumbens, and central nucleus of the amygdala, together with the upregulation of CRF and norepinephrine systems in the central nucleus of the amygdala and ventral tegmental area, may underlie excessive nicotine intake, driven by negative reinforcement in dependent subjects.

TRANSLATIONAL ASPECTS OF THE NEUROBIOLOGY OF NEGATIVE REINFORCEMENT

Three medications are currently on the market for the treatment of tobacco addiction: nicotine replacement therapy (gum, lozenge, and patch), bupropion (Zyban), and varenicline (Chantix). These medications have actions that can be considered relevant to treating the withdrawal/negative affect stage of the addiction cycle and thus the negative reinforcement processes associated with nicotine withdrawal. There are a number of neurotransmitter systems that are implicated in the negative reinforcing effects of nicotine withdrawal, may contribute to the development of dependence, and can be targeted to develop new medications for smoking cessation.

The vulnerability to nicotine addiction may be related to initial sensitivity to the reinforcing effects of nicotine, but recent conceptualizations regarding the development of addiction have introduced the hypothesis that vulnerability may engage other aspects of the addiction process (Koob & Le Moal, 1997, 2001, 2005, 2006; Robinson & Berridge, 1993). Under this framework, incentive salience via a sensitization-like process (Robinson & Berridge, 1993) may be initially engaged, but compulsive nicotine seeking and taking likely involve negative reinforcement that is driven by the loss of reward system activity and recruitment of brain stress system activity (Koob & Le Moal, 2005). The combination of excellent and validated animal models that incorporate the negative reinforcement processes that are associated with nicotine withdrawal and a better understanding of the neurocircuitry and neuropharmacological mechanisms that underlie nicotine motivational withdrawal has provided viable targets for future drug development. Human laboratory models of the withdrawal/negative affect stage permit the proof-of-concept testing of potential therapeutics and the clinical validation of relevant pharmacological targets. The results of such studies can loop back to validate the animal models. Such a domain approach rather than syndrome approach to drug development has the potential to reveal pharmacogenetic approaches to drug development and utility, and thus should fit well with new concepts related to precision medicine.

References

Agaku, I. T., King, B. A., & Dube, S. R. (2014). Current cigarette smoking among adults: United States, 2005–2012. *Morbidity and Mortality Weekly Report, 63*, 29–34.

American Psychiatric Association. (2000). *Diagnostic and statistical manual of mental disorders* (4th ed., text revision). Washington, DC: American Psychiatric Press.

Azam, L., Winzer-Serhan, U. H., Chen, Y., & Leslie, F. M. (2002). Expression of neuronal nicotinic acetylcholine receptor subunit mRNAs within midbrain dopamine neurons. *Journal of Comparative Neurology, 444*, 260–274.

Balfour, D. J. (1984). Nicotine and the tobacco smoking habit. In D. J. K. Balfour (Ed.), *Nicotine and the tobacco smoking habit. Series title: International encyclopedia of pharmacology and therapeutics* (Vol. 114, pp. 61–74). New York: Pergamon Press.

Benowitz, N. L. (1988). Drug therapy: pharmacologic aspects of cigarette smoking and nicotine addiction. *The New England Journal of Medicine, 319*, 1318–1330.

Benowitz, N. L. (1996). Pharmacology of nicotine: addiction and therapeutics. *Annual Review of Pharmacology and Toxicology, 36*, 597–613.

Benowitz, N. L., & Jacob, P., 3rd. (1984). Nicotine and carbon monoxide intake from high- and low-yield cigarettes. *Clinical Pharmacology and Therapeutics, 36*, 265–270.

Benowitz, N. L., Porchet, H., Sheiner, L., & Jacob, P., 3rd. (1988). Nicotine absorption and cardiovascular effects with smokeless tobacco use: comparison with cigarettes and nicotine gum. *Clinical Pharmacology and Therapeutics, 44*, 23–28.

Benwell, M. E., & Balfour, D. J. (1979). Effects of nicotine administration and its withdrawal on plasma corticosterone and brain 5-hydroxyindoles. *Psychopharmacology, 63*, 7–11.

Bruijnzeel, A. W., & Gold, M. S. (2005). The role of corticotropin-releasing factor-like peptides in cannabis, nicotine, and alcohol dependence. *Brain Research Reviews, 49*, 505–528.

Carboni, E., Acquas, E., Leone, P., & Di Chiara, G. (1989). 5HT3 receptor antagonists block morphine- and nicotine- but not amphetamine-induced reward. *Psychopharmacology, 97,* 175–178.

Clarke, P. B. S., & Pert, A. (1985). Autoradiographic evidence for nicotine receptors on nigrostriatal and mesolimbic dopaminergic neurons. *Brain Research, 348,* 355–358.

Cohen, A., & George, O. (2013). Animal models of nicotine exposure: relevance to secondhand smoking, electronic cigarette use, and compulsive smoking. *Frontiers in Psychiatry, 4,* 41.

Cohen, A., Koob, G. F., & George, O. (2012). Robust escalation of nicotine intake with extended access to nicotine self-administration and intermittent periods of abstinence. *Neuropsychopharmacology, 37,* 2153–2160.

Cohen, A., Treweek, J., Edwards, S., Leão, R. M., Schulteis, G., Koob, G. F., et al. (2015). Extended access to nicotine leads to a CRF$_1$ receptor dependent increase in anxiety-like behavior and hyperalgesia in rats. *Addiction Biology, 20,* 56–68.

Corrigall, W. A. (1999). Nicotine self-administration in animals as a dependence model. *Nicotine and Tobacco Research, 1,* 11–20.

Corrigall, W. A., & Coen, K. M. (1989). Nicotine maintains robust self-administration in rats on a limited-access schedule. *Psychopharmacology, 99,* 473–478.

Corrigall, W. A., & Coen, K. M. (1991). Selective dopamine antagonists reduce nicotine self-administration. *Psychopharmacology, 104,* 171–176.

Corrigall, W. A., Coen, K. M., & Adamson, K. L. (1994). Self-administered nicotine activates the mesolimbic dopamine system through the ventral tegmental area. *Brain Research, 653,* 278–284.

Corrigall, W. A., Coen, K. M., Adamson, K. L., Chow, B. L., & Zhang, J. (2000). Response of nicotine self-administration in the rat to manipulations of mu-opioid and γ-aminobutyric acid receptors in the ventral tegmental area. *Psychopharmacology, 149,* 107–114.

Corrigall, W. A., Coen, K. M., Zhang, J., & Adamson, K. L. (2001). GABA mechanisms in the pedunculopontine tegmental nucleus influence particular aspects of nicotine self-administration selectively in the rat. *Psychopharmacology, 158,* 190–197.

Corrigall, W. A., Franklin, K. B. J., Coen, K. M., & Clarke, P. B. S. (1992). The mesolimbic dopaminergic system is implicated in the reinforcing effects of nicotine. *Psychopharmacology, 107,* 285–289.

Davis, J. A., Kenney, J. W., & Gould, T. J. (2007). Hippocampal alpha4beta2 nicotinic acetylcholine receptor involvement in the enhancing effect of acute nicotine on contextual fear conditioning. *The Journal of Neuroscience, 27,* 10870–10877.

Dewey, S. L., Brodie, J. D., Gerasimov, M., Horan, B., Gardner, E. L., & Ashby, C. R., Jr. (1999). A pharmacologic strategy for the treatment of nicotine addiction. *Synapse, 31,* 76–86.

Donny, E. C., Caggiula, A. R., Knopf, S., & Brown, C. (1995). Nicotine self-administration in rats. *Psychopharmacology, 122,* 390–394.

Enrico, P., Sirca, D., Mereu, M., Peana, A. T., Mercante, B., & Diana, M. (2013). Acute restraint stress prevents nicotine-induced mesolimbic dopaminergic activation via a corticosterone-mediated mechanism: a microdialysis study in the rat. *Drug and Alcohol Dependence, 127,* 8–14.

Epping-Jordan, M. P., Watkins, S. S., Koob, G. F., & Markou, A. (1998). Dramatic decreases in brain reward function during nicotine withdrawal. *Nature, 393,* 76–79.

Faraday, M. M., Blakeman, K. H., & Grunberg, N. E. (2005). Strain and sex alter effects of stress and nicotine on feeding, body weight, and HPA axis hormones. *Pharmacology, Biochemistry, and Behavior, 80,* 577–589.

Forget, B., Wertheim, C., Mascia, P., Pushparaj, A., Goldberg, S. R., & Le Foll, B. (2010). Noradrenergic α$_1$ receptors as a novel target for the treatment of nicotine addiction. *Neuropsychopharmacology, 35,* 1751–1760 [erratum: 35(9): 2006].

Fowler, C. D., & Kenny, P. J. (2014). Nicotine aversion: neurobiological mechanisms and relevance to tobacco dependence vulnerability. *Neuropharmacology, 76*(Pt B), 533–544.

Fowler, C. D., Lu, Q., Johnson, P. M., Marks, M. J., & Kenny, P. J. (2011). Habenular α5 nicotinic receptor subunit signalling controls nicotine intake. *Nature, 471*, 597–601.

Fu, Y., Matta, S. G., Brower, V. G., & Sharp, B. M. (2001). Norepinephrine secretion in the hypothalamic paraventricular nucleus of rats during unlimited access to self-administered nicotine: an in vivo microdialysis study. *The Journal of Neuroscience, 21*, 8979–8989.

Fu, Y., Matta, S. G., Kane, V. B., & Sharp, B. M. (2003). Norepinephrine release in amygdala of rats during chronic nicotine self-administration: an in vivo microdialysis study. *Neuropharmacology, 45*, 514–523.

George, O., Ghozland, S., Azar, M. R., Cottone, P., Zorrilla, E. P., Parsons, L. H., et al. (2007). CRF-CRF$_1$ system activation mediates withdrawal-induced increases in nicotine self-administration in nicotine-dependent rats. *Proceedings of the National Academy of Sciences of the USA, 104*, 17198–17203.

George, O., Grieder, T. E., Cole, M., & Koob, G. F. (2010). Exposure to chronic intermittent nicotine vapor induces nicotine dependence. *Pharmacology Biochemistry and Behavior, 96*, 104–107.

Ghozland, S., Zorrilla, E., Parsons, L. H., & Koob, G. F. (2004). Mecamylamine increases extracellular CRF levels in the central nucleus of the amygdala or nicotine-dependent rats. *Society for Neuroscience, 30* abstract# 708.8.

Gilpin, N. W., Whitaker, A. M., Baynes, B., Abdel, A. Y., Weil, M. T., & George, O. (2014). Nicotine vapor inhalation escalates nicotine self-administration. *Addiction Biology, 19*, 587–592.

Goldberg, S. R., & Henningfield, J. E. (1988). Reinforcing effects of nicotine in humans and experimental animals responding under intermittent schedules of i.v. drug injection. *Pharmacology, Biochemistry, and Behavior, 30*, 227–234.

Goldberg, S. R., & Spealman, R. D. (1982). Maintenance and suppression of behavior by intravenous nicotine injections in squirrel monkeys. *Federation Proceedings, 41*, 216–220.

Goldberg, S. R., & Spealman, R. D. (1983). Suppression of behavior by intravenous injections of nicotine or by electric shocks in squirrel monkeys: effects of chlordiazepoxide and mecamylamine. *The Journal of Pharmacology and Experimental Therapeutics, 224*, 334–340.

Goldberg, S. R., Spealman, R. D., & Goldberg, D. M. (1981). Persistent behavior at high rates maintained by intravenous self-administration of nicotine. *Science, 214*, 573–575.

Goldberg, S. R., Spealman, R. D., Risner, M. E., & Henningfield, J. E. (1983). Control of behavior by intravenous nicotine injections in laboratory animals. *Pharmacology, Biochemistry, and Behavior, 19*, 1011–1020.

Goniewicz, M. L., Hajek, P., & McRobbie, H. (2014). Nicotine content of electronic cigarettes, its release in vapour and its consistency across batches: regulatory implications. *Addiction, 109*, 500–507.

Goodwin, A. K., Hiranita, T., & Paule, M. G. (2015). The reinforcing effects of nicotine in humans and nonhuman primates: a review of intravenous self-administration evidence and future directions for research. *Nicotine and Tobacco Research, 17*, 1297–1310.

Gould, T. J., & Leach, P. T. (2014). Cellular, molecular, and genetic substrates underlying the impact of nicotine on learning. *Neurobiology of Learning and Memory, 107*, 108–132.

Grieder, T. E., George, O., Tan, H., George, S. R., Le Foll, B., Laviolette, S. R., et al. (2012). Phasic D1 and tonic D2 dopamine receptor signaling double dissociate the motivational effects of acute nicotine and chronic nicotine withdrawal. *Proceedings of the National Academy of Sciences of the USA, 109*, 3101–3106.

Grieder, T. E., Herman, M. A., Contet, C., Tan, L. A., Vargas-Perez, H., Cohen, A., et al. (2014). VTA CRF neurons mediate the aversive effects of nicotine withdrawal and promote intake escalation. *Nature Neuroscience, 17*, 1751–1758.

Guillem, K., Vouillac, C., Azar, M. R., Parsons, L. H., Koob, G. F., Cador, M., et al. (2005). Monoamine oxidase inhibition dramatically increases the motivation to self-administer nicotine in rats. *The Journal of Neuroscience, 25*, 8593–8600.

Henningfield, J. E., Miyasato, K., & Jasinski, D. R. (1983). Cigarette smokers self-administer intravenous nicotine. *Pharmacology, Biochemistry, and Behavior, 19*, 887–890.

Hildebrand, B. E., Nomikos, G. G., Bondjers, C., Nisell, M., & Svensson, T. H. (1997). Behavioral manifestations of the nicotine abstinence syndrome in the rat: peripheral versus central mechanisms. *Psychopharmacology, 129,* 348–356.

Hildebrand, B. E., Nomikos, G. G., Hertel, P., Schilstrom, B., & Svensson, T. H. (1998). Reduced dopamine output in the nucleus accumbens but not in the medial prefrontal cortex in rats displaying a mecamylamine-precipitated nicotine withdrawal syndrome. *Brain Research, 779,* 214–225.

Hildebrand, B. E., Panagis, G., Svensson, T. H., & Nomikos, G. G. (1999). Behavioral and biochemical manifestations of mecamylamine-precipitated nicotine withdrawal in the rat: role of nicotinic receptors in the ventral tegmental area. *Neuropsychopharmacology, 21,* 560–574.

Houdi, A. A., Pierzchala, K., Marson, L., Palkovits, M., & Van Loon, G. R. (1991). Nicotine-induced alteration in Tyr-Gly-Gly and Met-enkephalin in discrete brain nuclei reflects altered enkephalin neuron activity. *Peptides, 12,* 161–166.

Hughes, J. R., Gust, S. W., Skoog, K., Keenan, R. M., & Fenwick, J. W. (1991). Symptoms of tobacco withdrawal: a replication and extension. *Archives of General Psychiatry, 48,* 52–59.

Hughes, J. R., Hatsukami, D. K., Pickens, R. W., Krahn, D., Malin, S., & Luknic, A. (1984). Effect of nicotine on the tobacco withdrawal syndrome. *Psychopharmacology, 83,* 82–87.

Isaac, P. F., & Rand, M. J. (1972). Cigarette smoking and plasma levels of nicotine. *Nature, 236,* 308–310.

Kaye, S., Gilsenan, J., Young, J. T., Carruthers, S., Allsop, S., Degenhardt, L., et al. (2014). Risk behaviours among substance use disorder treatment seekers with and without adult ADHD symptoms. *Drug and Alcohol Dependence, 144,* 70–77.

Koffarnus, M. N., & Winger, G. (2015). Individual differences in the reinforcing and punishing effects of nicotine in rhesus monkeys. *Psychopharmacology, 232,* 2393–2403.

Koob, G. F. (1999). Corticotropin-releasing factor, norepinephrine and stress. *Biological Psychiatry, 46,* 1167–1180.

Koob, G. F., & Bloom, F. E. (1988). Cellular and molecular mechanisms of drug dependence. *Science, 242,* 715–723.

Koob, G. F., & Le Moal, M. (1997). Drug abuse: hedonic homeostatic dysregulation. *Science, 278,* 52–58.

Koob, G. F., & Le Moal, M. (2001). Drug addiction, dysregulation of reward, and allostasis. *Neuropsychopharmacology, 24,* 97–129.

Koob, G. F., & Le Moal, M. (2005). Plasticity of reward neurocircuitry and the "dark side" of drug addiction. *Nature Neuroscience, 8,* 1442–1444.

Koob, G. F., & Le Moal, M. (2006). *Neurobiology of addiction.* London: Academic Press.

Koob, G. F., & Le Moal, M. (2008). Addiction and the brain antireward system. *Annual Review of Psychology, 59,* 29–53.

Koob, G. F., Markou, A., Weiss, F., & Schulteis, G. (1993). Opponent process and drug dependence: neurobiological mechanisms. *Seminars in Neuroscience, 5,* 351–358.

Koob, G. F., Sanna, P. P., & Bloom, F. E. (1998). Neuroscience of addiction. *Neuron, 21,* 467–476.

LeSage, M. G., Keyler, D. E., Collins, G., & Pentel, P. R. (2003). Effects of continuous nicotine infusion on nicotine self-administration in rats: relationship between continuously infused and self-administered nicotine doses and serum concentrations. *Psychopharmacology, 170,* 278–286.

LeSage, M. G., Keyler, D. E., Shoeman, D., Raphael, D., Collins, G., & Pentel, P. R. (2002). Continuous nicotine infusion reduces nicotine self-administration in rats with 23-h/day access to nicotine. *Pharmacology Biochemistry and Behavior, 72,* 279–289.

Lindstrom, J. (1997). Nicotinic acetylcholine receptors in health and disease. *Molecular Neurobiology, 15,* 193–222.

Madden, G. J., & Bickel, W. K. (1999). Abstinence and price effects on demand for cigarettes: a behavioral-economic analysis. *Addiction, 94,* 577–588.

Malin, D. H., Lake, J. R., Carter, V. A., Cunningham, J. S., Hebert, K. M., Conrad, D. L., et al. (1994). The nicotine antagonist mecamylamine precipitates nicotine abstinence syndrome in the rat. *Psychopharmacology, 115,* 180–184.

Malin, D. H., Lake, J. R., Carter, V. A., Cunningham, J. S., & Wilson, O. B. (1993). Naloxone precipitates nicotine abstinence syndrome in the rat. *Psychopharmacology, 112,* 339–342.

Malin, D. H., Lake, J. R., Newlin-Maultsby, P., Roberts, L. K., Lanier, J. G., Carter, V. A., et al. (1992). Rodent model of nicotine abstinence syndrome. *Pharmacology, Biochemistry, and Behavior, 43,* 779–784.

Markou, A., Kosten, T. R., & Koob, G. F. (1998). Neurobiological similarities in depression and drug dependence: a self-medication hypothesis. *Neuropsychopharmacology, 18,* 135–174.

Maskos, U., Molles, B. E., Pons, S., Besson, M., Guiard, B. P., Guilloux, J. P., et al. (2005). Nicotine reinforcement and cognition restored by targeted expression of nicotinic receptors. *Nature, 436,* 103–107.

Matta, S. G., Beyer, H. S., McAllen, K. M., & Sharp, B. M. (1987). Nicotine elevates rat plasma ACTH by a central mechanism. *The Journal of Pharmacology and Experimental Therapeutics, 243,* 217–226.

Matta, S. G., Fu, Y., Valentine, J. D., & Sharp, B. M. (1998). Response of the hypothalamo-pituitary-adrenal axis to nicotine. *Psychoneuroendocrinology, 23,* 103–113.

Matta, S. G., Valentine, J. D., & Sharp, B. M. (1997). Nicotinic activation of CRH neurons in extrahypothalamic regions of the rat brain. *Endocrine, 7,* 245–253.

McGehee, D. S., Heath, M. J., Gelber, S., Devay, P., & Role, L. W. (1995). Nicotine enhancement of fast excitatory synaptic transmission in CNS by presynaptic receptors. *Science, 269,* 1692–1696.

Mendelson, J. H., Sholar, M. B., Goletiani, N., Siegel, A. J., & Mello, N. K. (2005). Effects of low- and high-nicotine cigarette smoking on mood states and the HPA axis in men. *Neuropsychopharmacology, 30,* 1751–1763.

Morel, C., Fattore, L., Pons, S., Hay, Y. A., Marti, F., Lambolez, B., et al. (2014). Nicotine consumption is regulated by a human polymorphism in dopamine neurons. *Molecular Psychiatry, 19,* 930–936.

Nil, R., Woodson, P. P., & Battig, K. (1987). Effects of smoking deprivation on smoking behavior and heart rate response in high and low CO absorbing smokers. *Psychopharmacology, 92,* 465–469.

Nisell, M., Marcus, M., Nomikos, G. G., & Svensson, T. H. (1997). Differential effects of acute and chronic nicotine on dopamine output in the core and shell of the rat nucleus accumbens. *Journal of Neural Transmission, 104,* 1–10.

Nisell, M., Nomikos, G. G., & Svensson, T. H. (1994). Systemic nicotine-induced dopamine release in the rat nucleus accumbens is regulated by nicotinic receptors in the ventral tegmental area. *Synapse, 16,* 36–44.

Nomikos, G. G., Hildebrand, B. E., Panagis, G., & Svensson, T. H. (1999). Nicotine withdrawal in the rat: role of α7 nicotinic receptors in the ventral tegmental area. *Neuroreport, 10,* 697–702.

Oakman, S. A., Faris, P. L., Kerr, P. E., Cozzari, C., & Hartman, B. K. (1995). Distribution of pontomesencephalic cholinergic neurons projecting to substantia nigra differs significantly from those projecting to ventral tegmental area. *The Journal of Neuroscience, 15,* 5859–5869.

Okada, S., Shimizu, T., & Yokotani, K. (2003). Extrahypothalamic corticotropin-releasing hormone mediates (-)-nicotine-induced elevation of plasma corticosterone in rats. *European Journal of Pharmacology, 473,* 217–223.

Orejarena, M. J., Herrera-Solis, A., Pons, S., Maskos, U., Maldonado, R., & Robledo, P. (2012). Selective re-expression of β2 nicotinic acetylcholine receptor subunits in the ventral tegmental area of the mouse restores intravenous nicotine self-administration. *Neuropharmacology, 63,* 235–241.

O'Dell, L. E., Bruijnzeel, A. W., Smith, R. T., Parsons, L. H., Merves, M. L., Goldberger, B. A., et al. (2006). Diminished nicotine withdrawal in adolescent rats: implications for vulnerability to addiction. *Psychopharmacology, 186,* 612–619.

O'Dell, L. E., Chen, S. A., Smith, R. T., Specio, S. E., Balster, R. L., Paterson, N. E., et al. (2007). Extended access to nicotine self-administration leads to dependence: circadian measures, withdrawal measures, and extinction behavior in rats. *The Journal of Pharmacology and Experimental Therapeutics, 320,* 180–193.

Palazzolo, D. L. (2013). Electronic cigarettes and vaping: a new challenge in clinical medicine and public health: a literature review. *Frontiers in Public Health, 1,* 56.

Panagis, G., Hildebrand, B. E., Svensson, T. H., & Nomikos, G. G. (2000). Selective c-fos induction and decreased dopamine release in the central nucleus of amygdala in rats displaying a mecamylamine-precipitated nicotine withdrawal syndrome. *Synapse, 35,* 15–25.

Pandey, S. C., Roy, A., Xu, T., & Mittal, N. (2001). Effects of protracted nicotine exposure and withdrawal on the expression and phosphorylation of the CREB gene transcription factor in rat brain. *Journal of Neurochemistry, 77,* 943–952.

Panin, F., Lintas, A., & Diana, M. (2014). Nicotine-induced increase of dopaminergic mesoac-cumbal neuron activity is prevented by acute restraint stress: in vivo electrophysiology in rats. *European Neuropsychopharmacology, 24,* 1175–1180.

Paterson, N. E., & Markou, A. (2004). Prolonged nicotine dependence associated with extended access to nicotine self-administration in rats. *Psychopharmacology, 173,* 64–72.

Pomerleau, O. F., & Pomerleau, C. S. (1984). Neuroregulators and the reinforcement of smoking: towards a biobehavioral explanation. *Neuroscience and Biobehavioral Reviews, 8,* 503–513.

Pomerleau, C. S., & Pomerleau, O. F. (1992). Euphoriant effects of nicotine in smokers. *Psychopharmacology, 108,* 460–465.

Pons, S., Fattore, L., Cossu, G., Tolu, S., Porcu, E., McIntosh, J. M., et al. (2008). Crucial role of α4 and α6 nicotinic acetylcholine receptor subunits from ventral tegmental area in systemic nicotine self-administration. *The Journal of Neuroscience, 28,* 12318–12327.

Pontieri, F. E., Passarelli, F., Calo, L., & Caronti, B. (1998). Functional correlates of nicotine administration: similarity with drugs of abuse. *Journal of Molecular Medicine, 76,* 193–201.

Pontieri, F. E., Tanda, G., Orzi, F., & Di Chiara, G. (1996). Effects of nicotine on the nucleus accumbens and similarity to those of addictive drugs. *Nature, 382,* 255–257.

Risner, M. E., & Goldberg, S. R. (1983). A comparison of nicotine and cocaine self-administration in the dog: fixed-ratio and progressive-ratio schedules of intravenous drug infusion. *The Journal of Pharmacology and Experimental Therapeutics, 224,* 319–326.

Robinson, T. E., & Berridge, K. C. (1993). The neural basis of drug craving: an incentive-sensitization theory of addiction. *Brain Research Reviews, 18,* 247–291.

Rose, J. E., & Corrigall, W. A. (1997). Nicotine self-administration in animals and humans: similarities and differences. *Psychopharmacology, 130,* 28–40.

Rusted, J. M., Mackee, A., Williams, R., & Willner, P. (1998). Deprivation state but not nicotine content of the cigarette affects responding by smokers on a progressive ratio task. *Psychopharmacology, 140,* 411–417.

Salin-Pascual, R. J., Moro-Lopez, M. L., Gonzalez-Sanchez, H., & Blanco-Centurion, C. (1999). Changes in sleep after acute and repeated administration of nicotine in the rat. *Psychopharmacology, 145,* 133–138.

Schilstrom, B., Nomikos, G. G., Nisell, M., Hertel, P., & Svensson, T. H. (1998). N-methyl-D-aspartate receptor antagonism in the ventral tegmental area diminishes the systemic nicotine-induced dopamine release in the nucleus accumbens. *Neuroscience, 82,* 781–789.

Semba, J., Wakuta, M., Maeda, J., & Suhara, T. (2004). Nicotine withdrawal induces subsensitivity of hypothalamic-pituitary-adrenal axis to stress in rats: implications for precipitation of depression during smoking cessation. *Psychoneuroendocrinology, 29,* 215–226.

Shahan, T. A., Bickel, W. K., Badger, G. J., & Giordano, L. A. (2001). Sensitivity of nicotine-containing and de-nicotinized cigarette consumption to alternative non-drug reinforcement: a behavioral economic analysis. *Behavioural Pharmacology, 12,* 277–284.

Shahan, T. A., Bickel, W. K., Madden, G. J., & Badger, G. J. (1999). Comparing the reinforcing efficacy of nicotine containing and de-nicotinized cigarettes: a behavioral economic analysis. *Psychopharmacology, 147,* 210–216.

Sharp, B. M., & Matta, S. G. (1993). Detection by in vivo microdialysis of nicotine-induced norepinephrine secretion from the hypothalamic paraventricular nucleus of freely moving rats: dose-dependency and desensitization. *Endocrinology, 133,* 11–19.

Shiffman, S. M., & Jarvik, M. E. (1976). Smoking withdrawal symptoms in two weeks of abstinence. *Psychopharmacology, 50,* 35–39.

Slawecki, C. J., Thorsell, A. K., Khoury, A. E., Mathe, A. A., & Ehlers, C. L. (2005). Increased CRF-like and NPY-like immunoreactivity in adult rats exposed to nicotine during adolescence: relation to anxiety-like and depressive-like behavior. *Neuropeptides, 39,* 369–377.

Stinus, L., Cador, M., Zorrilla, E. P., & Koob, G. F. (2005). Buprenorphine and a CRF1 antagonist block the acquisition of opiate withdrawal-induced conditioned place aversion in rats. *Neuropsychopharmacology, 30,* 90–98.

Stolerman, I. P. (1991). Behavioural pharmacology of nicotine: multiple mechanisms. *British Journal of Addiction, 86,* 533–536.

Stolerman, I. P., & Jarvis, M. J. (1995). The scientific case that nicotine is addictive. *Psychopharmacology, 117,* 2–10 (discussion 14–20).

Swanson, L. W., Simmons, D. M., Whiting, P. J., & Lindstrom, J. (1987). Immunohistochemical localization of neuronal nicotinic receptors in the rodent central nervous system. *The Journal of Neuroscience, 7,* 3334–3342.

Tago, H., McGeer, P. L., McGeer, E. G., Akiyama, H., & Hersh, L. B. (1989). Distribution of choline acetyltransferase immunopositive structures in the rat brainstem. *Brain Research, 495,* 271–297.

Tejeda, H. A., Natividad, L. A., Orfila, J. E., Torres, O. V., & O'Dell, L. E. (2012). Dysregulation of kappa-opioid receptor systems by chronic nicotine modulate the nicotine withdrawal syndrome in an age-dependent manner. *Psychopharmacology, 224,* 289–301.

Tolu, S., Eddine, R., Marti, F., David, V., Graupner, M., Pons, S., et al. (2013). Co-activation of VTA DA and GABA neurons mediates nicotine reinforcement. *Molecular Psychiatry, 18,* 382–393.

Tucci, S., Cheeta, S., Seth, P., & File, S. E. (2003). Corticotropin releasing factor antagonist, α-helical CRF$_{9-41}$, reverses nicotine-induced conditioned, but not unconditioned, anxiety. *Psychopharmacology, 167,* 251–256.

Valentine, J. D., Hokanson, J. S., Matta, S. G., & Sharp, B. M. (1997). Self-administration in rats allowed unlimited access to nicotine. *Psychopharmacology, 133,* 300–304.

Vendruscolo, L. F., Barbier, E., Schlosburg, J. E., Misra, K. K., Whitfield, T., Jr., Logrip, M. L., et al. (2012). Corticosterone-dependent plasticity mediates compulsive alcohol drinking in rats. *The Journal of Neuroscience, 32,* 7563–7571.

Watkins, S. S., Epping-Jordan, M. P., Koob, G. F., & Markou, A. (1999). Blockade of nicotine self-administration with nicotinic antagonists in rats. *Pharmacology, Biochemistry, and Behavior, 62,* 743–751.

Watkins, S. S., Koob, G. F., & Markou, A. (2000). Neural mechanisms underlying nicotine addiction: acute positive reinforcement and withdrawal. *Nicotine and Tobacco Research, 2,* 19–37.

Watkins, S. S., Stinus, L., Koob, G. F., & Markou, A. (2000). Reward and somatic changes during precipitated nicotine withdrawal in rats: centrally and peripherally mediated effects. *The Journal of Pharmacology and Experimental Therapeutics, 292,* 1053–1064.

Young, J. W., Finlayson, K., Spratt, C., Marston, H. M., Crawford, N., Kelly, J. S., et al. (2004). Nicotine improves sustained attention in mice: evidence for involvement of the α7 nicotinic acetylcholine receptor. *Neuropsychopharmacology, 29*, 891–900.

Young, J. W., Meves, J. M., & Geyer, M. A. (2013). Nicotinic agonist-induced improvement of vigilance in mice in the 5-choice continuous performance test. *Behavioural Brain Research, 240*, 119–133.

Zhao-Shea, R., DeGroot, S. R., Liu, L., Vallaster, M., Pang, X., Su, Q., et al. (2015). Increased CRF signalling in a ventral tegmental area-interpeduncular nucleus-medial habenula circuit induces anxiety during nicotine withdrawal. *Nature Communications, 6*, 6770.

Nicotine Withdrawal and Attentional Deficit Studies Across Species: Conflation With Attentional Dysfunction in Psychiatric Patients

J. van Enkhuizen[1], J.W. Young[2,3]

[1]Utrecht University, Utrecht, The Netherlands; [2]University of California San Diego, La Jolla, CA, United States; [3]VA San Diego Healthcare System, San Diego, CA, United States

NICOTINE USE, WITHDRAWAL, AND COGNITION

An estimated 40 million adults in the United States currently smoke cigarettes, and this high smoking incidence helps to make smoking the leading cause of preventable disease and health problems in the United States and worldwide (CDC, 2014). Despite a strong desire in many smokers to quit, quitting remains extremely difficult even with the aid of approved pharmacotherapies (Ray, Schnoll, & Lerman, 2009). For example, more than half of those who attempt to quit relapse in the first week of trying (Garvey, Bliss, Hitchcock, Heinold, & Rosner, 1992). This early cessation period is therefore a critical window for people to successfully abstain from smoking. Cessation from smoking results in nicotine withdrawal and is associated with unpleasant physiological, psychological, and cognitive symptoms (Ashare, Falcone, & Lerman, 2014). This complex nicotine withdrawal syndrome drives the high relapse rate of smokers attempting to quit. Despite earlier focus on the physiological and anxiogenic symptoms resulting from withdrawal, the cognitive deficits emerging from

Negative Affective States and Cognitive Impairments in Nicotine Dependence
http://dx.doi.org/10.1016/B978-0-12-802574-1.00002-8

smoking abstinence have increasingly gained interest because they have predicted relapse [reviewed by Hall et al., 2015], and developing treatments for such dysfunction could improve quit rates (Ashare & Schmidt, 2014). Withdrawal-related cognitive deficits are multifaceted and include problems with executive function, working memory, and response inhibition. Perhaps most importantly contributing to smoking relapse are the attentional deficits experienced by people, anecdotally reported as having "difficulty concentrating" during withdrawal (Hughes, 2007), and quantified using numerous attentional tasks (discussed in detail later). Attentional deficits are also commonplace across numerous psychiatric disorders (Evans & Drobes, 2009) and may therefore share abnormal neural mechanisms with nicotine withdrawal (Evans, Park, Maxfield, & Drobes, 2009). In this chapter, we therefore focus on studies investigating attentional deficits resulting from nicotine withdrawal, and where overlap occurs in psychiatric disorders. For this purpose, we will describe evidence of these withdrawal-related deficits in attention from both human and animal studies.

ATTENTIONAL DEFICITS RESULTING FROM NICOTINE WITHDRAWAL IN HUMANS

Sustained attention or vigilance refers to the process that facilitates the ability to discriminate between relevant (target) stimuli and irrelevant distractors (non-target stimuli) (Sarter & Paolone, 2011). There are numerous behavioral tasks available to objectively measure sustained attention in humans. The most widely used test for assaying attention in clinical trials is the Continuous Performance Test (CPT), an umbrella term for a variety of tasks where the common denominator is that they all require a subject to respond to certain target stimuli, but withhold from responding to specified non-target stimuli (eg, when the letter "X" appears in the X-CPT). Some versions are more complex, requiring a sequence of target alphanumeric numbers to appear, such as in the Rapid Visual Information Processing test [RVIP (Lawrence, Ross, Hoffmann, Garavan, & Stein, 2003)]. Irrespective of the version and its complexity, however, all CPTs require responses to target stimuli and the inhibition of responding from non-target stimuli.

Many CPT versions have been used to measure attentive performance of people during smoking abstinence. For example, both male and female adults abstinent from smoking for 17, but not 5h, made more omission errors and reacted slower in the Connors' CPT (Harrison, Coppola, & McKee, 2009). In adolescent children, however, no change in performance was observed on two CPT versions after 24h of abstinence (Jacobsen et al., 2005). In other studies, overnight abstinence resulted in reduced correct responses and increased response time variability in adults performing the CPT (Myers, Taylor, Moolchan, & Heishman, 2008), but no change in discriminability (d-prime), a calculated measure reflecting attention, in the Connors' CPT (Ashare & Hawk, 2012). A more thorough longitudinal examination importantly demonstrated that inhibitory control as measured by CPT commission errors predicted relapse at 1 and 3 months after quitting [see Fig. 2.1; (Powell, Dawkins, West, Powell, & Pickering, 2010)]. A slower reaction time on the RVIP task was observed as quickly as 30 min after smoking cessation (Hendricks, Ditre, Drobes, & Brandon, 2006). Hence, it is clear that adults undergoing smoking abstinence demonstrate impaired attentional performance as measured by CPTs and CPT-like tasks, aspects of which predict smoking relapse.

Other indirect support for nicotine withdrawal causing attentional deficits comes from studies demonstrating that nicotinic treatments attenuate these deficits. Wesnes and Warburton demonstrated decades ago the potential for nicotine to improve attention, specifically so in individuals that are undergoing withdrawal (Wesnes & Warburton, 1983; Wesnes, Warburton, & Matz, 1983). More recent studies support these initial findings demonstrating that following overnight cigarette abstinence, nicotine replacement therapy improved the number of target responses compared to placebo in the Conners CPT and RVIP (Atzori, Lemmonds, Kotler, Durcan, & Boyle, 2008; Myers et al., 2008). Such nicotine replacement therapy also improved attention (as measured by d-prime) compared to placebo in an identical

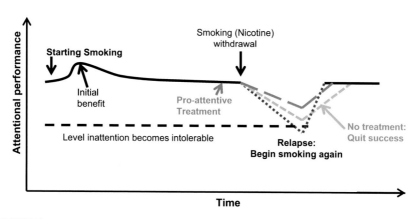

FIGURE 2.1 **Theoretical representation of relapse driven by smoking abstinence–induced inattention.** A small nicotine-induced benefit in attention beyond normal performance is initially observed in healthy subjects, although this effect is attenuated over time. During withdrawal, however, a deficit in attention is observed. While nicotine withdrawal–induced deficient attention may prove tolerable to some (*green dashes*), its effects may be intolerable to others, leading to relapse (*red dots*). By providing a pro-attentive treatment (*blue lines*) prior to withdrawal, however, intolerable inattention could be avoided and relapse prevented.

pair version of the CPT (Dawkins, Powell, West, Powell, & Pickering, 2007). Transdermal nicotine also increased attentional measures in female smokers performing the CPT (Poltavski, Petros, & Holm, 2012) and alcohol-dependent individuals compared to placebo (Boissoneault, Gilbertson, Prather, & Nixon, 2011). These studies provided sufficient evidence that more selective treatments targeting specific nicotinic acetylcholine receptor (nAChR) subunits might provide alleviation of attentional deficits without the need to utilize the prototypical nAChR ligand nicotine.

Other nicotinic agents have demonstrated efficacy at blocking smoking withdrawal–induced inattention in humans. The full $\alpha 7$ and partial $\alpha 4\beta 2$ nAChR agonist varenicline increased the number of correct responses and reduced reaction times compared with placebo following 72 h of abstinence (Patterson et al., 2009). Varenicline also improved reaction times during the Connors' CPT following overnight abstinence (Ashare & McKee, 2012). The weak norepinephrine/dopamine reuptake inhibitor and $\alpha 3\beta 4$ nAChR antagonist buproprion (Bondarev, Bondareva, Young, & Glennon, 2003; Foley, DeSanty, & Kast, 2006) also alleviated withdrawal-induced inattention (Perkins, Karelitz, Jao, Gur, & Lerman, 2013). Other studies have also demonstrated nicotinic agents can improve attention, especially during periods of withdrawal (Dawkins et al., 2007). Although some differences in findings have been reported, these differences are likely a result of altered abstinence duration protocols and specific task parameters (Ashare, Falcone, et al., 2014). Importantly, nAChR agents and dopaminergic agents can alleviate withdrawal-induced inattention.

In addition to nicotine-induced improvement in attention in subjects undergoing nicotine withdrawal, nicotine-induced improved attention has also been observed in nonsmoking healthy adults. These improvements were driven by increased target responding (Levin et al., 1998) and/or reduced commission errors (Myers, Taylor, Salmeron, Waters, & Heishman, 2013) in the CPT. This nicotine-induced enhancement in attention drove theories that the high rate of smoking in psychiatric patients is for self-medication purposes, a self-driven attempt to improve their cognitive functioning (Evans & Drobes, 2009). This point is of importance because various mentally ill patients exhibit attentional deficits, with reduced cognition in general being closely linked to functional outcome (Green, 2006). Hence, many researchers have attempted to understand the neural mechanisms underlying such attentional deficits in psychiatric patients to develop procognitive treatments. Subsequently, nAChRs have become an important target for procognitive enhancement in psychiatric disorders (Bidwell, McClernon, & Kollins, 2011; Demeter & Sarter, 2013; Martin et al., 2007; Young & Geyer, 2013), in part given the overlap of attentional deficits and improvements associated with nicotine use already described.

ATTENTIONAL DYSFUNCTION IN PSYCHIATRIC PATIENTS: OVERLAP WITH NICOTINIC RESEARCH

Among mental disorders, it is most obvious that inattentiveness is experienced by patients with attention deficit hyperactive disorder (ADHD). Several other psychiatric populations also suffer from attentional deficits, however, including those diagnosed with schizophrenia and bipolar disorder. Interestingly, the NIMH has provided a novel framework (Research Domain Criteria; RDoC) for investigating and looking at mental disorders, advocating a bottom-up transdiagnostic biological approach where behavioral domains such as inattention overlap in several psychiatric populations (Insel, 2014). Attentional deficits, as part of the overarching cognitive symptoms, have gained an increasing interest in the field as these deficits negatively affect patients' quality of life. Where mood-stabilizers, sedatives, and antipsychotics are often used in treating the extremes of a disorder such as psychosis or in alleviating a euphoric mood in bipolar disorder, cognitive symptoms largely remain untreated and therefore continue to limit everyday functioning (Green, 2006).

There is particularly a high prevalence of nicotine usage among psychiatric populations, such as those with schizophrenia (Kumari & Postma, 2005), bipolar disorder (Thomson et al., 2015), and major depressive disorder (Lasser et al., 2000; Ziedonis et al., 2008). As mentioned, psychiatric patients may be heavier tobacco smokers than the general population to self-medicate attentional deficits associated with the disorder (Potter & Newhouse, 2008). Indeed, nicotine ameliorated various attentional deficits in psychiatric patients as assessed by different controlled laboratory tasks (Barr et al., 2008; George et al., 2002). Importantly, cigarette smoking had selective effects on attention performance in the CPT in patients with schizophrenia compared to healthy controls (Sacco et al., 2005). Moreover, the nonselective nAChR antagonist mecamylamine blocked this reversal of abstinence-related deficits on sustained attention by smoking reinstatement only in patients with schizophrenia. These results therefore suggest that schizophrenia patients' attempt to alleviate attentional deficits associated with the disorder by smoking cigarettes could be driven by stimulation of central nAChRs. When directly compared, however, it was observed that schizophrenia patients exhibited no larger benefits of nicotine or ad libitum smoking on attentional performance compared to healthy controls as both benefitted equally (Hahn et al., 2013), hence the continued proposition that the attentional enhancing properties of nicotine may underlie cigarette use in healthy subjects. Supporting evidence for self-medication in another patient population, nicotine improved attention in male ADHD nonsmokers in the CPT compared to placebo, with more pronounced effects in a subgroup selected for low baseline attention (Poltavski & Petros, 2006). These nicotine-induced effects support higher smoking rates among anxiety, Alzheimer's Disease, and Parkinson's Disease sufferers, who also exhibit poor attention (Evans & Drobes, 2009).

Consistent with healthy subjects, withdrawal of nicotine potentiates deficits in attention in psychiatric patients. Specifically, smokers with a history of depression exhibited greater abstinence-induced cognitive deficits compared to non-depressed abstinent smokers (Ashare, Strasser, Wileyto, Cuevas, & Audrain-McGovern, 2014). Furthermore, there is a correlation between the severity of inattention symptoms in patients with ADHD and their attentional deficits caused by nicotine withdrawal (Ameringer & Leventhal, 2012). This withdrawal-induced attentional deficit is not selective to psychiatric patients, however, as smoking abstinence decreased inhibitory control and increased reaction time variability on the CPT in adults, regardless of ADHD diagnosis (Kollins et al., 2013). Nevertheless, nicotine replacement therapy may be particularly useful for ADHD patients with high levels of inattention during an attempt to quit smoking. The potentiated attentional deficits of psychiatric patients arising from smoking withdrawal suggest that the neural mechanisms underlying attentional deficits from each may not overlap. This observation is important given that treatments based on nAChR mechanisms can affect attentional functioning in patients.

MECHANISMS UNDERLYING NICOTINIC EFFECTS ON ATTENTION

It has long been clear that acetylcholine (ACh) serves a predominant role in attentional functioning. Lesions of the basal forebrain—the site for primary ACh efflux into the prefrontal cortex (PFC)—impair attention in rats in the 5-choice serial reaction time task (5-CSRTT) and sustained attention task [SAT (McGaughy & Sarter, 1998; Muir, Bussey, Everitt, & Robbins, 1996)]. When similar lesions were conducted in the PFC, similar deficits in attention were observed (Dalley et al., 2004; McGaughy, Ross, & Eichenbaum, 2008). Thus, there is evidence for the importance of PFC ACh in mediating attentional functioning. In further support of these findings, microdialysis studies have reported ACh efflux into the PFC during the performance of the 5-CSRTT (Dalley et al., 2001; Passetti, Dalley, O'Connell, Everitt, & Robbins, 2000). These PFC ACh efflux findings represent a general escalation in ACh, as these levels can only be recorded over minutes as opposed to smaller timescales in response to specific events. In vivo, voltammetry can record ACh in the millisecond range, however, and there is complementary evidence that ACh spikes occur following the appearance of signal targets, but not signal targets missed (Parikh, Kozak, Martinez, & Sarter, 2007). To date in 2016, it is unclear whether such ACh spikes also arise in response to non-target stimuli, which occur in human CPTs, the RVIP, and the rodent 5-choice (5C-)CPT (see later). Further details on cholinergic innervation of attention are reviewed elsewhere (Proulx, Piva, Tian, Bailey, & Lambe, 2014). It remains unclear, however, what cholinergic factors exactly contribute to impaired attention after chronic nicotine intake via smoking or in psychiatric patients.

Differences in smoking prevalence among psychiatric populations and normal individuals and related differences in attention may be the result of various factors. For instance, disease-specific changes in receptor expression, particularly aberrations in the cholinergic/cortical attention system, may underlie attentional deficits in patients. Alternatively, given that nicotine improves attention in patients, and withdrawal from nicotine can impair attention further in patients (see earlier), the direct mechanisms of action are unlikely to overlap. Furthermore, long-term smoking-induced changes in nicotinic receptor availability (Brasic et al., 2012) could also explain additional detrimental effects on attention (Counotte, Smit, & Spijker, 2012). With links to observed frontal importance in attention, fMRI studies have demonstrated decreased activation in right frontal regions after 24h of nicotine abstinence (Kozink, Lutz, Rose, Froeliger, & McClernon, 2010) that are ameliorated with nicotine treatment (Beaver et al., 2011). Beyond non-psychiatric smokers, nicotine also improved attention during withdrawal in patients with schizophrenia (Hahn et al., 2013). The main effect of nicotine seems to be on enhancing alerting attention (Myers et al., 2013), corresponding with voltammetry studies demonstrating that ACh spikes occur after presentation of target signals (Parikh et al., 2007).

Unlike nicotinic and dopaminergic agents (nicotine, varenicline, and bupropion) the anxiolytic agent pregabalin reduced anxiety-related effects of nicotine withdrawal, but not attentional deficits (Herman, Waters, McKee, & Sofuoglu, 2012). Given that pregabalin acts on $\alpha2\delta$ auxiliary subunits, not nicotinic or dopaminergic mechanisms (Frampton, 2014), these data implicate the latter in remediating deficits in attention but not the former. Furthermore, these data offer a dissociation of mechanisms for nicotine withdrawal effects on anxiety vs. attention, narrowing the focus on identifying treatments selective for withdrawal-induced inattention. Ultimately, developing more selective treatments for inattention in both nicotine withdrawal and psychiatric disorders will require appropriate models in animals to test potential therapeutic compounds.

ATTENTIONAL DEFICITS FROM NICOTINE WITHDRAWAL IN ANIMALS

Conducting nicotine withdrawal studies in animals enables the opportunity to hold many other factors constant (more so than can be done in humans) to delineate mechanisms underlying withdrawal effects as well as test putative treatments for that withdrawal. Approaches vary on how to treat animals with chronic nicotine, from self-administration to chronic treatment via osmotic mini-pumps. Irrespective of method, the important observation is what effect removal of that nicotine has on behavior (enforced abstinence). Attentional deficits have been observed in rats undergoing nicotine withdrawal via osmotic mini-pumps driven by missed responding to target stimuli [omissions (Semenova, Stolerman, & Markou, 2007; Shoaib & Bizarro, 2005)]. Attention was quantified in this study by using the 5-CSRTT, a commonly used attentional test for rats and mice (Carli, Robbins, Evenden, & Everitt, 1983; Lustig, Kozak, Sarter, Young, & Robbins, 2013; Passetti, Dalley, & Robbins, 2003). Consistent with some human studies, nicotine withdrawal thus reduced target responding in rats. Additionally, temporal consistency with human attentional deficits in performance has also been observed, whereby rats exhibited deficits early in testing (10 and 16 h after withdrawal), but in later testing (34 and 106 h) performance recovered and normalized (Shoaib & Bizarro, 2005). Hence, similarities are observed between human withdrawal-induced inattention and data from rodent studies conducted to date.

In addition to withdrawal studies, subunit selective antagonist treatment studies have also been used to determine whether they recreate attentional deficits. For example, treatment with the α4β2 nAChR antagonist DHβE and the dopamine D1 receptor antagonist SCH 23390 replicated nicotine withdrawal–induced impairments in the 5-CSRTT (Shoaib & Bizarro, 2005), although a similar study could not replicate these findings (Hahn, Shoaib, & Stolerman, 2011). The α7 nAChR antagonist methyllycaconitine (MLA) impaired 5-CSRTT performance in rats after nicotine treatment in one study (Hahn et al., 2011), but not in another (Blondel, Sanger, & Moser, 2000). Hence, nicotine withdrawal study effects have been consistent, but conflicting evidence has been generated to date on the effects of nAChR antagonists.

In other nAChR-related attentional studies, both nicotine and the selective α4β4 subtype nAChR agonist SIB-1553A improved aspects of attentional functioning in nonhuman primates after treatment with an attention deficit–inducing neurotoxin (Decamp & Schneider, 2006). The full α7 and partial α4β2 nAChR agonist varenicline improved signal detection in the SAT, specifically under challenging conditions (Rollema et al., 2009). Other approaches to investigating nAChR contribution to attention have included the use of genetic knockout studies. For example, mice with a null mutation of the α7 (Hoyle, Genn, Fernandes, & Stolerman, 2006; Young et al., 2004) and α5 (Bailey, De Biasi, Fletcher, & Lambe, 2010) nAChRs exhibit impaired attention, driven largely by increased misses to target stimuli. The fact that these mice have a constitutive null mutation complicates the interpretation of these findings, however, given putative developmental alterations on attentional performance. For example, chronic nicotine treatment during adolescence in rats resulted in attentional deficits as measured by the 5-CSRTT, which could be due to enhanced dopamine release in the medial prefrontal cortex (mPFC) (Counotte et al., 2009). Certainly dopamine levels are elevated during 5-CSRTT performance (Robbins, 2002), and they can be affected by nicotine treatment in both striatal and PFC structures (Faure, Tolu, Valverde, & Naude, 2014). Another mechanism possibly associated with adolescent nicotine-induced deficits is reduced metabotropic glutamate receptor 2 (mGluR2) proteins and function on presynaptic terminals of PFC glutamatergic synapses (Counotte et al., 2011). Again, nAChR activation interacts with glutamatergic function (Marchi, Grilli, & Pittaluga, 2015; Pistillo, Clementi, Zoli, & Gotti, 2015). These data therefore indicate that multiple nAChRs and their interaction with dopamine and glutamate could underlie performance of rodents in the attentional 5-CSRTT.

While commonly used to study attention, the 5-CSRTT and SAT have some limitations as to how attention is measured compared to CPTs. Only target trials are used in the 5-CSRTT, with presence or lack of targets in the SAT, unlike human CPTs and the RVIP task that include stimuli for which subjects must inhibit from responding (Lustig et al., 2013; Young, Light, Marston, Sharp, & Geyer, 2009). Hence, it is unclear whether the reduced target responding of the rats in these studies (Semenova et al., 2007; Shoaib & Bizarro, 2005) resulted in reduced overall responding (which would require non-target stimuli) or was selective to target trials only. The lack of information on non-target responding could also limit the validity of treatment studies, given that withdrawal-induced inattention driven by non-target responding (response disinhibition) in the CPT predicted relapse rates (Powell et al., 2010). Initial studies of a rodent CPT, the 5C-CPT, which includes target and non-target trials consistent with human CPTs (Young et al., 2009), demonstrated that withdrawal from nicotine in mice resulted in attentional deficits driven by reduced target responding in addition to elevated non-target responding (Young, van Enkhuizen, Markou, Eyler, & Geyer, 2012). These studies are therefore consistent with human CPTs. Expansion of this work is required, however, to determine the mechanism(s) underlying this effect.

IMPLICATIONS AND FUTURE STUDIES

This review of the literature highlights that abstinence from nicotine (smoking cessation) results in cognitive deficits in general and impaired attention specifically. That these attentional deficits predict relapse into smoking underscores the premise that treating inattention arising from withdrawal is a viable target for reducing relapse and hence smoking rates. The evidence covered here also indicates that treating inattention from withdrawal could reduce relapse rates in both healthy subjects and psychiatric patients. Because inattention is commonplace in psychiatric disorders, and patients exhibit additive impairments during withdrawal, the mechanisms driving inattention in these two instances may not overlap.

Interestingly, allelic variation in the 15q25 gene cluster that includes several nAChR subunit genes is associated with nicotine dependence, schizophrenia, and bipolar disorder (Jackson, Fanous, Chen, Kendler, & Chen, 2013). To date in 2016, this gene cluster has not been specifically examined with regard to inattention, so while it may relate to dependence and psychiatric traits, dissociable downstream mechanisms underlying inattention during withdrawal and psychiatric disorders may yet exist. This genetic association supports epidemiological evidence suggesting that people who smoke during adolescence have an increased risk of psychosis (McGrath et al., 2015; Saha et al., 2011), although again direction of effect cannot be ascertained. Further investigation indicates that the majority of patients with schizophrenia smoke (59%) by the time of their first episode (Myles et al., 2012). Hence, the elevated smoking rates in patients may not be driven by self-treatment (as discussed earlier), but by comorbidity. Delineating the differences between comorbidity and self-treatment across individuals will be important for future research.

Future studies should be conducted with the aim of understanding the role of specific nAChR, glutamatergic, and dopaminergic receptors underlying nicotine withdrawal–induced inattention. These studies could be conducted using selective knockout of these receptors, preferably conditional knockouts, to eliminate the confounding factor of developmental compensatory changes. These studies should be conducted in conjunction with studies determining the role that psychiatry-relevant pathology (mechanisms associated with psychiatric conditions) has on inattention (Barnes, Young, & Neill, 2012; Young et al., 2015) so that the relationship between receptor mechanisms and this pathology can be systematically evaluated.

CONCLUSIONS

Despite widespread acceptance of the ill-effects of smoking on health, it continues to be a problem for many individuals in the 21st century. Knowledge of the role that nicotine withdrawal has in relapse-based studies of somatic symptoms has not resulted in better treatments to date. Recent evidence that nicotine withdrawal induces inattention that predicts relapse re-energizes research in the field toward novel drug treatment targets for preventing relapse during quit attempts (Fig. 2.1). Identifying the mechanism(s) underlying withdrawal-induced inattention—preferably using cross-species relevant tests—will provide specific targets for developing novel treatments. Because inattention is commonplace in patients with psychiatric disorders, with putatively conflated underlying mechanisms with withdrawal, such novel treatments could also aid in treating patients. Future research should determine the epidemiological and genetic contributions to nicotine withdrawal–induced inattention.

Acknowledgments

We thank Drs. Berend Olivier and Mark Geyer for their support. This work was supported by NIH grant R01-MH071916, R01-MH104344 and the Veteran's Administration VISN 22 Mental Illness Research, Education, and Clinical Center.

References

Ameringer, K. J., & Leventhal, A. M. (2012). Symptom dimensions of attention deficit hyperactivity disorder and nicotine withdrawal symptoms. *Journal of Addictive Diseases, 31*, 363–375.

Ashare, R. L., & Hawk, L. W., Jr. (2012). Effects of smoking abstinence on impulsive behavior among smokers high and low in ADHD-like symptoms. *Psychopharmacology, 219*, 537–547.

Ashare, R. L., & McKee, S. A. (2012). Effects of varenicline and bupropion on cognitive processes among nicotine-deprived smokers. *Experimental and Clinical Psychopharmacology, 20*, 63–70.

Ashare, R. L., & Schmidt, H. D. (2014). Optimizing treatments for nicotine dependence by increasing cognitive performance during withdrawal. *Expert Opinion on Drug Discovery, 9*, 579–594.

Ashare, R., Strasser, A. A., Wileyto, E. P., Cuevas, J., & Audrain-McGovern, J. (2014). Cognitive deficits specific to depression-prone smokers during abstinence. *Experimental and Clinical Psychopharmacology, 22*, 323–331.

Ashare, R. L., Falcone, M., & Lerman, C. (2014). Cognitive function during nicotine withdrawal: implications for nicotine dependence treatment. *Neuropharmacology, 76*(Pt B), 581–591.

Atzori, G., Lemmonds, C. A., Kotler, M. L., Durcan, M. J., & Boyle, J. (2008). Efficacy of a nicotine (4 mg)-containing lozenge on the cognitive impairment of nicotine withdrawal. *Journal of Clinical Psychopharmacology, 28*, 667–674.

Bailey, C. D., De Biasi, M., Fletcher, P. J., & Lambe, E. K. (2010). The nicotinic acetylcholine receptor alpha5 subunit plays a key role in attention circuitry and accuracy. *The Journal of Neuroscience: the Official Journal of the Society for Neuroscience, 30*, 9241–9252.

Barnes, S. A., Young, J. W., & Neill, J. C. (2012). Rats tested after a washout period from subchronic PCP administration exhibited impaired performance in the 5-Choice Continuous Performance Test (5C-CPT) when the attentional load was increased. *Neuropharmacology, 62*, 1432–1441.

Barr, R. S., Culhane, M. A., Jubelt, L. E., Mufti, R. S., Dyer, M. A., Weiss, A. P., et al. (2008). The effects of transdermal nicotine on cognition in nonsmokers with schizophrenia and nonpsychiatric controls. *Neuropsychopharmacology: Official Publication of the American College of Neuropsychopharmacology, 33*, 480–490.

Beaver, J. D., Long, C. J., Cole, D. M., Durcan, M. J., Bannon, L. C., Mishra, R. G., et al. (2011). The effects of nicotine replacement on cognitive brain activity during smoking withdrawal studied with simultaneous fMRI/EEG. *Neuropsychopharmacology: Official Publication of the American College of Neuropsychopharmacology, 36*, 1792–1800.

Bidwell, L. C., McClernon, F. J., & Kollins, S. H. (2011). Cognitive enhancers for the treatment of ADHD. *Pharmacology, Biochemistry, and Behavior, 99*, 262–274.

Blondel, A., Sanger, D. J., & Moser, P. C. (2000). Characterisation of the effects of nicotine in the five-choice serial reaction time task in rats: antagonist studies. *Psychopharmacology, 149*, 293–305.

Boissoneault, J., Gilbertson, R., Prather, R., & Nixon, S. J. (2011). Contrasting behavioral effects of acute nicotine and chronic smoking in detoxified alcoholics. *Addictive Behaviors, 36*, 1344–1348.

Bondarev, M. L., Bondareva, T. S., Young, R., & Glennon, R. A. (2003). Behavioral and biochemical investigations of bupropion metabolites. *European Journal of Pharmacology, 474*, 85–93.

Brasic, J. R., Cascella, N., Kumar, A., Zhou, Y., Hilton, J., Raymont, V., et al. (2012). Positron emission tomography experience with 2-[(1)(8)F]fluoro-3-(2(S)-azetidinylmethoxy)pyridine (2-[(1)(8)F]FA) in the living human brain of smokers with paranoid schizophrenia. *Synapse, 66*, 352–368.

Carli, M., Robbins, T. W., Evenden, J. L., & Everitt, B. J. (1983). Effects of lesions to ascending noradrenergic neurones on performance of a 5-choice serial reaction task in rats; implications for theories of dorsal noradrenergic bundle function based on selective attention and arousal. *Behavioural Brain Research, 9*, 361–380.

CDC. (2014). The health consequences of smoking—50 years of progress: a report of the Surgeon General. In Services USDoHaH (Ed.), *Centers for Disease Control and Prevention*.

Counotte, D. S., Spijker, S., Van de Burgwal, L. H., Hogenboom, F., Schoffelmeer, A. N., De Vries, T. J., et al. (2009). Long-lasting cognitive deficits resulting from adolescent nicotine exposure in rats. *Neuropsychopharmacology: Official Publication of the American College of Neuropsychopharmacology, 34*, 299–306.

Counotte, D. S., Goriounova, N. A., Li, K. W., Loos, M., van der Schors, R. C., Schetters, D., et al. (2011). Lasting synaptic changes underlie attention deficits caused by nicotine exposure during adolescence. *Nature Neuroscience, 14*, 417–419.

Counotte, D. S., Smit, A. B., & Spijker, S. (2012). The Yin and Yang of nicotine: harmful during development, beneficial in adult patient populations. *Frontiers in Pharmacology, 3*, 180.

Dalley, J. W., McGaughy, J., O'Connell, M. T., Cardinal, R. N., Levita, L., & Robbins, T. W. (2001). Distinct changes in cortical acetylcholine and noradrenaline efflux during contingent and noncontingent performance of a visual attentional task. *The Journal of Neuroscience: the Official Journal of the Society for Neuroscience, 21*, 4908–4914.

Dalley, J. W., Theobald, D. E., Bouger, P., Chudasama, Y., Cardinal, R. N., & Robbins, T. W. (2004). Cortical cholinergic function and deficits in visual attentional performance in rats following 192 IgG-saporin-induced lesions of the medial prefrontal cortex. *Cerebral Cortex, 14*, 922–932.

Dawkins, L., Powell, J. H., West, R., Powell, J., & Pickering, A. (2007). A double-blind placebo-controlled experimental study of nicotine: II–effects on response inhibition and executive functioning. *Psychopharmacology, 190*, 457–467.

Decamp, E., & Schneider, J. S. (2006). Effects of nicotinic therapies on attention and executive functions in chronic low-dose MPTP-treated monkeys. *The European Journal of Neuroscience, 24*, 2098–2104.

Demeter, E., & Sarter, M. (2013). Leveraging the cortical cholinergic system to enhance attention. *Neuropharmacology, 64*, 294–304.

Evans, D. E., & Drobes, D. J. (2009). Nicotine self-medication of cognitive-attentional processing. *Addiction Biology, 14*, 32–42.

Evans, D. E., Park, J. Y., Maxfield, N., & Drobes, D. J. (2009). Neurocognitive variation in smoking behavior and withdrawal: genetic and affective moderators. *Genes Brain Behavior, 8*, 86–96.

Faure, P., Tolu, S., Valverde, S., & Naude, J. (2014). Role of nicotinic acetylcholine receptors in regulating dopamine neuron activity. *Neuroscience, 282C*, 86–100.

Foley, K. F., DeSanty, K. P., & Kast, R. E. (2006). Bupropion: pharmacology and therapeutic applications. *Expert Review of Neurotherapeutics, 6*, 1249–1265.

Frampton, J. E. (2014). Pregabalin: a review of its use in adults with generalized anxiety disorder. *CNS Drugs, 28*, 835–854.

Garvey, A. J., Bliss, R. E., Hitchcock, J. L., Heinold, J. W., & Rosner, B. (1992). Predictors of smoking relapse among self-quitters: a report from the normative aging study. *Addictive Behaviors, 17*, 367–377.

George, T. P., Vessicchio, J. C., Termine, A., Sahady, D. M., Head, C. A., Pepper, W. T., et al. (2002). Effects of smoking abstinence on visuospatial working memory function in schizophrenia. *Neuropsychopharmacology: Official Publication of the American College of Neuropsychopharmacology, 26*, 75–85.

Green, M. F. (2006). Cognitive impairment and functional outcome in schizophrenia and bipolar disorder. *Journal of Clinical Psychiatry, 67*, e12.

Hahn, B., Shoaib, M., & Stolerman, I. P. (2011). Selective nicotinic receptor antagonists: effects on attention and nicotine-induced attentional enhancement. *Psychopharmacology, 217*, 75–82.

Hahn, B., Harvey, A. N., Concheiro-Guisan, M., Huestis, M. A., Holcomb, H. H., & Gold, J. M. (2013). A test of the cognitive self-medication hypothesis of tobacco smoking in schizophrenia. *Biological Psychiatry, 74*, 436–443.

Hall, F. S., Der-Avakian, A., Gould, T. J., Markou, A., Shoaib, M., & Young, J. W. (2015). Negative affective states and cognitive impairments in nicotine dependence. *Neuroscience and Biobehavioral Review, 58*, 168–185.

Harrison, E. L., Coppola, S., & McKee, S. A. (2009). Nicotine deprivation and trait impulsivity affect smokers' performance on cognitive tasks of inhibition and attention. *Experimental and Clinical Psychopharmacology, 17*, 91–98.

Hendricks, P. S., Ditre, J. W., Drobes, D. J., & Brandon, T. H. (2006). The early time course of smoking withdrawal effects. *Psychopharmacology, 187*, 385–396.

Herman, A. I., Waters, A. J., McKee, S. A., & Sofuoglu, M. (2012). Effects of pregabalin on smoking behavior, withdrawal symptoms, and cognitive performance in smokers. *Psychopharmacology, 220*, 611–617.

Hoyle, E., Genn, R. F., Fernandes, C., & Stolerman, I. P. (2006). Impaired performance of alpha7 nicotinic receptor knockout mice in the five-choice serial reaction time task. *Psychopharmacology, 189*, 211–223.

Hughes, J. R. (2007). Effects of abstinence from tobacco: valid symptoms and time course. *Nicotine & Tobacco Research: Official Journal of the Society for Research on Nicotine and Tobacco, 9*, 315–327.

Insel, T. R. (2014). The NIMH research domain criteria (RDoC) project: precision medicine for psychiatry. *The American Journal of Psychiatry, 171*, 395–397.

Jackson, K. J., Fanous, A. H., Chen, J., Kendler, K. S., & Chen, X. (2013). Variants in the 15q25 gene cluster are associated with risk for schizophrenia and bipolar disorder. *Psychiatric Genetics, 23*, 20–28.

Jacobsen, L. K., Krystal, J. H., Mencl, W. E., Westerveld, M., Frost, S. J., & Pugh, K. R. (2005). Effects of smoking and smoking abstinence on cognition in adolescent tobacco smokers. *Biological Psychiatry, 57*, 56–66.

Kollins, S. H., English, J. S., Roley, M. E., O'Brien, B., Blair, J., Lane, S. D., et al. (2013). Effects of smoking abstinence on smoking-reinforced responding, withdrawal, and cognition in adults with and without attention deficit hyperactivity disorder. *Psychopharmacology, 227*, 19–30.

Kozink, R. V., Lutz, A. M., Rose, J. E., Froeliger, B., & McClernon, F. J. (2010). Smoking withdrawal shifts the spatiotemporal dynamics of neurocognition. *Addiction Biology, 15*, 480–490.

Kumari, V., & Postma, P. (2005). Nicotine use in schizophrenia: the self medication hypotheses. *Neuroscience and Biobehavioral Reviews, 29*, 1021–1034.

Lasser, K., Boyd, J. W., Woolhandler, S., Himmelstein, D. U., McCormick, D., & Bor, D. H. (2000). Smoking and mental illness: a population-based prevalence study. *JAMA, 284*, 2606–2610.

Lawrence, N. S., Ross, T. J., Hoffmann, R., Garavan, H., & Stein, E. A. (2003). Multiple neuronal networks mediate sustained attention. *Journal of Cognitive Neuroscience, 15*, 1028–1038.

Levin, E. D., Conners, C. K., Silva, D., Hinton, S. C., Meck, W. H., March, J., et al. (1998). Transdermal nicotine effects on attention. *Psychopharmacology, 140*, 135–141.

Lustig, C., Kozak, R., Sarter, M., Young, J. W., & Robbins, T. W. (2013). CNTRICS final animal model task selection: control of attention. *Neuroscience and Biobehavioral Reviews, 37*, 2099–2110.

Marchi, M., Grilli, M., & Pittaluga, A. M. (2015). Nicotinic modulation of glutamate receptor function at nerve terminal level: a fine-tuning of synaptic signals. *Frontiers in Pharmacology, 6*, 89.

Martin, L. F., Leonard, S., Hall, M. H., Tregellas, J. R., Freedman, R., & Olincy, A. (2007). Sensory gating and alpha-7 nicotinic receptor gene allelic variants in schizoaffective disorder, bipolar type. *American Journal of Medical Genetics. Part B, Neuropsychiatric Genetics: the Official Publication of the International Society of Psychiatric Genetics, 144B*, 611–614.

McGaughy, J., & Sarter, M. (1998). Sustained attention performance in rats with intracortical infusions of 192 IgG-saporin-induced cortical cholinergic deafferentation: effects of physostigmine and FG 7142. *Behavioral Neuroscience, 112*, 1519–1525.

McGaughy, J., Ross, R. S., & Eichenbaum, H. (2008). Noradrenergic, but not cholinergic, deafferentation of prefrontal cortex impairs attentional set-shifting. *Neuroscience, 153*, 63–71.

McGrath, J. J., Alati, R., Clavarino, A., Williams, G. M., Bor, W., Najman, J. M., et al. (2015). Age at first tobacco use and risk of subsequent psychosis-related outcomes: a birth cohort study. *The Australian and New Zealand Journal of Psychiatry, 50*(6), 577–583.

Muir, J. L., Bussey, T. J., Everitt, B. J., & Robbins, T. W. (1996). Dissociable effects of AMPA-induced lesions of the vertical limb diagonal band of Broca on performance of the 5-choice serial reaction time task and on acquisition of a conditional visual discrimination. *Behavioural Brain Research, 82*, 31–44.

Myers, C. S., Taylor, R. C., Moolchan, E. T., & Heishman, S. J. (2008). Dose-related enhancement of mood and cognition in smokers administered nicotine nasal spray. *Neuropsychopharmacology: Official Publication of the American College of Neuropsychopharmacology, 33*, 588–598.

Myers, C. S., Taylor, R. C., Salmeron, B. J., Waters, A. J., & Heishman, S. J. (2013). Nicotine enhances alerting, but not executive, attention in smokers and nonsmokers. *Nicotine & Tobacco Research: Official Journal of the Society for Research on Nicotine and Tobacco, 15*, 277–281.

Myles, N., Newall, H. D., Curtis, J., Nielssen, O., Shiers, D., & Large, M. (2012). Tobacco use before, at, and after first-episode psychosis: a systematic meta-analysis. *Journal of Clinical Psychiatry, 73*, 468–475.

Parikh, V., Kozak, R., Martinez, V., & Sarter, M. (2007). Prefrontal acetylcholine release controls cue detection on multiple timescales. *Neuron, 56*, 141–154.

Passetti, F., Dalley, J. W., O'Connell, M. T., Everitt, B. J., & Robbins, T. W. (2000). Increased acetylcholine release in the rat medial prefrontal cortex during performance of a visual attentional task. *The European Journal of Neuroscience, 12*, 3051–3058.

Passetti, F., Dalley, J. W., & Robbins, T. W. (2003). Double dissociation of serotonergic and dopaminergic mechanisms on attentional performance using a rodent five-choice reaction time task. *Psychopharmacology, 165*, 136–145.

Patterson, F., Jepson, C., Strasser, A. A., Loughead, J., Perkins, K. A., Gur, R. C., et al. (2009). Varenicline improves mood and cognition during smoking abstinence. *Biological Psychiatry, 65*, 144–149.

Perkins, K. A., Karelitz, J. L., Jao, N. C., Gur, R. C., & Lerman, C. (2013). Effects of bupropion on cognitive performance during initial tobacco abstinence. *Drug and Alcohol Dependence, 133*, 283–286.

Pistillo, F., Clementi, F., Zoli, M., & Gotti, C. (2015). Nicotinic, glutamatergic and dopaminergic synaptic transmission and plasticity in the mesocorticolimbic system: focus on nicotine effects. *Progress in Neurobiology, 124*, 1–27.

Poltavski, D. V., & Petros, T. (2006). Effects of transdermal nicotine on attention in adult nonsmokers with and without attentional deficits. *Physiology & Behavior, 87*, 614–624.

Poltavski, D. V., Petros, T. V., & Holm, J. E. (2012). Lower but not higher doses of transdermal nicotine facilitate cognitive performance in smokers on gender non-preferred tasks. *Pharmacology, Biochemistry, and Behavior, 102*, 423–433.

Potter, A. S., & Newhouse, P. A. (2008). Acute nicotine improves cognitive deficits in young adults with attention-deficit/hyperactivity disorder. *Pharmacology, Biochemistry, and Behavior, 88*, 407–417.

Powell, J., Dawkins, L., West, R., Powell, J., & Pickering, A. (2010). Relapse to smoking during unaided cessation: clinical, cognitive and motivational predictors. *Psychopharmacology, 212*, 537–549.

Proulx, E., Piva, M., Tian, M. K., Bailey, C. D., & Lambe, E. K. (2014). Nicotinic acetylcholine receptors in attention circuitry: the role of layer VI neurons of prefrontal cortex. *Cellular and Molecular Life Sciences: CMLS, 71*, 1225–1244.

Ray, R., Schnoll, R. A., & Lerman, C. (2009). Nicotine dependence: biology, behavior, and treatment. *Annual Review of Medicine, 60*, 247–260.

Robbins, T. W. (2002). The 5-choice serial reaction time task: behavioral pharmacology and functional neurochemistry. *Psychopharmacology, 163*(3–4), 362–380.

Rollema, H., Hajos, M., Seymour, P. A., Kozak, R., Majchrzak, M. J., Guanowsky, V., et al. (2009). Preclinical pharmacology of the alpha4beta2 nAChR partial agonist varenicline related to effects on reward, mood and cognition. *Biochemical Pharmacology, 78*, 813–824.

Sacco, K. A., Termine, A., Seyal, A., Dudas, M. M., Vessicchio, J. C., Krishnan-Sarin, S., et al. (2005). Effects of cigarette smoking on spatial working memory and attentional deficits in schizophrenia: involvement of nicotinic receptor mechanisms. *Archives of General Psychiatry, 62*, 649–659.

Saha, S., Scott, J. G., Varghese, D., Degenhardt, L., Slade, T., & McGrath, J. J. (2011). The association between delusional-like experiences, and tobacco, alcohol or cannabis use: a nationwide population-based survey. *BMC Psychiatry, 11*, 202.

Sarter, M., & Paolone, G. (2011). Deficits in attentional control: cholinergic mechanisms and circuitry-based treatment approaches. *Behavioral Neuroscience, 125*, 825–835.

Semenova, S., Stolerman, I. P., & Markou, A. (2007). Chronic nicotine administration improves attention while nicotine withdrawal induces performance deficits in the 5-choice serial reaction time task in rats. *Pharmacology, Biochemistry, and Behavior, 87*, 360–368.

Shoaib, M., & Bizarro, L. (2005). Deficits in a sustained attention task following nicotine withdrawal in rats. *Psychopharmacology, 178*, 211–222.

Thomson, D., Berk, M., Dodd, S., Rapado-Castro, M., Quirk, S. E., Ellegaard, P. K., et al. (2015). Tobacco use in bipolar disorder. *Clinical Psychopharmacology and Neuroscience, 13*, 1–11.

Wesnes, K., & Warburton, D. M. (1983). Smoking, nicotine and human performance. *Pharmacology & Therapeutics, 21*, 189–208.

Wesnes, K., Warburton, D. M., & Matz, B. (1983). Effects of nicotine on stimulus sensitivity and response bias in a visual vigilance task. *Neuropsychobiology, 9*, 41–44.

Young, J. W., & Geyer, M. A. (2013). Evaluating the role of the alpha-7 nicotinic acetylcholine receptor in the pathophysiology and treatment of schizophrenia. *Biochemical Pharmacology, 86*, 1122–1132.

Young, J. W., Finlayson, K., Spratt, C., Marston, H. M., Crawford, N., Kelly, J. S., et al. (2004). Nicotine improves sustained attention in mice: evidence for involvement of the alpha7 nicotinic acetylcholine receptor. *Neuropsychopharmacology: Official Publication of the American College of Neuropsychopharmacology, 29*, 891–900.

Young, J. W., Light, G. A., Marston, H. M., Sharp, R., & Geyer, M. A. (2009). The 5-choice continuous performance test: evidence for a translational test of vigilance for mice. *PLoS One, 4*, e4227.

Young, J. W., van Enkhuizen, J., Markou, A., Eyler, L. T., & Geyer, M. A. (2012). Withdrawal from chronic nicotine impairs attention in mice and humans as measured by the 5-choice continuous performance test: a model for identifying treatments. *Society for Neuroscience*, 696–704.

Young, J. W., Kamenski, M. E., Higa, K. K., Light, G. A., Geyer, M. A., & Zhou, X. (2015). GlyT-1 inhibition attenuates attentional but not learning or motivational deficits of the Sp4 hypomorphic mouse model relevant to psychiatric disorders. *Neuropsychopharmacology: Official Publication of the American College of Neuropsychopharmacology, 40*, 2715–2726.

Ziedonis, D., Hitsman, B., Beckham, J. C., Zvolensky, M., Adler, L. E., Audrain-McGovern, J., et al. (2008). Tobacco use and cessation in psychiatric disorders: National Institute of Mental Health report. *Nicotine & Tobacco Research: Official Journal of the Society for Research on Nicotine and Tobacco, 10*, 1691–1715.

Preclinical Models of Nicotine Withdrawal: Targeting Impaired Cognition

M. Shoaib[1], F.S. Hall[2]

[1]Newcastle University, Newcastle, United Kingdom; [2]University of Toledo, Toledo, OH, United States

INTRODUCTION

In humans, abrupt cessation of tobacco use produces cognitive, affective, and physical symptoms that include severe craving for nicotine, irritability, anxiety, poor concentration, restlessness, decreased heart rate, dysphoria, impatience, insomnia, increased appetite, and weight gain (Hughes & Hatsukami, 1986). Withdrawal symptoms begin within a few hours of cessation, typically peak in 1–4 days, and last for 3–4 weeks. Deficits in cognitive performance are observed within 4h and peak 12–48h later (Snyder, Davis, & Henningfield, 1989). Cognitive deficits impair performance in a variety of tasks that are relevant to daily life, due in part to deficits in sustained attention (Heimstra, Bancroft, & DeKock, 1967; Tarriere & Hartmann, 1964). The restlessness, agitation, and depression that accompany tobacco withdrawal are relieved by nicotine self-administration (Walker, Hall, & Hurst, 1990). Consequently, it has been suggested that nicotine and other drugs are used for "self-medication" of withdrawal-induced deficits, as well as similar premorbid conditions (Markou, Kosten, & Koob, 1998). Depressed smokers experience greater nicotine withdrawal than nondepressed smokers and have a higher incidence of relapse, and their depressive symptomatology may drive them to self-medicate with nicotine (Murphy et al., 2003). This may be, in part, why some antidepressants work as smoking cessation aids. One implication of the self-medication hypothesis is that different underlying causes of depressive symptoms

Negative Affective States and Cognitive Impairments in Nicotine Dependence
http://dx.doi.org/10.1016/B978-0-12-802574-1.00003-X

could potentially determine how they react to different smoking cessation agents and antidepressant drugs as cessation aids (Markou et al., 1998). Similar arguments could be made for cognitive impairments. For example, cognitive deficits in nonsmoking schizophrenia patients are ameliorated by nicotine (D'Souza & Markou, 2012; Jubelt et al., 2008; Young & Geyer, 2013), consistent with the self-medication hypothesis.

A number of psychiatric conditions have a high comorbidity with nicotine dependence. It remains to be seen what proportion of smoking is driven by premorbid symptomatology versus the exacerbation of nicotine withdrawal symptoms. In any case, cognitive deficits are certainly seen to result from nicotine withdrawal, including deficits in attention (Gross, Jarvik, & Rosenblatt, 1993; Hughes, Keenan, & Yellin, 1989) and working memory (Carlson et al., 2009; Sweet et al., 2010). Nicotine improves performance on a variety of attentional, mnemonic, and cognitive tasks in which smokers show deficits (Atzori, Lemmonds, Kotler, Durcan, & Boyle, 2008; George et al., 2002; Hatsukami, Fletcher, Morgan, Keenan, & Amble, 1989; Kollins, McClernon, & Epstein, 2009; Loughead et al., 2010; Myers, Taylor, Moolchan, & Heishman, 2008; Sacco et al., 2005; Snyder & Henningfield, 1989). Procognitive effects are observed in both smokers and nonsmokers, but these effects are greater in smokers (Froeliger, Gilbert, & McClernon, 2009). Overall, there is a substantial literature suggesting that smoking alleviates withdrawal-associated cognitive deficits (see review by Heishman, Taylor, & Henningfield, 1994), although the importance of this factor in relapse and response to treatment needs further assessment. There is, however, at least some evidence that the decline in cognitive performance during enforced abstinence is associated with smoking relapse (Patterson et al., 2010).

NICOTINE WITHDRAWAL IN LABORATORY RODENTS

Most quit attempts fail very early in abstinence (Hughes, Keely, & Naud, 2004), and preclinical models allow various aspects of withdrawal to be investigated that are observed during early abstinence in human smokers (Butler, Rusted, Gard, & Jackson, 2011). Although weaker than the physical withdrawal observed with other major classes of abused drugs (Corrigall, Herling, & Coen, 1989), behavioral effects of nicotine withdrawal have been demonstrated following chronic infusion of nicotine delivered via osmotic minipumps (Malin et al., 1992). Nicotine withdrawal is evaluated by means of direct observation of changes in behavior after termination of nicotine infusion or after challenge with mecamylamine. The most frequent physical signs during withdrawal include teeth chattering and chewing, writhes, yawns, ptosis, piloerection, wet dog shakes, paw tremor, body tremor, and scratches (Berrendero et al., 2005; Castane et al., 2002; Malin et al., 1992), more subtle effects than were observed for other drugs. Subsequently, more objective and robust nicotine withdrawal–dependent measures have been developed, such as increases in auditory startle responses (Helton, Tizzano, Monn, Schoepp, & Kallman, 1997) and increases in the threshold for rewarding brain stimulation (Epping-Jordan, Watkins, Koob, & Markou, 1998).

NICOTINE EXPOSURE TO INDUCE PHYSICAL DEPENDENCE IN RODENTS

The use of osmotic minipumps has provided a simple means to produce chronic exposure to nicotine for periods of 1–4 weeks to induce "physiological" (or somatic) dependence, demonstrated by either spontaneous withdrawal (abstinence) or precipitated withdrawal induced by administration of a nicotinic receptor antagonist. It is the nature of the slow, prolonged nicotine exposure that allows adaptations to develop that do not develop as easily with repeated systemic injections of nicotine (Corrigall et al., 1989). The constant infusion of nicotine via minipumps achieves plasma levels comparable to those found in smokers (Henningfield, London, & Benowitz, 1990; Jansson, Andersson, Fuxe, Bjelke, & Eneroth, 1989). In addition to the somatic signs of nicotine dependence, other behavioral consequences of dependence and withdrawal have been measured, including changes in locomotion, rearing, motor coordination, startle, temperature, heart rate, and operant responding for food reinforcement (Marks & Collins, 1985; Marks, Romm, Gaffney, & Collins, 1986; Marks, Stitzel, & Collins, 1986; McCallum, Collins, Paylor, & Marks, 2006; Naylor, Quarta, Fernandes, & Stolerman, 2005). The rate of the development of dependence, and the magnitude of dependence, varies across outcomes and differs among rodent strains (Marks et al., 1986; Marks, Stitzel, et al., 1986).

Although providing a quantifiable measure of nicotine withdrawal, somatic signs of withdrawal may have little association with resumption of nicotine intake, and thus it will be important to measure other outcomes that may be more relevant to the symptoms that humans report during initial abstinence and withdrawal. Of more relevance to affective consequences of spontaneous nicotine withdrawal, removal of an osmotic minipump delivering nicotine produces a short-lasting conditioned place aversion (Grieder et al., 2010), and mecamylamine-precipitated withdrawal induces a place aversion after a period of chronic forced consumption of nicotine (Scott & Hiroi, 2011). One could speculate that nicotine self-administration at this time would produce negative reinforcement. Indeed, a tone paired with the mecamylamine-induced withdrawal state was then used as a conditioned stimulus to reinstate nicotine conditioned place preference (Scott & Hiroi, 2010), indicative of such negative reinforcement.

Studies on the neurobiological substrates of nicotine withdrawal in rodents suggest that dopamine may be a critical neurotransmitter. Nicotine abstinence precipitated by systemic mecamylamine results in reduced dopamine release in the nucleus accumbens (Carboni, Bortone, Giua, & Di Chiara, 2000; Hildebrand, Nomikos, Hertel, Schilstrom, & Svensson, 1998), an effect that is also observed when mecamylamine is administered in the ventral tegmentum of nicotine-dependent rats (Hildebrand, Panagis, Svensson, & Nomikos, 1999). By contrast, dopamine levels have been shown to increase in the medial prefrontal cortex following mecamylamine administration to nicotine-dependent or saline-treated rats (Hildebrand et al., 1998). These observations, together with analogous increases in electrical brain stimulation thresholds (Epping-Jordan et al., 1998), have been proposed to explain certain behavioral phenomena such as the anhedonia that often accompanies smoking cessation (Warner & Shoaib, 2005). Alterations in dopamine function may also be involved in impaired cognitive performance during nicotine withdrawal.

Methods used to map and quantify the changes following nicotine exposure in rodent brains initially utilized *ex vivo* approaches. The 2-deoxyglucose (2-DG) method found increases in both striatal and limbic dopamine turnover following acute administration of nicotine (London, Connolly, Szikszay, Wamsley, & Dam, 1988, 1990), consistent with observations of increased dopamine release measured using *in vivo* microdialysis (Imperato, Mulas, & Di Chiara, 1986). A host of other brain nuclei has also been implicated using the 2-DG method after administration of behaviorally relevant doses of nicotine (London et al., 1988). Cerebrometabolic consequences of nicotine withdrawal have also been assessed using 2-DG in rodents. Schrock and Kuschinsky (1991) reported on significant short-lasting decreases in glucose utilization due to nicotine withdrawal in the anterior hypothalamus, inferior colliculus, and superior olivary nucleus.

The expression of c-fos, an immediate-early gene, has also served as a marker of neuronal activity in the context of nicotine dependence. Acutely administered nicotine elevates c-fos expression in various brain regions, including dopaminergic target areas (Matta, Foster, & Sharp, 1993; Panagis, Nisell, Nomikos, Chergui, & Svensson, 1996). Similarly, c-fos expression is also elevated when nicotine is actively self-administered by rats (Pagliusi, Tessari, DeVevey, Chiamulera, & Pich, 1996; Pich et al., 1997). The pattern of activation changes during nicotine withdrawal. Panagis et al. (1996) have shown in nicotine-dependent rats that mecamylamine-precipitated withdrawal leads to an increase in the number of Fos-positive nuclei in the central nucleus of the amygdala. However, no changes were observed in the basolateral areas of the amygdala, the nucleus accumbens core or shell, the dorsolateral striatum, or the prefrontal cortex (Panagis, Hildebrand, Svensson, & Nomikos, 2000; Salminen, Seppa, Gaddnas, & Ahtee, 2000). Spontaneous withdrawal produces an alteration in response to acute nicotine challenge. Nicotine does not alter Fos immunostaining in the caudate, nucleus accumbens, or cingulate, interpreted as desensitization, but continues to increase Fos in the central nucleus of the amygdala (Salminen et al., 2000).

Advances in rapid neuroimaging techniques have led to a revolution in mapping brain function, including structural and functional changes accompanying pharmacological manipulations. In particular, functional magnetic resonance imaging (fMRI) has been utilized to reveal changes in the oxygen extraction fraction index of neuronal activity following administration of abused substances (Jenkins, Chen, & Mandeville, 2003). In an innovative study, fMRI was used to capture changes in neural activity following mecamylamine-precipitated withdrawal in nicotine-dependent rats (Shoaib, Lowe, & Williams, 2004). Using a relatively small dose of mecamylamine, this antagonist precipitated regionally specific increases in BOLD contrast that were confined to the nucleus accumbens, while significant negative BOLD contrast changes were observed in cortical regions (Fig. 3.1). These changes

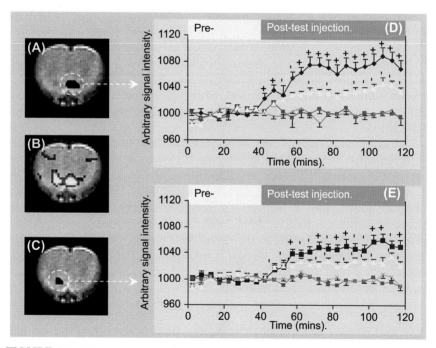

FIGURE 3.1   Time–course plots for signal intensity changes for a region of interest within the right nucleus accumbens (A and D) and the left nucleus accumbens (C and E). The group SPM ($n = 5$) for the respective regions is provided for comparison (B). Signal intensities have been averaged into five volume bins, then scaled to arbitrary units and grand mean scaled to the mean of each time series. Time–course plots of changes in arbitrary signal intensity (±sem) for pre-treatment/test condition groups ($n = 5$): ■ nicotine/1 mg/kg mecamylamine; saline/1 mg/kg mecamylamine; ■ nicotine/saline; and × saline/saline. Dunnett multiple comparison analyses: * indicates scores that the nicotine/mecamylamine group is significantly different from all other groups at each time point ($p < 0.05$); † for scores that are significantly different between ■ and ■ or × groups ($p < 0.05$); and ‡ for scores that are significantly different between ▲ and ■ or × groups ($p < 0.05$). *Reproduced from Shoaib, M., Lowe, A.S., Williams, S.C. (2004). Imaging localised dynamic changes in the nucleus accumbens following nicotine withdrawal in rats. NeuroImage, 22, 847–854.*

were pharmacologically specific since the same dose of mecamylamine elicited a smaller response in saline-treated controls, although these changes were less defined around the NAc. These findings are consistent with previous reports of decreases in extracellular dopamine levels in the NAc during nicotine withdrawal (Rahman, Zhang, Engleman, & Corrigall, 2004).

PHARMACOLOGICAL SCREENING

The effects of an array of pharmacological compounds have been evaluated on the somatic signs of nicotine withdrawal in rats using the methodology described by Malin et al. (1992). Selective dopamine receptor subtype agonists for the D1/5 and D2/3 subtypes differentially attenuate somatic signs of nicotine withdrawal (Ohmura, Jutkiewicz, Zhang, & Domino, 2011), and L-DOPA attenuates withdrawal-induced behaviors (Ohmura, Jutkiewicz, & Domino, 2011). 5-HTP is also effective in attenuating somatic signs of nicotine withdrawal (Ohmura, Jutkiewicz, Yoshioka, & Domino, 2011). Targeting the catabolism enzymes for catecholamines, notably with the selective monoamine oxidase B (MAO-B) inhibitor deprenyl, attenuates nicotine withdrawal, while clorgyline, a MAO-A selective inhibitor, exacerbates the somatic signs of nicotine withdrawal (Malin et al., 2013).

The glutamate system represents another important neurotransmitter system that is implicated in nicotine dependence. Blockade of glutamatergic neurotransmission by dizocilpine, a noncompetitive NMDA receptor antagonist, has been shown to block both behavioral and biochemical adaptations to repeated nicotine exposure (Shoaib, Benwell, Akbar, Stolerman, & Balfour, 1994, 1997; Shoaib & Stolerman, 1992). Studies utilizing acoustic startle as the dependent measure of nicotine dependence have shown that the Group II mGluR selective agonist LY354740 ameliorates the increase in acoustic startle response observed in rats during nicotine withdrawal (Helton et al., 1997).

MEASURES OF COGNITION IN RODENT MODELS OF NICOTINE WITHDRAWAL

The involvement of monoaminergic and glutamatergic systems in nicotine withdrawal, and cortical activity changes from imaging studies, would be expected to also be involved in cognitive aspects of withdrawal. However, most research in this area has focused on establishing cognitive-enhancing effects of nicotine in noncompromised subjects. It has been well established that, depending on which cognitive domain is investigated, both the α_7 and $\alpha_4\beta_2$ subunits mediate pro-cognitive effects of nicotine. The α_7 subtype mediates effects on working memory (Levin et al., 2009), some aspects of associative learning (Young, Meves, Tarantino, Caldwell, & Geyer, 2011), attention (Hoyle, Genn, Fernandes, & Stolerman, 2006; Young et al., 2004), and fear conditioning (Davis & Gould, 2009; Raybuck & Gould, 2009). Effects of the β_2 subunit are also observed (Guillem et al., 2011; Hahn, Shoaib, & Stolerman, 2002). A full review of the cognitive-enhancing effects of nicotine in all species is outside the scope of this review chapter, and thus this review will focus on cognitive deficits following abstinence from nicotine or following precipitation of withdrawal by nicotinic receptor antagonists in laboratory rodents.

ANIMAL MODELS OF NICOTINE DEPENDENCE: WITHDRAWAL EFFECTS ON ATTENTION

The effects of nicotine on visuospatial attention have been studied using the five-choice serial reaction time task (5CSRTT). Nicotine improves attentional performance in the 5CSRTT (Hahn et al., 2002; Stolerman, Mirza, Hahn, & Shoaib, 2000; Young et al., 2004), although chronic nicotine treatment may be necessary to produce attentional improvements under some circumstances (Pattij et al., 2007). Furthermore, as would be anticipated within a homeostasis model of adaptation to chronic nicotine exposure, spontaneous or precipitated nicotine withdrawal impairs attention in this task (Semenova, Stolerman, & Markou, 2007; Shoaib & Bizarro, 2005). Despite the evidence discussed here, these effects did not seem to involve α_7 nicotinic receptors, as the selective antagonist methyllycaconitine did not induce attentional deficits, in contrast to the nonselective antagonist dihydro-β-erythroidine (Fig. 3.2). The profile of the attentional deficits was similar to those produced by the D2/D3 receptor antagonist raclopride (Shoaib & Bizarro, 2005) and 6-hydroxydopamine lesions to the nucleus accumbens (Cole & Robbins, 1989). In a similar study, nicotine withdrawal impaired vigilance in the five-choice continuous performance task, a task that incorporates nontarget trials as well as target trials (Young, van Enkhuizen, Markou, Eyler, & Geyer, 2012). Interestingly, although acute nicotine treatment improves attention by increasing target responding in this task, withdrawal from nicotine impairs performance by increasing response disinhibition (eg, responding to nontarget signals and reducing accuracy as seen in the task). Hence, differing mechanisms may contribute to the initial beneficial effects of nicotine on cognition compared with the impairing effects of nicotine withdrawal.

Nicotine and nicotine withdrawal may also influence attentional mechanisms by influencing preattentional mechanisms, or sensory-motor

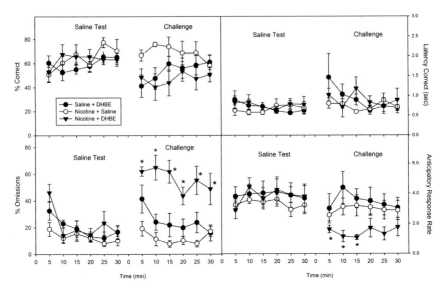

FIGURE 3.2 Precipitation of nicotine withdrawal by DHβE (5.0 mg/kg SC) on 5-CSRTT performance. The four segments of the graph depict the variables used to assess attention in three groups of rats: (●) saline treated–DHBE challenged, (○) nicotine treated–saline challenged, and (▼) nicotine treated–DHBE challenged. Results are expressed as mean ± SEM. In each segment, baseline performance following saline injection is shown on the left for comparison with results obtained following challenge with the antagonist or vehicle, shown in the right section. Significant differences between groups were tested using two-way ANOVA for repeated measures followed by Tukey B *post hoc* tests (asterisk denotes a significant difference of $p < 0.05$). *Reproduced from Shoaib, M., Bizarro, L. (2005). Deficits in a sustained attention task following nicotine withdrawal in rats.* Psychopharmacology, 178, 211–222.

gating, such as prepulse inhibition of acoustic startle. Nicotine withdrawal impairs prepulse inhibition of acoustic startle in DBA2J mice (Semenova, Bespalov, & Markou, 2003) and in human subjects (Kumari & Gray, 1999). However, effects of nicotine withdrawal were not observed in another study that used C57BL6/J mice (Andre, Gulick, Portugal, & Gould, 2008). It would appear that genetic background and some predisposition to such deficits are important factors, as appears to be the case for other cognitive effects of nicotine.

Nicotine and nicotine withdrawal also affect a number of other cognitive and mnemonic processes, particularly certain aspects of fear conditioning (for review, see Hall et al. (2012, 2015), and Chapter 4 by Kutlu, Holliday and Gould in this volume). Importantly, only certain types of fear conditioning are affected by chronic nicotine exposure, suggesting that these effects might be different across anatomical circuits underlying these different types of conditioned responses. Importantly for the present argument, nicotine cessation treatments reverse nicotine withdrawal-associated impairments in contextual fear conditioning (Davis, James, Siegel, & Gould, 2005; Portugal & Gould, 2007; Raybuck, Portugal, Lerman, & Gould, 2008). The withdrawal-induced deficits in contextual fear conditioning in these studies have been compared to cognitive deficits in ADHD and are reversed by atomoxetine as well (Davis & Gould, 2007). This is of interest given the high comorbidity of smoking and ADHD.

PHARMACOLOGICAL TREATMENT OF NICOTINE DEPENDENCE

The medications currently available for the treatment of nicotine dependence differ substantially in their mechanisms of action. Given the various motivations reported by tobacco smokers, it seems likely that each medication may only be effective in a subset of smokers. Nicotine replacement therapy (Silagy, Lancaster, Stead, Mant, & Fowler, 2004) does not differentiate among the potential underlying mechanisms, nor really does the partial agonist varenicline (Gonzales et al., 2006; Nides et al., 2006). Other pharmacological treatments that have been extensively investigated include antidepressants such as bupropion and nortripty-line, which would obviously focus on affective symptoms but perhaps not affect other symptoms, including cognition. Various other drugs are also being investigated as potential smoking cessation treatments (Elrashidi & Ebbert, 2014), some of which may be more effective for cognitive symptoms, including atomoxetine, baclofen, carvedilol, labetalol, lobeline, mecamylamine, naltrexone, reboxetine, rimonabant, surinabant, selegi-line, EVT 302, Tiagabine, topiramate, vigabatrin, cytosine, buspirone, and D-cycloserine. Given the different mechanisms of action of these drugs, it might be thought that some may be effective in treating the cognitive symptoms of withdrawal. Nicotine has only a moderate efficacy in smoking cessation trials (Jorenby et al., 1999), suggesting that other approaches are certainly needed.

Bupropion is an effective smoking cessation treatment (Goldstein, 1998) that is more effective when combined with nicotine replacement (Jorenby et al., 1999), suggesting that they work through different mechanisms. Bupropion does not alter many acute effects of nicotine, including self-administration, drug discrimination, and conditioned taste aversion (Shoaib, Sidhpura, & Shafait, 2003), prompting those authors to suggest that the effects of bupropion may be primarily on withdrawal-associated effects, as other studies have demonstrated (Warner & Shoaib, 2005; Wing & Shoaib, 2007), in particular withdrawal-induced anhedonia (Cryan, Bruijnzeel, Skjei, & Markou, 2003; Paterson, Balfour, & Markou, 2007) and aversion (Malin et al., 2006). This is consistent with reduced affective symptoms during bupropion treatment but not reduced nicotine craving (Shiffman et al., 2000).

For similar reasons, other antidepressant compounds have been examined in both preclinical and clinical studies. For example, nortriptyline, like bupropion, reduces somatic signs of nicotine withdrawal (Prochazka et al., 1998; Wing & Shoaib, 2007). Fluoxetine reverses nicotine withdrawal-induced ICSS threshold elevations (ie, anhedonia) when co-administered with p-MPPI [4-(2'-methoxy-phenyl)-1-[2'-(n-(2"-pyridinyl)-p-iodobenzamido]-ethylpiperazine], a 5-HT1A receptor antagonist (Harrison, Liem, & Markou, 2001). Similarly, paroxetine reverses amphetamine withdrawal-induced anhedonia when co-administered with p-MPPI (Markou, Harrison, Chevrette, & Hoyer, 2005). These drug combinations act to enhance serotonergic transmission rapidly, suggesting that nicotine withdrawal-induced anhedonia may be mediated by decreased serotonergic function, as is hypothesized for depression. Interestingly, fluoxetine and p-MPPI did not alleviate somatic signs of nicotine withdrawal (Harrison et al., 2001), indicating a clear dissociation between affective and somatic signs, and demonstrating that it is not somatic discomfort that induces anhedonia. The effects of these drugs on cognitive symptoms of nicotine withdrawal are unknown, but it seems likely that other approaches will be needed for treatment of these symptoms.

SUMMARY

In reviewing the preclinical literature on nicotine withdrawal and associated cognitive deficits, our approaches in developing new pharmacological treatments do not address all circumstances. The majority of preclinical studies have largely focused on physical signs of dependence; some studies have addressed affective symptoms, but few have addressed cognitive symptoms. This is a clear limitation since one of the key aspects of the tobacco withdrawal syndrome is cognitive impairment. The improved clinical success of varenicline suggests that this partial agonist may provide some cognitive restoration in addition to acting, essentially, as a nicotine replacement to affect craving and relapse. Cognitive deficits can play a role, perhaps by acting as drivers of relapse or by reducing resistance to factors that trigger relapse in former smokers. In some studies, cognitive deficits have been found to be predictors of relapse (eg, Powell, Dawkins, West, Powell, & Pickering, 2010), while in others, superior cognitive performance has been associated with successful quitting (eg, Nestor, McCabe, Jones, Clancy, & Garavan, 2011). Therefore, future preclinical studies on nicotine withdrawal should be designed with more clinically relevant measures of cognition in mind and consider evaluating cognitive enhancers as putative smoking cessation compounds.

References

Andre, J. M., Gulick, D., Portugal, G. S., & Gould, T. J. (2008). Nicotine withdrawal disrupts both foreground and background contextual fear conditioning but not pre-pulse inhibition of the acoustic startle response in C57BL/6 mice. *Behavioural Brain Research, 190*, 174–181.

Atzori, G., Lemmonds, C. A., Kotler, M. L., Durcan, M. J., & Boyle, J. (2008). Efficacy of a nicotine (4 mg)-containing lozenge on the cognitive impairment of nicotine withdrawal. *Journal of Clinical Psychopharmacology, 28*, 667–674.

Berrendero, F., Mendizabal, V., Robledo, P., Galeote, L., Bilkei-Gorzo, A., Zimmer, A., et al. (2005). Nicotine-induced antinociception, rewarding effects, and physical dependence are decreased in mice lacking the preproenkephalin gene. *The Journal of Neuroscience: The Official Journal of the Society for Neuroscience, 25*, 1103–1112.

Butler, K., Rusted, J., Gard, P., & Jackson, A. (2011). Probabilistic reversal learning behaviour in current, former and never smokers. In *European Meeting of the Society for research on nicotine and tobacco, Turkey*.

Carboni, E., Bortone, L., Giua, C., & Di Chiara, G. (2000). Dissociation of physical abstinence signs from changes in extracellular dopamine in the nucleus accumbens and in the prefrontal cortex of nicotine dependent rats. *Drug and Alcohol Dependence, 58*, 93–102.

Carlson, J. M., Gilbert, D. G., Riise, H., Rabinovich, N. E., Sugai, C., & Froeliger, B. (2009). Serotonin transporter genotype and depressive symptoms moderate effects of nicotine on spatial working memory. *Experimental and Clinical Psychopharmacology, 17*, 173–180.

Castane, A., Valjent, E., Ledent, C., Parmentier, M., Maldonado, R., & Valverde, O. (2002). Lack of CB1 cannabinoid receptors modifies nicotine behavioural responses, but not nicotine abstinence. *Neuropharmacology, 43*, 857–867.

Cole, B. J., & Robbins, T. W. (1989). Effects of 6-hydroxydopamine lesions of the nucleus accumbens septi on performance of a 5-choice serial reaction time task in rats: implications for theories of selective attention and arousal. *Behavioural Brain Research, 33*, 165–179.

Corrigall, W. A., Herling, S., & Coen, K. M. (1989). Evidence for a behavioral deficit during withdrawal from chronic nicotine treatment. *Pharmacology, Biochemistry, and Behavior, 33*, 559–562.

Cryan, J. F., Bruijnzeel, A. W., Skjei, K. L., & Markou, A. (2003). Bupropion enhances brain reward function and reverses the affective and somatic aspects of nicotine withdrawal in the rat. *Psychopharmacology, 168*, 347–358.

D'Souza, M. S., & Markou, A. (2012). Schizophrenia and tobacco smoking comorbidity: nAChR agonists in the treatment of schizophrenia-associated cognitive deficits. *Neuropharmacology, 62*, 1564–1573.

Davis, J. A., & Gould, T. J. (2007). Atomoxetine reverses nicotine withdrawal-associated deficits in contextual fear conditioning. *Neuropsychopharmacology, 32*, 2011–2019.

Davis, J. A., & Gould, T. J. (2009). Hippocampal nAChRs mediate nicotine withdrawal-related learning deficits. *European Neuropsychopharmacology: The Journal of the European College of Neuropsychopharmacology, 19*, 551–561.

Davis, J. A., James, J. R., Siegel, S. J., & Gould, T. J. (2005). Withdrawal from chronic nicotine administration impairs contextual fear conditioning in C57BL/6 mice. *The Journal of Neuroscience: The Official Journal of the Society for Neuroscience, 25*, 8708–8713.

Elrashidi, M. Y., & Ebbert, J. O. (2014). Emerging drugs for the treatment of tobacco dependence: 2014 update. *Expert Opinion on Emerging Drugs, 19*, 243–260.

Epping-Jordan, M. P., Watkins, S. S., Koob, G. F., & Markou, A. (1998). Dramatic decreases in brain reward function during nicotine withdrawal. *Nature, 393*, 76–79.

Froeliger, B., Gilbert, D. G., & McClernon, F. J. (2009). Effects of nicotine on novelty detection and memory recognition performance: double-blind, placebo-controlled studies of smokers and nonsmokers. *Psychopharmacology, 205*, 625–633.

George, T. P., Vessicchio, J. C., Termine, A., Sahady, D. M., Head, C. A., Pepper, W. T., et al. (2002). Effects of smoking abstinence on visuospatial working memory function in schizophrenia. *Neuropsychopharmacology, 26*, 75–85.

Goldstein, M. G. (1998). Bupropion sustained release and smoking cessation. *The Journal of Clinical Psychiatry, 59*(Suppl. 4), 66–72.

Gonzales, D., Rennard, S. I., Nides, M., Oncken, C., Azoulay, S., Billing, C. B., et al. (2006). Varenicline, an alpha4beta2 nicotinic acetylcholine receptor partial agonist, vs sustained-release bupropion and placebo for smoking cessation: a randomized controlled trial. *The Journal of the American Medical Association, 296*, 47–55.

Grieder, T. E., Sellings, L. H., Vargas-Perez, H., Ting, A. K. R., Siu, E. C., Tyndale, R. F., et al. (2010). Dopaminergic signaling mediates the motivational response underlying the opponent process to chronic but not acute nicotine. *Neuropsychopharmacology, 35*, 943–954.

Gross, T. M., Jarvik, M. E., & Rosenblatt, M. R. (1993). Nicotine abstinence produces content-specific stroop interference. *Psychopharmacology, 110*, 333–336.

Guillem, K., Bloem, B., Poorthuis, R. B., Loos, M., Smit, A. B., Maskos, U., et al. (2011). Nicotinic acetylcholine receptor beta2 subunits in the medial prefrontal cortex control attention. *Science, 333*, 888–891.

Hahn, B., Shoaib, M., & Stolerman, I. P. (2002). Nicotine-induced enhancement of attention in the five-choice serial reaction time task: the influence of task demands. *Psychopharmacology, 162*, 129–137.

Hall, F. S., Der-Avakian, A., Gould, T. J., Markou, A., Shoaib, M., & Young, J. W. (2015). Negative affective states and cognitive impairments in nicotine dependence. *Neuroscience and Biobehavioral Reviews, 58*, 168–185.

Hall, F. S., Markou, A., Levin, E. D., & Uhl, G. R. (2012). Mouse models for studying genetic influences on factors determining smoking cessation success in humans. *Annals of the New York Academy of Sciences, 1248*, 39–70.

Harrison, A. A., Liem, Y. T., & Markou, A. (2001). Fluoxetine combined with a serotonin-1A receptor antagonist reversed reward deficits observed during nicotine and amphetamine withdrawal in rats. *Neuropsychopharmacology, 25*, 55–71.

Hatsukami, D., Fletcher, L., Morgan, S., Keenan, R., & Amble, P. (1989). The effects of varying cigarette deprivation duration on cognitive and performance tasks. *Journal of Substance Abuse Treatment, 1*, 407–416.

Heimstra, N. W., Bancroft, N. R., & DeKock, A. R. (1967). Effects of smoking upon sustained performance in a simulated driving task. *Annals of the New York Academy of Sciences, 142*, 345–395.

Heishman, S. J., Taylor, R. C., & Henningfield, J. E. (1994). Nicotine and smoking: a review of effects on nicotine performance. *Experimental and Clinical Psychopharmacology, 2*, 345–395.

Helton, D. R., Tizzano, J. P., Monn, J. A., Schoepp, D. D., & Kallman, M. J. (1997). LY354740: a metabotropic glutamate receptor agonist which ameliorates symptoms of nicotine withdrawal in rats. *Neuropharmacology, 36*, 1511–1516.

Henningfield, J. E., London, E. D., & Benowitz, N. L. (1990). Arterial-venous differences in plasma concentrations of nicotine after cigarette smoking. *The Journal of the American Medical Association, 263*, 2049–2050.

Hildebrand, B. E., Nomikos, G. G., Hertel, P., Schilstrom, B., & Svensson, T. H. (1998). Reduced dopamine output in the nucleus accumbens but not in the medial prefrontal cortex in rats displaying a mecamylamine-precipitated nicotine withdrawal syndrome. *Brain Research, 779*, 214–225.

Hildebrand, B. E., Panagis, G., Svensson, T. H., & Nomikos, G. G. (1999). Behavioral and biochemical manifestations of mecamylamine-precipitated nicotine withdrawal in the rat: role of nicotinic receptors in the ventral tegmental area. *Neuropsychopharmacology, 21*, 560–574.

Hoyle, E., Genn, R. F., Fernandes, C., & Stolerman, I. P. (2006). Impaired performance of alpha7 nicotinic receptor knockout mice in the five-choice serial reaction time task. *Psychopharmacology, 189*, 211–223.

Hughes, J. R., & Hatsukami, D. (1986). Signs and symptoms of tobacco withdrawal. *Archives of General Psychiatry, 43*, 289–294.

Hughes, J. R., Keely, J., & Naud, S. (2004). Shape of the relapse curve and long-term abstinence among untreated smokers. *Addiction, 99*, 29–38.

Hughes, J. R., Keenan, R. M., & Yellin, A. (1989). Effect of tobacco withdrawal on sustained attention. *Addictive Behaviors, 14*, 577–580.

Imperato, A., Mulas, A., & Di Chiara, G. (1986). Nicotine preferentially stimulates dopamine release in the limbic system of freely moving rats. *European Journal of Pharmacology, 132*, 337–338.

Jansson, A., Andersson, K., Fuxe, K., Bjelke, B., & Eneroth, P. (1989). Effects of combined pre- and postnatal treatment with nicotine on hypothalamic catecholamine nerve terminal systems and neuroendocrine function in the 4-week old and adult male and female diestrous rat. *Journal of Neuroendocrinology, 1*, 455–464.

Jenkins, B. G., Chen, Y. I., & Mandeville, J. B. (2003). Pharmacologic magnetic resonance imaging (phMRI). In N. van Bruggen, & T. Roberts (Eds.), *Biomedical imaging in experimental neuroscience* (pp. 155–210). Boca Raton: CRC Press.

Jorenby, D. E., Leischow, S. J., Nides, M. A., Rennard, S. I., Johnston, J. A., Hughes, A. R., et al. (1999). A controlled trial of sustained-release bupropion, a nicotine patch, or both for smoking cessation. *The New England Journal of Medicine, 340*, 685–691.

Jubelt, L. E., Barr, R. S., Goff, D. C., Logvinenko, T., Weiss, A. P., & Evins, A. E. (2008). Effects of transdermal nicotine on episodic memory in non-smokers with and without schizophrenia. *Psychopharmacology, 199*, 89–98.

Kollins, S. H., McClernon, F. J., & Epstein, J. N. (2009). Effects of smoking abstinence on reaction time variability in smokers with and without ADHD: an ex-Gaussian analysis. *Drug and Alcohol Dependence, 100*, 169–172.

Kumari, V., & Gray, J. A. (1999). Smoking withdrawal, nicotine dependence and prepulse inhibition of the acoustic startle reflex. *Psychopharmacology, 141*, 11–15.

Levin, E. D., Petro, A., Rezvani, A. H., Pollard, N., Christopher, N. C., Strauss, M., et al. (2009). Nicotinic alpha7- or beta2-containing receptor knockout: effects on radial-arm maze learning and long-term nicotine consumption in mice. *Behavioural Brain Research, 196*, 207–213.

London, E. D., Connolly, R. J., Szikszay, M., Wamsley, J. K., & Dam, M. (1988). Effects of nicotine on local cerebral glucose utilization in the rat. *The Journal of Neuroscience: the Official Journal of the Society for Neuroscience, 8*, 3920–3928.

London, E. D., Fanelli, R. J., Kimes, A. S., & Moses, R. L. (1990). Effects of chronic nicotine on cerebral glucose utilization in the rat. *Brain Research, 520*, 208–214.

Loughead, J., Ray, R., Wileyto, E. P., Ruparel, K., Sanborn, P., Siegel, S., et al. (2010). Effects of the alpha4beta2 partial agonist varenicline on brain activity and working memory in abstinent smokers. *Biological Psychiatry, 67*, 715–721.

Malin, D. H., Lake, J. R., Newlin-Maultsby, P., Roberts, L. K., Lanier, J. G., Carter, V. A., et al. (1992). Rodent model of nicotine abstinence syndrome. *Pharmacology, Biochemistry, and Behavior, 43*, 779–784.

Malin, D. H., Lake, J. R., Smith, T. D., Khambati, H. N., Meyers-Paal, R. L., Montellano, A. L., et al. (2006). Bupropion attenuates nicotine abstinence syndrome in the rat. *Psychopharmacology, 184*, 494–503.

Malin, D. H., Moon, W. D., Goyarzu, P., Barclay, E., Magallanes, N., Vela, A. J., et al. (2013). Inhibition of monoamine oxidase isoforms modulates nicotine withdrawal syndrome in the rat. *Life Sciences, 93*, 448–453.

Markou, A., Harrison, A. A., Chevrette, J., & Hoyer, D. (2005). Paroxetine combined with a 5-HT(1A) receptor antagonist reversed reward deficits observed during amphetamine withdrawal in rats. *Psychopharmacology, 178*, 133–142.

Markou, A., Kosten, T. R., & Koob, G. F. (1998). Neurobiological similarities in depression and drug dependence: a self-medication hypothesis. *Neuropsychopharmacology, 18*, 135–174.

Marks, M. J., & Collins, A. C. (1985). Tolerance, cross-tolerance, and receptors after chronic nicotine or oxotremorine. *Pharmacology, Biochemistry, and Behavior, 22,* 283–291.

Marks, M. J., Romm, E., Gaffney, D. K., & Collins, A. C. (1986). Nicotine-induced tolerance and receptor changes in four mouse strains. *The Journal of Pharmacology and Experimental Therapeutics, 237,* 809–819.

Marks, M. J., Stitzel, J. A., & Collins, A. C. (1986). Dose-response analysis of nicotine tolerance and receptor changes in two inbred mouse strains. *The Journal of Pharmacology and Experimental Therapeutics, 239,* 358–364.

Matta, S. G., Foster, C. A., & Sharp, B. M. (1993). Nicotine stimulates the expression of cFos protein in the parvocellular paraventricular nucleus and brainstem catecholaminergic regions. *Endocrinology, 132,* 2149–2156.

McCallum, S. E., Collins, A. C., Paylor, R., & Marks, M. J. (2006). Deletion of the beta2 nicotinic acetylcholine receptor subunit alters development of tolerance to nicotine and eliminates receptor upregulation. *Psychopharmacology, 184,* 314–327.

Murphy, J. M., Horton, N. J., Monson, R. R., Laird, N. M., Sobol, A. M., & Leighton, A. H. (2003). Cigarette smoking in relation to depression: historical trends from the Stirling County Study. *The American Journal of Psychiatry, 160,* 1663–1669.

Myers, C. S., Taylor, R. C., Moolchan, E. T., & Heishman, S. J. (2008). Dose-related enhancement of mood and cognition in smokers administered nicotine nasal spray. *Neuropsychopharmacology, 33,* 588–598.

Naylor, C., Quarta, D., Fernandes, C., & Stolerman, I. P. (2005). Tolerance to nicotine in mice lacking alpha7 nicotinic receptors. *Psychopharmacology, 180,* 558–563.

Nestor, L., McCabe, E., Jones, J., Clancy, L., & Garavan, H. (2011). Differences in "bottom-up" and "top-down" neural activity in current and former cigarette smokers: evidence for neural substrates which may promote nicotine abstinence through increased cognitive control. *NeuroImage, 56,* 2258–2275.

Nides, M., Oncken, C., Gonzales, D., Rennard, S., Watsky, E. J., Anziano, R., et al. (2006). Smoking cessation with varenicline, a selective alpha4beta2 nicotinic receptor partial agonist: results from a 7-week, randomized, placebo- and bupropion-controlled trial with 1-year follow-up. *Archives of Internal Medicine, 166,* 1561–1568.

Ohmura, Y., Jutkiewicz, E. M., & Domino, E. F. (2011a). L-DOPA attenuates nicotine withdrawal-induced behaviors in rats. *Pharmacology, Biochemistry, and Behavior, 98,* 552–558.

Ohmura, Y., Jutkiewicz, E. M., Yoshioka, M., & Domino, E. F. (2011b). 5-Hydroxytryptophan attenuates somatic signs of nicotine withdrawal. *Journal of Pharmacological Sciences, 117,* 121–124.

Ohmura, Y., Jutkiewicz, E. M., Zhang, A., & Domino, E. F. (2011c). Dopamine D1/5 and D2/3 agonists differentially attenuate somatic signs of nicotine withdrawal in rats. *Pharmacology, Biochemistry, and Behavior, 99,* 552–556.

Pagliusi, S. R., Tessari, M., DeVevey, S., Chiamulera, C., & Pich, E. M. (1996). The reinforcing properties of nicotine are associated with a specific patterning of c-fos expression in the rat brain. *The European Journal of Neuroscience, 8,* 2247–2256.

Panagis, G., Hildebrand, B. E., Svensson, T. H., & Nomikos, G. G. (2000). Selective c-fos induction and decreased dopamine release in the central nucleus of amygdala in rats displaying a mecamylamine-precipitated nicotine withdrawal syndrome. *Synapse, 35,* 15–25.

Panagis, G., Nisell, M., Nomikos, G. G., Chergui, K., & Svensson, T. H. (1996). Nicotine injections into the ventral tegmental area increase locomotion and Fos-like immunoreactivity in the nucleus accumbens of the rat. *Brain Research, 730,* 133–142.

Paterson, N. E., Balfour, D. J., & Markou, A. (2007). Chronic bupropion attenuated the anhedonic component of nicotine withdrawal in rats via inhibition of dopamine reuptake in the nucleus accumbens shell. *The European Journal of Neuroscience, 25,* 3099–3108.

Patterson, F., Jepson, C., Loughead, J., Perkins, K., Strasser, A. A., Siegel, S., et al. (2010). Working memory deficits predict short-term smoking resumption following brief abstinence. *Drug and Alcohol Dependence, 106,* 61–64.

Pattij, T., Janssen, M. C., Loos, M., Smit, A. B., Schoffelmeer, A. N., & van Gaalen, M. M. (2007). Strain specificity and cholinergic modulation of visuospatial attention in three inbred mouse strains. *Genes, Brain and Behavior, 6,* 579–587.

Pich, E. M., Pagliusi, S. R., Tessari, M., Talabot-Ayer, D., Hooft van Huijsduijnen, R., & Chiamulera, C. (1997). Common neural substrates for the addictive properties of nicotine and cocaine. *Science, 275,* 83–86.

Portugal, G. S., & Gould, T. J. (2007). Bupropion dose-dependently reverses nicotine withdrawal deficits in contextual fear conditioning. *Pharmacology, Biochemistry, and Behavior, 88,* 179–187.

Powell, J., Dawkins, L., West, R., Powell, J., & Pickering, A. (2010). Relapse to smoking during unaided cessation: clinical, cognitive and motivational predictors. *Psychopharmacology, 212,* 537–549.

Prochazka, A. V., Weaver, M. J., Keller, R. T., Fryer, G. E., Licari, P. A., & Lofaso, D. (1998). A randomized trial of nortriptyline for smoking cessation. *Archives of Internal Medicine, 158,* 2035–2039.

Rahman, S., Zhang, J., Engleman, E. A., & Corrigall, W. A. (2004). Neuroadaptive changes in the mesoaccumbens dopamine system after chronic nicotine self-administration: a microdialysis study. *Neuroscience, 129,* 415–424.

Raybuck, J. D., & Gould, T. J. (2009). Nicotine withdrawal-induced deficits in trace fear conditioning in C57BL/6 mice–a role for high-affinity beta2 subunit-containing nicotinic acetylcholine receptors. *The European of Neuroscience, 29,* 377–387.

Raybuck, J. D., Portugal, G. S., Lerman, C., & Gould, T. J. (2008). Varenicline ameliorates nicotine withdrawal-induced learning deficits in C57BL/6 mice. *Behavioral Neuroscience, 122,* 1166–1171.

Sacco, K. A., Termine, A., Seyal, A., Dudas, M. M., Vessicchio, J. C., Krishnan-Sarin, S., et al. (2005). Effects of cigarette smoking on spatial working memory and attentional deficits in schizophrenia: involvement of nicotinic receptor mechanisms. *Archives of General Psychiatry, 62,* 649–659.

Salminen, O., Seppa, T., Gaddnas, H., & Ahtee, L. (2000). Effect of acute nicotine on Fos protein expression in rat brain during chronic nicotine and its withdrawal. *Pharmacology, Biochemistry, and Behavior, 66,* 87–93.

Schrock, H., & Kuschinsky, W. (1991). Effects of nicotine withdrawal on the local cerebral glucose utilization in conscious rats. *Brain Research, 545,* 234–238.

Scott, D., & Hiroi, N. (2010). Emergence of dormant conditioned incentive approach by conditioned withdrawal in nicotine addiction. *Biological Psychiatry, 68,* 726–732.

Scott, D., & Hiroi, N. (2011). Deconstructing craving: dissociable cortical control of cue reactivity in nicotine addiction. *Biological Psychiatry, 69,* 1052–1059.

Semenova, S., Bespalov, A., & Markou, A. (2003). Decreased prepulse inhibition during nicotine withdrawal in DBA/2J mice is reversed by nicotine self-administration. *European Journal of Pharmacology, 472,* 99–110.

Semenova, S., Stolerman, I. P., & Markou, A. (2007). Chronic nicotine administration improves attention while nicotine withdrawal induces performance deficits in the 5-choice serial reaction time task in rats. *Pharmacology, Biochemistry, and Behavior, 87,* 360–368.

Shiffman, S., Johnston, J. A., Khayrallah, M., Elash, C. A., Gwaltney, C. J., Paty, J. A., et al. (2000). The effect of bupropion on nicotine craving and withdrawal. *Psychopharmacology, 148,* 33–40.

Shoaib, M., Benwell, M. E., Akbar, M. T., Stolerman, I. P., & Balfour, D. J. (1994). Behavioural and neurochemical adaptations to nicotine in rats: influence of NMDA antagonists. *British Journal of Pharmacology, 111,* 1073–1080.

Shoaib, M., & Bizarro, L. (2005). Deficits in a sustained attention task following nicotine withdrawal in rats. *Psychopharmacology, 178,* 211–222.

Shoaib, M., Lowe, A. S., & Williams, S. C. (2004). Imaging localised dynamic changes in the nucleus accumbens following nicotine withdrawal in rats. *NeuroImage, 22,* 847–854.

Shoaib, M., Schindler, C. W., Goldberg, S. R., & Pauly, J. R. (1997). Behavioural and biochemical adaptations to nicotine in rats: influence of MK801, an NMDA receptor antagonist. *Psychopharmacology, 134*, 121–130.

Shoaib, M., Sidhpura, N., & Shafait, S. (2003). Investigating the actions of bupropion on dependence-related effects of nicotine in rats. *Psychopharmacology, 165*, 405–412.

Shoaib, M., & Stolerman, I. P. (1992). MK801 attenuates behavioural adaptation to chronic nicotine administration in rats. *British Journal of Pharmacology, 105*, 514–515.

Silagy, C., Lancaster, T., Stead, L., Mant, D., & Fowler, G. (2004). Nicotine replacement therapy for smoking cessation. *The Cochrane Database of Systematic Reviews*, CD000146.

Snyder, F. R., Davis, F. C., & Henningfield, J. E. (1989). The tobacco withdrawal syndrome: performance decrements assessed on a computerized test battery. *Drug and Alcohol Dependence, 23*, 259–266.

Snyder, F. R., & Henningfield, J. E. (1989). Effects of nicotine administration following 12 h of tobacco deprivation: assessment on computerized performance tasks. *Psychopharmacology, 97*, 17–22.

Stolerman, I. P., Mirza, N. R., Hahn, B., & Shoaib, M. (2000). Nicotine in an animal model of attention. *European Journal of Pharmacology, 393*, 147–154.

Sweet, L. H., Mulligan, R. C., Finnerty, C. E., Jerskey, B. A., David, S. P., Cohen, R. A., et al. (2010). Effects of nicotine withdrawal on verbal working memory and associated brain response. *Psychiatry Research, 183*, 69–74.

Tarriere, H. C., & Hartmann, F. (1964). Investigations into the effects of tobacco smoke on a visual vigilance task. In *Proceedings of the 2nd International Congress on Ergonomics* (pp. 525–530).

Walker, H. K., Hall, W. D., & Hurst, J. W. (1990). *Clinical methods*. Boston: Butterworths.

Warner, C., & Shoaib, M. (2005). How does bupropion work as a smoking cessation aid? *Addiction Biology, 10*, 219–231.

Wing, V. C., & Shoaib, M. (2007). Examining the clinical efficacy of bupropion and nortriptyline as smoking cessation agents in a rodent model of nicotine withdrawal. *Psychopharmacology, 195*, 303–313.

Young, J. W., Finlayson, K., Spratt, C., Marston, H. M., Crawford, N., Kelly, J. S., et al. (2004). Nicotine improves sustained attention in mice: evidence for involvement of the alpha7 nicotinic acetylcholine receptor. *Neuropsychopharmacology, 29*, 891–900.

Young, J. W., & Geyer, M. A. (2013). Evaluating the role of the alpha-7 nicotinic acetylcholine receptor in the pathophysiology and treatment of schizophrenia. *Biochemical Pharmacology, 86*, 1122–1132.

Young, J. W., Meves, J. M., Tarantino, I. S., Caldwell, S., & Geyer, M. A. (2011). Delayed procedural learning in alpha7-nicotinic acetylcholine receptor knockout mice. *Genes, Brain, and Behavior, 10*, 720–733.

Young, J. W., van Enkhuizen, J., Markou, A., Eyler, L. T., & Geyer, M. A. (2012). *Withdrawal from chronic nicotine impairs attention in mice and humans as measured by the 5-choice continuous performance test: A model for identifying treatments society for neuroscience* pp. 696.604.

4

Genetic, Developmental, and Receptor-Level Influences on Nicotine Withdrawal-Associated Deficits in Learning

M.G. *Kutlu*, E. *Holliday*, T.J. *Gould*

Temple University, Philadelphia, PA, United States

INTRODUCTION

Tobacco use has been declining in the United States, from 42% in the 1960s to 20% in 2004 (http://www.cdc.gov/tobacco/data_statistics/tables/trends/cig_smoking). However, these rates have remained relatively stable since then and smoking is still the leading cause of preventable death in the United States, responsible for over 440,000 deaths per year in the United States alone (CDC, 2004; Mokdad, Marks, Stroup, & Gerberding, 2004). While these numbers show an overwhelming problem of nicotine addiction, the majority of smokers indicate that they want to quit smoking (70%). Unfortunately, however, only a small percentage of the quitting attempts (42%) are actually successful (3–5%; Nides, 2008). Although the reasons why quitting smoking is so difficult are unknown, there are several potential environmental and genetic factors that may contribute to the development and maintenance of nicotine addiction. One possibility is that a subset of smokers are composed of individuals with mental or cognitive difficulties that increase their vulnerability for nicotine addiction. In support of this idea, increasing evidence links nicotine addiction with mental illness and cognitive impairments. For example, nicotine has been shown to alleviate symptoms associated with anxiety disorders, depression, attention deficit/hyperactivity disorder, and schizophrenia (see Kutlu, Parikh, & Gould, 2015, for a review). Also, there

Negative Affective States and Cognitive Impairments in Nicotine Dependence
http://dx.doi.org/10.1016/B978-0-12-802574-1.00004-1

is evidence showing that cognitive impairment is a serious problem during nicotine withdrawal. Nicotine withdrawal has been linked to difficulty concentrating (Pomerleau, Marks, & Pomerleau, 2000), working memory deficits (Jacobsen et al., 2005; Mendrek et al., 2006), deficits in verbal memory (Jacobsen et al., 2005), increased response time (Bell, Taylor, Singleton, Henningfield, & Heishman, 1999; Snyder, Davis, & Henningfield, 1989), and deficits in paired-associate learning (Kleinman, Vaughn, & Christ, 1973) in humans. Furthermore, the severity of cognitive deficits during abstinence has been shown to predict relapse of smoking (Patterson et al., 2010; Rukstalis, Jepson, Patterson, & Lerman, 2005). Overall, these results suggest that difficulty quitting smoking may be associated with cognitive and affective changes that arise as a result of nicotine withdrawal.

Although in humans there is anecdotal as well as clinical evidence suggesting cognitive changes during abstinence, animal models have advanced understanding of the neurobiological mechanisms underlying nicotine withdrawal-induced alterations in cognition. There are several behavioral paradigms for animals that enable researchers to study the effects of nicotine withdrawal on cognition in the laboratory setting. One such paradigm is contextual and cued fear conditioning, which models both cognitive and affective components of human behavior. Fear conditioning is a behavioral paradigm in which a conditioned stimulus (CS) is presented with an aversive, unconditioned stimulus (US), such as a foot shock. The CS can be either a simple discrete stimulus such as an auditory or visual cue or a complex stimulus such as a context. In a typical fear-conditioning session, two forms of association are learned, CS-US (cued conditioning) and Context-US (contextual conditioning). After the conditioning session, the conditioned response (CR) to the context, such as freezing, is measured 24 h later to assess long-term memory. Following the contextual test, CR to the CS is measured in a novel context to test for cued conditioning. The strength of the CR is an indicator of the strength of the cued or contextual fear memories. For cued fear conditioning, there are also two different temporal arrangements. In delayed fear conditioning, the offset of the CS coincides with the US, whereas in trace fear conditioning there is a time period between the offset of the CS and the onset of the US, in which a memory trace of the CS must be maintained. While contextual and trace conditioning depend on the hippocampus, delayed conditioning (cued conditioning) is a hippocampus-independent form of learning (Clark & Squire, 1998; Kim & Fanselow, 1992; Logue, Paylor, & Wehner, 1997; McEchron, Bouwmeester, Tseng, Weiss, & Disterhoft, 1998; Phillips & LeDoux, 1992).

Another behavioral paradigm widely used to study animal cognition is object recognition. During training, animals are allowed to explore objects in an arena. Then, in the spatial version of the task, spatial object recognition (SOR), one of the objects is displaced while the other one stays in the same place. In contrast, in novel object recognition (NOR), one of the objects is replaced with a new object during testing. During testing, animals are allowed to explore the objects again, and the time they spend exploring the displaced object in SOR, or replaced object in NOR, is measured as the indicator of learning strength. Whereas SOR is hippocampus dependent, NOR is hippocampus independent (Barker & Warburton, 2011). In the present chapter, we review the existing literature of studies investigating the effects of nicotine withdrawal on hippocampus-dependent learning using fear-conditioning and object recognition paradigms, the neurobiological and genetic mechanisms underlying the withdrawal effects, and the effects of age as the mediator for nicotine withdrawal.

HIPPOCAMPUS-DEPENDENT LEARNING IS MORE SENSITIVE TO THE EFFECTS OF NICOTINE WITHDRAWAL THAN HIPPOCAMPUS-INDEPENDENT LEARNING

As explained in this chapter, nicotine withdrawal results in a variety of cognitive deficits. A large body of literature has used rodent models to investigate the effects of nicotine withdrawal on the hippocampus-dependent forms of learning and memory (Davis, Porter, & Gould, 2006; Gould, 2003; Gould, Feiro, & Moore, 2004; Gould & Stephen Higgins, 2003; Gould & Wehner, 1999; Wehner et al., 2004). The results from these studies have consistently shown that intraperitoneal injections of acute nicotine enhance hippocampus-dependent contextual fear conditioning but have no effect on hippocampus-independent cued fear conditioning (Gould & Stephen Higgins, 2003; Gould & Wehner, 1999). These changes in learning were in long-term memory and not short-term memory (Gould et al., 2014). There is also evidence showing that acute nicotine enhances contextual processing in the contextual pre-exposure facilitation paradigm (Kenney & Gould, 2008), which may contribute to acute nicotine's enhancing effects on contextual fear conditioning. Contextual fear conditioning is not the only hippocampus-dependent form of learning that is altered by nicotine. As described here, trace fear conditioning also requires the hippocampus and it is enhanced by systemic injections of acute nicotine (Raybuck & Gould, 2009). Furthermore, there is evidence suggesting that acute nicotine enhances hippocampus-dependent SOR while hippocampus-independent NOR is impaired (Kenney, Adoff, Wilkinson, & Gould, 2011). Finally, several studies have shown that acute nicotine improves hippocampus-dependent spatial learning in the Morris Water Maze (Abdulla et al., 1996; Sharifzadeh, Sharifzadeh, Naghdi, Ghahremani, & Roghani, 2005) and spatial working memory in the Radial Arm Maze (Levin, Bettegowda, Weaver, & Christopher 1998; Levin, Kaplan, & Boardman, 1997; Levin & Torry, 1996).

While acute nicotine administration models the initial effects of smoking, chronic nicotine administration is employed by studies investigating the effects of long-term nicotine dependence on cognition. Several studies from our laboratory have found no effects of subcutaneous chronic nicotine administration via osmotic minipumps on hippocampus-dependent contextual fear conditioning and trace fear conditioning as well as hippocampus-independent cued fear learning; learning took place during chronic nicotine administration (André, Gulick, Portugal, & Gould, 2008; Davis, James, Siegel, & Gould, 2005; Portugal & Gould, 2009; Portugal, Wilkinson, Turner, Blendy, & Gould, 2012; Raybuck & Gould, 2009). Nevertheless, there is evidence showing that chronic nicotine may have effects on other hippocampus-dependent learning paradigms. For example, there is evidence that chronic nicotine administration enhances spatial working memory (Abdulla et al., 1996; Bernal, Vicens, Carrasco, & Redolat, 1999; Socci, Sanberg, & Arendash, 1995). In contrast to these studies, Scerri, Stewart, Breen, and Balfour (2006) found deficits in spatial working memory as a result of chronic nicotine exposure. However, while Scerri et al. (2006) used continuous administration of nicotine, other studies showing enhancement of spatial working memory used repeated nicotine injections, a discrepancy that may explain the contradictory results.

Although chronic nicotine may have minimal effects on hippocampus-dependent learning, withdrawal from chronic nicotine results in major changes in cognition, which is also an indicator that during chronic nicotine the systems responsible for some aspects of learning and memory are altered. Central to this discussion, Davis et al. (2005) showed that withdrawal from chronic nicotine leads to deficits in the hippocampus-dependent contextual fear conditioning. However, the same study showed no effect of withdrawal on hippocampus-independent cued fear conditioning. Subsequently, Raybuck and Gould (2009) demonstrated that trace fear conditioning is also impaired during nicotine withdrawal. Adding to the other hippocampus-dependent tasks, there is also evidence that withdrawal from chronic nicotine disrupts hippocampus-dependent SOR but not hippocampus-independent NOR. Interestingly, there is also evidence showing that nicotine withdrawal impairs new contextual learning but not recall of the previously learned contextual associations (Portugal & Gould, 2009). In addition, the same study showed that mice trained before chronic nicotine exposure and tested during withdrawal show normal retrieval of contextual fear. These results suggest that withdrawal disrupts encoding and/or consolidation of the hippocampus-dependent long-term memory but not the retrieval of already consolidated memories. Overall, these studies show that nicotine alters neurobiological mechanisms underlying long-term memory formation and consolidation, where acute nicotine boosts hippocampus-dependent learning, withdrawal from chronic nicotine disrupts it, but chronic nicotine largely has no effects.

Nevertheless, during chronic nicotine administration, tolerance to nicotine develops and the mechanisms that underlie tolerance may contribute to withdrawal deficits.

CHRONIC NICOTINE ACTS DIRECTLY IN THE HIPPOCAMPUS TO CHANGE NACHR FUNCTION AND DISRUPT LEARNING DURING WITHDRAWAL

Although nicotine withdrawal effects on hippocampus-dependent learning and memory are evident in animal models, the underlying mechanisms responsible for these effects are just becoming clear. Numerous studies investigating these mechanisms converged on a potential model for the effects of chronic nicotine on hippocampal function. Importantly, activation and desensitization of the hippocampal nicotinic acetylcholine receptors (nAChRs) may play a central role in associated withdrawal deficits. The hippocampus is the locus of many forms of learning and memory, including episodic memory, spatial learning, contextual learning, and spatial working memory (Aggleton, Hunt, & Rawlins, 1986; Burgess, Maguire, & O'Keefe, 2002; Daumas, Halley, Francés, & Lassalle, 2005; Jung & McNaughton, 1993). Furthermore, nicotine-induced activation of the hippocampal nAChRs has been shown repeatedly to both enhance (Fujii, Ji, Morita, Sumikawa, 1999; Fujii, Ji, & Sumikawa, 2000; Ji, Lape, & Dani, 2001; Mann & Greenfield, 2003; Welsby, Rowan, & Anwyl, 2007, 2009) and directly induce (He, Deng, Chen, Zhu, & Yu, 2000; Matsuyama & Matsumoto, 2003; Matsuyama, Matsumoto, Enomoto, & Nishizaki, 2000) synaptic plasticity in the form of long-term potentiation, which is suggested to be a mechanism underlying part of long-term memory formation (Bliss & Lømo, 1973; Bliss & Collingridge, 1993). Critically, as a response to chronic nicotine exposure, nAChRs desensitize in order to adapt to the increased nicotine binding, which leads to upregulation of the receptors that is region and cell-type specific, affecting select nAChR subtypes (Dani & Heinemann, 1996; Gould et al., 2012; Marks, Grady, & Collins, 1993; Marks et al., 2014; Mugnaini et al., 2006; Perry et al., 2007; Schwartz & Kellar, 1983). This process has been shown to result in a hypersensitive cholinergic system as the upregulated nAChRs resensitize rapidly when nicotine is withdrawn (Gould et al., 2012), which may be responsible for the deficits in cognition during this stage. In line with this hypothesis, Gould et al. (2012) first found that the duration of withdrawal effects on contextual fear conditioning is temporally correlated with the upregulation of hippocampal high-affinity nAChRs. Second, Gould et al. (2014) showed that withdrawal-associated deficits in learning require the same length of chronic nicotine administration as is required for hippocampal nAChR upregulation. These results clearly suggest that withdrawal deficits emerge with nAChR upregulation and disappear as upregulation goes back to baseline. Also supporting the role of hypersensitive nAChRs in withdrawal effects, Wilkinson and Gould (2013) showed that nicotine administration during acute nicotine withdrawal results in even greater enhancement of contextual fear conditioning compared to acute nicotine's enhancing effects in nicotine-naïve mice. This result is in agreement with the hypersensitive cholinergic system model and also suggests that high levels of relapse in smokers may be explained by the alleviation of cognitive deficits with the reintroduction of nicotine. Finally, Gould et al. (2014) showed that the effects of withdrawal and tolerance are two separate processes, as tolerance to the nicotine behavioral effects occurred before withdrawal effects and before nAChR upregulation developed. This result is also consistent with other results showing that somatic withdrawal signs are reduced in mutant mice lacking α7 nAChRs but these mice exhibited normal tolerance to nicotine-induced hypolocomotion (Salas, Main, Gangitano, & De Biasi, 2007). Moreover, there is evidence suggesting that different strains of mice developed tolerance to the enhancing effects of acute nicotine on contextual fear conditioning, whereas not all strains exhibited withdrawal deficits in the same learning task (Portugal, Wilkinson, Kenney, Sullivan, & Gould, 2012). In addition, in humans, several studies demonstrated that nondependent smokers showed tolerance to the effects of nicotine but did not exhibit withdrawal effects upon cessation (Perkins, 2002; Perkins et al., 2001). Therefore, it is possible that while nAChR upregulation is required for withdrawal effects, desensitization may be responsible for nicotine tolerance as it occurs faster than nAChR upregulation (Bullock et al., 1997; Collins, Luo, Selvaag, & Marks, 1994; Ochoa, Chattopadhyay, & McNamee, 1989).

The effects of withdrawal on hippocampus-dependent learning and memory are also associated with certain subtypes of nAChRs. nAChRs are structured as either homomeric (α7–α10) or heteromeric receptors, the latter containing a combination of α (α2–α6) and β (β2–β4) subunits (Decker, Brioni, Bannon, & Arneric, 1995; Hogg, Raggenbass, & Bertrand, 2003; Jones, Sudweeks, & Yakel, 1999; McGhee, 1999). These receptors are expressed in both the peripheral and central nervous systems (Cordero-Erausquin, Marubio, Klink, Changeux, 2000; Le Noverre, Grutter, Changeux, 2002; Léna & Changeux, 1998; Rush, Kuryatov, Nelson, & Lindstrom, 2002). Among possible combinations of nAChR subtypes, α7 and α4β2* (the asterisk * denotes an additional subunit) nAChRs are the most commonly expressed in the central nervous system and the hippocampus (Marks & Collins, 1982; Marks, Stitzel, Romm, Wehner, & Collins, 1986). α7 and α4β2* nAChRs display different characteristics in terms of affinity for nicotine binding and localization. For example, while α7 nAChRs show low affinity for nicotine binding, they desensitize rapidly. In contrast, α4β2* nAChRs show high affinity for nicotine but desensitize relatively slowly (Marks, Stitzel, & Collins, 1985; Olale, Gerzanich, Kuryatov, Wang, & Lindstrom, 1997). Regarding the hippocampal localization of these receptors, low-affinity α7 nAChRs are mainly located in the granule and pyramidal cell layers of the hippocampus (Fabian-Fine et al., 2001; Seguela et al., 1993; del Toro, Juiz, Peng, Lindstrom, & Criado, 1994), whereas high-affinity α4β2* nAChRs are mostly expressed in the dentate gyrus and CA1 subregions of the hippocampus (Perry et al., 2002). These different characteristics of the α7 and α4β2* nAChRs potentially suggest that they play differential roles in the modulation of cognition during nicotine withdrawal.

Several studies have investigated the role of specific subtypes of nAChRs in nicotine withdrawal effects on hippocampus-dependent learning (Davis & Gould, 2009; Portugal, Kenney, & Gould, 2008; Raybuck & Gould, 2009; Raybuck, Portugal, Lerman, & Gould, 2008). These studies overwhelmingly found that β2-containing high-affinity nAChRs are necessary for nicotine withdrawal effects on hippocampus-dependent learning. For example, Portugal et al. (2008) demonstrated that knockout (KO) mice that lack the β2 subunit of nAChRs did not show withdrawal deficits in contextual fear conditioning, whereas β2 wild-type (WT) littermates and α7 KO mice showed withdrawal-induced impairment of contextual fear learning. Furthermore, the same study showed that in C57BL/6 mice, systemic injections of the high-affinity nAChR antagonist dihydro-beta-erythroidine (DhβE) prior to training, but not testing, of contextual fear conditioning precipitated withdrawal deficits during chronic nicotine administration. Following up the Portugal et al. (2008) study, Davis and Gould (2009) chronically administered nicotine locally into the hippocampus. The results of this study indicated that while chronic intrahippocampal infusions of nicotine had no effect on contextual fear conditioning, withdrawal from chronic intrahippocampal nicotine resulted in impairment of learning. Davis and Gould (2009) also found that intrahippocampal injections of DhβE precipitated withdrawal deficits in the β2 WT but not β2 KO animals that received chronic nicotine systemically. Furthermore, Raybuck et al. (2008) investigated the role of high-affinity nAChRs in withdrawal deficits in contextual fear conditioning using varenicline, a partial agonist of the α4β2* nAChRs developed to aid smoking cessation in humans (Mihalak, Carroll, & Luetje, 2006). As a partial agonist of the α4β2* nAChRs, varenicline increases nAChR activity but maintains it at a submaximal level and therefore effectively desensitizes nAChRs by preventing endogenous acetylcholine binding (Mineur & Picciotto, 2010). Raybuck et al. (2008) found that while varenicline did not affect normal contextual fear conditioning in nicotine-naïve mice, it did prevent nicotine withdrawal deficits in the same learning paradigm. In addition to the studies investigating the roles of specific nAChRs in withdrawal effects on contextual fear conditioning, Raybuck and Gould (2009) implicated a role for the high-affinity β2-containing nAChRs in the withdrawal deficits in trace fear conditioning. This study showed that while the low-affinity nAChR antagonist methyllycaconitine had no effect on withdrawal deficits in trace fear conditioning, DhβE reversed the deficits. The same study also showed that the withdrawal deficits in trace fear conditioning are absent in the β2 KO mice. Overall, these studies show a major involvement of the β2-containing nAChRs in the withdrawal-induced deficits in hippocampus-dependent contextual and trace fear conditioning, whereas α7 nAChRs seemingly have no observed effect on the process.

GENETIC BACKGROUND MODULATES NICOTINE WITHDRAWAL EFFECTS ON LEARNING

In humans, there is strong evidence suggesting that genetic factors play a major role in smoking behavior (Carmelli, Swan, Robinette, & Fabsitz, 1992; Sabol et al., 1999; see Portugal & Gould, 2008, for a review). According to a study investigating the influence of genetic factors on smoking behavior in Dutch adolescents and young adults, genetic factors account for 39% of the variance in smoking initiation, and once smoking, the genetic component of severity of nicotine dependence accounts for 86% of the variance (Koopmans, Slutske, Heath, Neale, & Boomsma, 1999). Furthermore, heritability can account for 26–53% of behavioral nicotine withdrawal symptoms in humans (Pergadia, Heath, Martin, & Madden, 2006).

In animals, many studies have investigated the role of genetics in the effects of nicotine and withdrawal on hippocampus-dependent learning (Portugal, Wilkinson, Kenny et al., 2012; Wilkinson, Turner, Blendy, & Gould, 2013). One approach commonly used to detect genetic influences on behavior in animal studies is to test behavioral differences between different lines of inbred mice. As inbred mice within a line are highly genetically homogeneous after repeated breeding (Lyon & Searle, 1989), differences between inbred lines may be attributed to genetic dissimilarities. Taking advantage of this methodology using eight inbred mouse strains, Portugal, Wilkinson, Kenny et al. (2012) investigated the strain differences in the effects of acute nicotine, chronic nicotine, and withdrawal from chronic nicotine on contextual fear conditioning. Results showed a clear effect of genetic background on acute nicotine and nicotine withdrawal effects on contextual fear conditioning. No genetic effect was observed in chronic nicotine-administered animals. Based on these results, we calculated the heritability of the withdrawal deficits in the contextual fear-conditioning phenotype using within- and between-strain variances (Owen, Christensen, Paylor, & Wehner, 1997; Rai et al., 2012).

Our analysis showed that the heritability of the withdrawal phenotype was moderate to strong, $h^2 = 0.43$. Moreover, no genetic correlation was detected between the strain-dependent effects of acute nicotine and withdrawal from chronic nicotine for contextual fear conditioning, which suggests that these effects are controlled by independent groups of genes. Wilkinson et al. (2013) also examined the strain-dependent differences in the effects of withdrawal on learning and high-affinity nAChR receptor binding in the ventral and dorsal hippocampus. The results of the study demonstrated that while C57BL/6NTac mice showed both withdrawal-induced deficits in contextual fear conditioning and associated nAChR upregulation in the dorsal hippocampus, 129S6/SvEvTac mice showed neither of the effects. Interestingly, B6129SF1/Tac mice, a hybrid of the C57BL/6NTac and 129S6/SvEvTac lines, exhibited no effects of withdrawal on contextual fear conditioning but showed nAChR upregulation in the ventral hippocampus. This suggests that changes in dorsal hippocampus nAChRs, but not ventral hippocampus nAChRs, contribute to the withdrawal learning deficits. Taken together, the impairing effects of nicotine withdrawal on hippocampus-dependent learning are strongly influenced by genetic background and altered nAChR upregulation in the hippocampus may be responsible for these strain-dependent differences.

EFFECTS OF NICOTINE WITHDRAWAL ON LEARNING VARY WITH AGE

Adolescence represents a transition from childhood to adulthood and is preserved across most mammalian species. In rodents, it is defined as being between postnatal day (PND) 20 and PND40, which corresponds to 12–20 years of age in humans (Spear, 2000). Some defining characteristics of adolescence are the maturation of several neurotransmitter systems involved in learning and reward, an increase in impulsivity and risk-taking behavior likely due to a mature limbic system coupled with an immature executive function system, and increased sensitivity to the rewarding effects of drugs of abuse (Spear, 2000; Steinberg, 2010; Willoughby, Good, Adachi, Hamza, & Tavernier, 2013). Due to increased risk-taking and impulsive behaviors coupled with the increased sensitivity to reward, it is no surprise that adolescence represents a vulnerable time for the initiation of nicotine abuse. Additionally, research has demonstrated that adolescents show decreased withdrawal symptoms after nicotine treatment, which, when coupled with increased reward saliency, may underlie accelerated transition between casual use, abuse, and compulsive use (Kota et al., 2007; O'Dell et al., 2004). Finally, adolescence represents a critical period for the development of long-term consequences resulting from adolescent nicotine use (Brielmaier, McDonald, & Smith, 2007; Portugal, Wilkinson, Turner et al., 2012). This section will examine the short-term and long-term consequences of adolescent nicotine use on cognition.

Adolescence represents a unique window for the development of nicotine addiction. One reason for this may be due to adolescent mice demonstrating enhanced sensitivity to the acute effects of nicotine while simultaneously showing reduced nicotine withdrawal (Portugal, Wilkinson, Turner et al., 2012). Thus, the rewarding aspects of nicotine are unopposed by aversive withdrawal symptoms, increasing the odds of continued use into adulthood. Early adolescent (PND23), late adolescent (PND38), and adult (PND54) mice were given a range of acute doses during training and testing for contextual fear conditioning (Portugal, Wilkinson, Turner et al., 2012). Early adolescent mice showed enhancement of contextual fear conditioning at all doses of nicotine (0.045, 0.09, and 0.18 mg/kg), late adolescent mice showed enhancement at the two highest doses, and adult mice showed enhancement at the two lowest doses. This suggests that early adolescent mice are especially sensitive to the acute cognitive-enhancing properties of nicotine, while the dose response is shifted in late adolescence compared to adult animals receiving the same doses of nicotine. Furthermore, when early adolescent, late adolescent, and adult animals were given varying doses of chronic nicotine (3, 6.3, and 12 mg/kg/day) and trained and tested in contextual fear conditioning, late adolescent and adult animals developed tolerance, evident by no change in contextual fear conditioning compared to saline controls, while early adolescent mice showed enhancement to the highest dose. This effect was not due to increases in anxiety or changes in locomotion, as freezing behaviors during baseline measures were unaffected and young animals are particularly resistant to the hypolocomotor effects of nicotine (Belluzzi et al., 2004). In addition, withdrawal from chronic nicotine produced deficits in adult animals at the two highest doses, in late adolescence at all doses, and only with the highest dose for early adolescents. Finally, because adolescent mice displayed disrupted contextual fear conditioning at all doses administered, an additional two lower doses of nicotine (0.5 and 1.1 mg/kg/day) were given to PND38 mice. It was found that the 1.1 mg/kg/day dose also led to withdrawal-related deficits in contextual fear conditioning, further suggesting that adolescence is a very vulnerable time to the cognitive impairments produced by chronic nicotine treatment and that the hippocampus is especially sensitive to the effects of nicotine during this age period. However, it is likely that the lack of tolerance and subsequent withdrawal-related deficits in early adolescents is due to the lack of α4β2 upregulation, since withdrawal symptoms are mediated by the upregulation of α4β2 subunits (Portugal, Wilkinson, Turner et al., 2012). Thus, it appears that early adolescence is a very sensitive time for the acute effects of nicotine while displaying virtually no aversive behaviors during nicotine cessation. Conversely, withdrawal-related deficits begin to emerge in late adolescence at doses that did not elicit withdrawal deficits in younger animals. In addition, the lack of tolerance to chronic nicotine observed during early adolescence suggests that the cholinergic system is functionally different compared to later developmental time points. Taken together, it is possible that continued nicotine use during the transition from early adolescence to late adolescence represents the ontogeny of developing nicotine dependence, as cognitive impairments, which were observed at all doses in midadolescent animals, are often cited as a reason to continue smoking (Cole et al., 2010; Parrott & Roberts, 1991; Patterson et al., 2010).

Unlike early adolescent nicotine exposure, exposure to nicotine during mid- to late-adolescence causes both persistent upregulation of nAChRs and changes in hippocampal function that can be observed into adulthood, and it likely underlies some of the enduring cognitive deficits as a result of adolescent nicotine treatment. For example, chronic nicotine administration causes an upregulation of nAChRs in the adolescent brain that can be observed up to 4 weeks after cessation (Trauth, Seidler, McCook, & Slotkin, 1999). Adolescent Sprague–Dawley rats were implanted with osmotic minipumps to chronically administer nicotine from PND30 to PND47 and brains were analyzed for nAChR upregulation. At the end of nicotine treatment, adults showed higher levels of binding specific to the hippocampus and cortex, while adolescents showed more global upregulation. However, only adolescents displayed nAChR upregulation 4 weeks after nicotine cessation, and this effect was limited to the cortex and the hippocampus. In a follow-up study, Trauth, Seidler, and Slotkin (2000) found that the same dosing regimen in the same ages of animals caused a persistent reduction in cholinergic activity in the hippocampus, coupled with increases in apoptosis-related genes, demonstrating permanent alterations to the structure and function of the hippocampus following adolescent nicotine use (Trauth et al., 2000). The persistent upregulation of nicotinic receptors coupled with decreases in cholinergic activity and alterations in gene expression in the hippocampus may contribute to both the development and subsequent maintenance of nicotine addiction. This dysregulation of the hippocampus by adolescent nicotine exposure increases the likelihood of continued nicotine abuse by creating conditions that ultimately lead to cognitive impairments as cognitive impairments are associated with addiction.

Studies that followed Trauth and colleagues' findings (ie, the adolescent hippocampus is especially vulnerable to the effects of nicotine) have demonstrated persisting deficits in learning tasks that are hippocampal dependent in animals exposed to nicotine during adolescence.

When examining contextual fear conditioning, a hippocampus-dependent task, in adolescent and adult mice, it is clear that chronic nicotine exposure during adolescence causes long-term impairments in cognition (Portugal, Wilkinson, Turner et al., 2012). Early adolescent (PND23), late adolescent (PND38), and adult (PND54) mice were administered nicotine (8.8 and 12 mg/kg) via mini-osmotic pumps for 12 days. Thirty days after nicotine cessation, animals were assessed in fear conditioning. Both early adolescent and late adolescent mice showed deficits in contextual fear conditioning, while adult mice did not, and cued conditioning remained unaffected in both age groups. Furthermore, early adolescent mice showed deficits at both doses (8.8 and 12 mg/kg) of nicotine, while late adolescents showed deficits only at the highest dose. These effects may be related to changes in CREB availability, as CREB expression was reduced in the hippocampus but increased in the cortex in early adolescent mice following chronic nicotine treatment, and this effect was not seen in adult mice. Thus, exposure to nicotine during adolescence alters hippocampal functioning that manifests as deficits in contextual fear conditioning. This in turn can increase the risk of addiction as nicotine use in adolescence leads to long-term cognitive impairments and cognitive impairments are correlated with higher rates of smoking relapse in adult clinical populations (Patterson et al., 2010).

CONCLUSION

Increasing evidence indicates that cognitive/learning-related deficits are a major component of nicotine addiction. Studies in mice have shown that the hippocampus is particularly sensitive to the effects of nicotine withdrawal. Specifically, while nicotine withdrawal disrupts formation of new hippocampus-dependent memories, memories formed before or during early nicotine exposure seem to be intact during nicotine withdrawal. Therefore, it is possible that the inability to change already-established context–drug associations may contribute to the persistence of nicotine addiction and, consequently, lead to relapse. The hippocampus seems to be especially sensitive to the modulation by nicotine withdrawal as effects of nicotine withdrawal on memory formation were associated with upregulation of high-affinity β2-containing nAChRs in the hippocampus. Furthermore, the withdrawal-associated modulation of hippocampal function is clearly influenced by genetic factors. Finally, age appears to be critical in determining the effects of nicotine withdrawal on hippocampus-dependent learning. While early adolescent mice are less affected by the negative effects of nicotine withdrawal, chronic nicotine exposure during this developmental stage results in deficits in learning and memory that emerge during adulthood. Overall, identification of the factors that contribute to the cognitive deficits associated with nicotine withdrawal is crucial in order to develop pharmacological and behavioral treatments for nicotine dependence.

Acknowledgment

This work was funded with grant support to TJG from the National Institute on Drug Abuse (grant no. DA017949).

References

Abdulla, F. A., Gray, J. A., Sinden, J. D., Bradbury, E., Calaminici, M. R., Lippiello, P. M., & Wonnacott, S. (1996). Relationship between up-regulation of nicotine binding sites in rat brain and delayed cognitive enhancement observed after chronic or acute nicotinic receptor stimulation. *Psychopharmacology, 124*(4), 323–331.

Aggleton, J. P., Hunt, P. R., & Rawlins, J. N. P. (1986). The effects of hippocampal lesions upon spatial and non-spatial tests of working memory. *Behavioural Brain Research, 19*(2), 133–146.

André, J. M., Gulick, D., Portugal, G. S., & Gould, T. J. (2008). Nicotine withdrawal disrupts both foreground and background contextual fear conditioning but not pre-pulse inhibition of the acoustic startle response in C57BL/6 mice. *Behavioural Brain Research, 190*(2), 174–181.

Barker, G. R., & Warburton, E. C. (2011). When is the hippocampus involved in recognition memory? *The Journal of Neuroscience, 31*(29), 10721–10731.

Bell, S. L., Taylor, R. C., Singleton, E. G., Henningfield, J. E., & Heishman, S. J. (1999). Smoking after nicotine deprivation enhances cognitive performance and decreases tobacco craving in drug abusers. *Nicotine & Tobacco Research, 1*(1), 45–52.

Belluzzi, J. D., Lee, A. G., Oliff, H. S., & Leslie, F. M. (2004). Age-dependent effects of nicotine on locomotor activity and conditioned place preference in rats. *Psychopharmacology, 174*(3), 389–395.

Bernal, M. C., Vicens, P., Carrasco, M. C., & Redolat, R. (1999). Effects of nicotine on spatial learning in C57BL mice. *Behavioural Pharmacology, 10*(3), 333–336.

Bliss, T. V., & Collingridge, G. L. (1993). A synaptic model of memory: long-term potentiation in the hippocampus. *Nature, 361*(6407), 31–39.

Bliss, T. V., & Lømo, T. (1973). Long-lasting potentiation of synaptic transmission in the dentate area of the anaesthetized rabbit following stimulation of the perforant path. *The Journal of Physiology, 232*(2), 331–356.

Brielmaier, J., McDonald, C., & Smith, R. (2007). Immediate and long-term behavioral effects of a single nicotine injection in adolescent and adult rats. *Neurotoxicology and Teratology, 29*(1), 74–80.

Bullock, A. E., Clark, A. L., Grady, S. R., Robinson, S. F., Slobe, B. S., Marks, M. J., & Collins, A. C. (1997). Neurosteroids modulate nicotinic receptor function in mouse striatal and thalamic synaptosomes. *Journal of Neurochemistry, 68*(6), 2412–2423.

Burgess, N., Maguire, E. A., & O'Keefe, J. (2002). The human hippocampus and spatial and episodic memory. *Neuron, 35*(4), 625–641.

Carmelli, D., Swan, G. E., Robinette, D., & Fabsitz, R. (1992). Genetic influence on smoking— a study of male twins. *New England Journal of Medicine, 327*(12), 829–833.

Centers for Disease Control and Prevention (CDC). (2004). Cigarette smoking among adults– United States, 2002. *MMWR. Morbidity and Mortality Weekly Report, 53*(20), 427.

Clark, R. E., & Squire, L. R. (1998). Classical conditioning and brain systems: the role of awareness. *Science, 280*(5360), 77–81.

Cole, D., Beckmann, C., Long, C., Matthews, P., Durcan, M., & Beaver, J. (2010). Nicotine replacement in abstinent smokers improves cognitive withdrawal symptoms with modulation of resting brain network dynamics. *Neuroimage, 52*(2), 590–599.

Collins, A. C., Luo, Y., Selvaag, S., & Marks, M. J. (1994). Sensitivity to nicotine and brain nicotinic receptors are altered by chronic nicotine and mecamylamine infusion. *Journal of Pharmacology and Experimental Therapeutics, 271*(1), 125–133.

Committee on Standardized Genetic Nomenclature for Mice. (1989). Rules for nomenclature of inbred strains. In M. F. Lyon, & A. G. Searle (Eds.), *Genetic variants and strains of the laboratory mouse* (pp. 632–635). New York: Oxford University Press.

Cordero-Erausquin, M., Marubio, L. M., Klink, R., & Changeux, J. P. (2000). Nicotinic receptor function: new perspectives from knockout mice. *Trends in Pharmacological Sciences, 21*(6), 211–217.

Dani, J. A., & Heinemann, S. (1996). Molecular and cellular aspects of nicotine abuse. *Neuron, 16*(5), 905–908.

Daumas, S., Halley, H., Francés, B., & Lassalle, J. M. (2005). Encoding, consolidation, and retrieval of contextual memory: differential involvement of dorsal CA3 and CA1 hippocampal subregions. *Learning & Memory, 12*(4), 375–382.

Davis, J. A., & Gould, T. J. (2009). Hippocampal nAChRs mediate nicotine withdrawal-related learning deficits. *European Neuropsychopharmacology, 19*(8), 551–561.

Davis, J. A., James, J. R., Siegel, S. J., & Gould, T. J. (2005). Withdrawal from chronic nicotine administration impairs contextual fear conditioning in C57BL/6 mice. *The Journal of Neuroscience, 25*(38), 8708–8713.

Davis, J. A., Porter, J., & Gould, T. J. (2006). Nicotine enhances both foreground and background contextual fear conditioning. *Neuroscience Letters, 394*(3), 202–205.

Decker, M. W., Brioni, J. D., Bannon, A. W., & Arneric, S. P. (1995). Diversity of neuronal nicotinic acetylcholine receptors: lessons from behavior and implications for CNS therapeutics. *Life Sciences, 56*(8), 545–570.

Fabian-Fine, R., Skehel, P., Errington, M. L., Davies, H. A., Sher, E., Stewart, M. G., & Fine, A. (2001). Ultrastructural distribution of the α7 nicotinic acetylcholine receptor subunit in rat hippocampus. *The Journal of Neuroscience, 21*(20), 7993–8003.

Fujii, S., Ji, X., Morita, N., & Sumikawa, K. (1999). Acute and chronic nicotine exposure differentially facilitate the induction of LTP. *Brain Research, 846*, 137–143.

Fujii, S., Ji, Z., & Sumikawa, K. (2000). Inactivation of α7 ACh receptors and activation of non-α7 ACh receptors both contribute to long term potentiation induction in the hippocampal CA1 region. *Neuroscience Letters, 286*(2), 134–138.

Gould, T. J. (2003). Nicotine produces a within-subject enhancement of contextual fear conditioning in C57BL/6 mice independent of sex. *Integrative Physiological & Behavioral Science, 38*(2), 124–132.

Gould, T. J., Feiro, O., & Moore, D. (2004). Nicotine enhances trace cued fear conditioning but not delay cued fear conditioning in C57BL/6 mice. *Behavioural Brain Research, 155*(1), 167–173.

Gould, T. J., Portugal, G. S., André, J. M., Tadman, M. P., Marks, M. J., Kenney, J. W., … Adoff, M. (2012). The duration of nicotine withdrawal-associated deficits in contextual fear conditioning parallels changes in hippocampal high affinity nicotinic acetylcholine receptor upregulation. *Neuropharmacology, 62*(5), 2118–2125.

Gould, T. J., & Stephen Higgins, J. (2003). Nicotine enhances contextual fear conditioning in C57BL/6J mice at 1 and 7 days post-training. *Neurobiology of Learning and Memory, 80*(2), 147–157.

Gould, T. J., & Wehner, J. M. (1999). Nicotine enhancement of contextual fear conditioning. *Behavioural Brain Research, 102*(1), 31–39.

Gould, T. J., Wilkinson, D. S., Yildirim, E., Poole, R. L., Leach, P. T., & Simmons, S. J. (2014). Nicotine shifts the temporal activation of hippocampal protein kinase A and extracellular signal-regulated kinase 1/2 to enhance long-term, but not short-term, hippocampus-dependent memory. *Neurobiology of Learning and Memory, 109*, 151–159.

He, J., Deng, C. Y., Chen, R. Z., Zhu, X. N., & Yu, J. P. (2000). Long-term potentiation induced by nicotine in CA1 region of hippocampal slice is Ca2+-dependent. *Acta Pharmacologica Sinica*, *21*, 429–432.

Hogg, R. C., Raggenbass, M., & Bertrand, D. (2003). Nicotinic acetylcholine receptors: from structure to brain function. In *Reviews of physiology, biochemistry and pharmacology* (pp. 1–46). Berlin Heidelberg: Springer.

Jacobsen, L. K., Krystal, J. H., Mencl, W. E., Westerveld, M., Frost, S. J., & Pugh, K. R. (2005). Effects of smoking and smoking abstinence on cognition in adolescent tobacco smokers. *Biological Psychiatry*, *57*(1), 56–66.

Ji, D., Lape, R., & Dani, J. A. (2001). Timing and location of nicotinic activity enhances or depresses hippocampal synaptic plasticity. *Neuron*, *31*, 131–141.

Jones, S., Sudweeks, S., & Yakel, J. L. (1999). Nicotinic receptors in the brain: correlating physiology with function. *Trends in Neurosciences*, *22*(12), 555–561.

Jung, M. W., & McNaughton, B. L. (1993). Spatial selectivity of unit activity in the hippocampal granular layer. *Hippocampus*, *3*(2), 165–182.

Kenney, J. W., Adoff, M. D., Wilkinson, D. S., & Gould, T. J. (2011). The effects of acute, chronic, and withdrawal from chronic nicotine on novel and spatial object recognition in male C57BL/6J mice. *Psychopharmacology*, *217*(3), 353–365.

Kenney, J. W., & Gould, T. J. (2008). Nicotine enhances context learning but not context-shock associative learning. *Behavioral Neuroscience*, *122*(5), 1158.

Kim, J. J., & Fanselow, M. S. (1992). Modality-specific retrograde amnesia of fear. *Science*, *256*(5057), 675–677.

Kleinman, K. M., Vaughn, R. L., & Christ, T. S. (1973). Effects of cigarette smoking and smoking deprivation on paired-associate learning of high and low meaningful nonsense syllables. *Psychological Reports*, *32*(3), 963–966.

Koopmans, J. R., Slutske, W. S., Heath, A. C., Neale, M. C., & Boomsma, D. I. (1999). The genetics of smoking initiation and quantity smoked in Dutch adolescent and young adult twins. *Behavior Genetics*, *29*(6), 383–393.

Kota, D., Martin, B. R., Robinson, S. E., & Damaj, M. I. (2007). Nicotine dependence and reward differ between adolescent and adult male mice. *Journal of Pharmacology and Experimental Therapeutics*, *322*(1), 399–407.

Kota, D., Sanjakdar, S., Marks, M., Khabour, O., Alzoubi, K., & Damaj, M. (2011). Exploring behavioral and molecular mechanisms of nicotine reward in adolescent mice. *Biochemical Pharmacology*, *82*(8), 1008–1014.

Kutlu, M. G., Parikh, V., & Gould, T. J. (2015). Nicotine addiction and psychiatric disorders. In M. De Biasi (Ed.). M. De Biasi (Ed.), *Tobacco & mental illness (pp. xxx-xxx). International review of Neurobiology: (Vol. x)*. New York, NY: Academic Press.

Le Novere, N., Grutter, T., & Changeux, J. P. (2002). Models of the extracellular domain of the nicotinic receptors and of agonist-and Ca2+-binding sites. *Proceedings of the National Academy of Sciences*, *99*(5), 3210–3215.

Léna, C., & Changeux, J. P. (1998). Allosteric nicotinic receptors, human pathologies. *Journal of Physiology-Paris*, *92*(2), 63–74.

Levin, E. D., Bettegowda, C., Weaver, T., & Christopher, N. C. (1998). Nicotine–dizocilpine interactions and working and reference memory performance of rats in the radial-arm maze. *Pharmacology Biochemistry and Behavior*, *61*(3), 335–340.

Levin, E. D., Kaplan, S., & Boardman, A. (1997). Acute nicotine interactions with nicotinic and muscarinic antagonists: working and reference memory effects in the 16-arm radial maze. *Behavioural Pharmacology*, *8*, 236–242.

Levin, E. D., & Torry, D. (1996). Acute and chronic nicotine effects on working memory in aged rats. *Psychopharmacology*, *123*(1), 88–97.

Logue, S. F., Paylor, R., & Wehner, J. M. (1997). Hippocampal lesions cause learning deficits in inbred mice in the Morris water maze and conditioned-fear task. *Behavioral Neuroscience*, *111*(1), 104.

Mann, E. O., & Greenfield, S. A. (2003). Novel modulatory mechanisms revealed by the sustained application of nicotine in the guinea-pig hippocampus in vitro. *Journal of Physiology, Paris, 551*, 539–550.

Marks, M. J., & Collins, A. C. (1982). Characterization of nicotine binding in mouse brain and comparison with the binding of alpha-bungarotoxin and quinuclidinyl benzilate. *Molecular Pharmacology, 22*(3), 554–564.

Marks, M. J., Grady, S. R., & Collins, A. C. (1993). Downregulation of nicotinic receptor function after chronic nicotine infusion. *Journal of Pharmacology and Experimental Therapeutics, 266*(3), 1268–1276.

Marks, M. J., Grady, S. R., Salminen, O., Paley, M. A., Wageman, C. R., McIntosh, J. M., & Whiteaker, P. (2014). α6β2*-subtype nicotinic acetylcholine receptors are more sensitive than α4β2*-subtype receptors to regulation by chronic nicotine administration. *Journal of Neurochemistry, 130*(2), 185–198.

Marks, M. J., Stitzel, J. A., & Collins, A. C. (1985). Time course study of the effects of chronic nicotine infusion on drug response and brain receptors. *Journal of Pharmacology and Experimental Therapeutics, 235*(3), 619–628.

Marks, M. J., Stitzel, J. A., Romm, E. , Wehner, J. M., & Collins, A. C. (1986). Nicotinic binding sites in rat and mouse brain: comparison of acetylcholine, nicotine, and alpha-bungarotoxin. *Molecular Pharmacology, 30*(5), 427–436.

Matsuyama, S., & Matsumoto, A. (2003). Epibatidine induces long-term potentiation (LTP) via activation of alpha4beta2 nicotinic acetylcholine receptors (nAChRs) in vivo in the intact mouse dentate gyrus: both alpha7 and alpha4beta2 nAChRs essential to nicotinic LTP. *Journal of Pharmacological Sciences, 93*(2), 180–187.

Matsuyama, S., Matsumoto, A., Enomoto, T., & Nishizaki, T. (2000). Activation of nicotinic acetylcholine receptors induces long-term potentiation in vivo in the intact mouse dentate gyrus. *European Journal of Neuroscience, 12*(10), 3741–3747.

McEchron, M. D., Bouwmeester, H., Tseng, W., Weiss, C., & Disterhoft, J. F. (1998). Hippocampectomy disrupts auditory trace fear conditioning and contextual fear conditioning in the rat. *Hippocampus, 8*(6), 638–646.

McGehee, D. S. (1999). Molecular diversity of neuronal nicotinic acetylcholine receptors. *Annals of the New York Academy of Sciences, 868*(1), 565–577.

Mendrek, A., Monterosso, J., Simon, S. L., Jarvik, M., Brody, A., Olmstead, R., … London, E. D. (2006). Working memory in cigarette smokers: comparison to non-smokers and effects of abstinence. *Addictive Behaviors, 31*(5), 833–844.

Mihalak, K. B., Carroll, F. I., & Luetje, C. W. (2006). Varenicline is a partial agonist at α4β2 and a full agonist at α7 neuronal nicotinic receptors. *Molecular Pharmacology, 70*(3), 801–805.

Mineur, Y. S., & Picciotto, M. R. (2010). Nicotine receptors and depression: revisiting and revising the cholinergic hypothesis. *Trends in Pharmacological Sciences, 31*(12), 580–586.

Mokdad, A. H., Marks, J. S., Stroup, D. F., & Gerberding, J. L. (2004). Actual causes of death in the United States, 2000. *JAMA: The Journal of the American Medical Association, 291*(10), 1238–1245.

Mugnaini, M., Garzotti, M., Sartori, I., Pilla, M., Repeto, P., Heidbreder, C. A., & Tessari, M. (2006). Selective down-regulation of [125I] Y 0-α-conotoxin MII binding in rat mesostriatal dopamine pathway following continuous infusion of nicotine. *Neuroscience, 137*(2), 565–572.

Nides, M. (2008). Update on pharmacologic options for smoking cessation treatment. *The American Journal of Medicine, 121*(4), S20–S31.

O'Dell, L., Bruijnzeel, A., Ghozland, S., Markou, A., & Koob, G. (2004). Nicotine withdrawal in adolescent and adult rats. *Annals of the New York Academy of Sciences, 1021*, 167–174.

Ochoa, E. L., Chattopadhyay, A., & McNamee, M. G. (1989). Desensitization of the nicotinic acetylcholine receptor: molecular mechanisms and effect of modulators. *Cellular and Molecular Neurobiology, 9*(2), 141–178.

Olale, F., Gerzanich, V., Kuryatov, A., Wang, F., & Lindstrom, J. (1997). Chronic nicotine exposure differentially affects the function of human α3, α4, and α7 neuronal nicotinic receptor subtypes. *Journal of Pharmacology and Experimental Therapeutics, 283*(2), 675–683.

Owen, E. H., Christensen, S. C., Paylor, R., & Wehner, J. M. (1997). Identification of quantitative trait loci involved in contextual and auditory-cued fear conditioning in BXD recombinant inbred strains. *Behavioral Neuroscience, 111*(2), 292.

Parrott, A., & Roberts, G. (1991). Smoking deprivation and cigarette reinstatement: effects upon visual attention. *Journal of Psychopharmacology, 5*(4), 404–409.

Patterson, F., Jepson, C., Loughead, J., Perkins, K., Strasser, A. A., Siegel, S., … Lerman, C. (2010). Working memory deficits predict short-term smoking resumption following brief abstinence. *Drug and Alcohol Dependence, 106*(1), 61–64.

Pergadia, M. L., Heath, A. C., Martin, N. G., & Madden, P. A. (2006). Genetic analyses of DSM-IV nicotine withdrawal in adult twins. *Psychological Medicine, 36*(07), 963–972.

Perkins, K. A. (2002). Chronic tolerance to nicotine in humans and its relationship to tobacco dependence. *Nicotine & Tobacco Research, 4*(4), 405–422.

Perkins, K. A., Gerlach, D., Broge, M., Grobe, J. E., Sanders, M., Fonte, C., … Wilson, A. (2001). Dissociation of nicotine tolerance from tobacco dependence in humans. *Journal of Pharmacology and Experimental Therapeutics, 296*(3), 849–856.

Perry, D. C., Mao, D., Gold, A. B., McIntosh, J. M., Pezzullo, J. C., & Kellar, K. J. (2007). Chronic nicotine differentially regulates α6-and β3-containing nicotinic cholinergic receptors in rat brain. *Journal of Pharmacology and Experimental Therapeutics, 322*(1), 306–315.

Perry, D. C., Xiao, Y., Nguyen, H. N., Musachio, J. L., Dávila-García, M. I., & Kellar, K. J. (2002). Measuring nicotinic receptors with characteristics of α4β2, α3β2 and α3β4 subtypes in rat tissues by autoradiography. *Journal of Neurochemistry, 82*(3), 468–481.

Phillips, R. G., & LeDoux, J. E. (1992). Differential contribution of amygdala and hippocampus to cued and contextual fear conditioning. *Behavioral Neuroscience, 106*(2), 274.

Pomerleau, C. S., Marks, J. L., & Pomerleau, O. F. (2000). Who gets what symptom? Effects of psychiatric cofactors and nicotine dependence on patterns of smoking withdrawal symptomatology. *Nicotine & Tobacco Research, 2*(3), 275–280.

Portugal, G. S., & Gould, T. J. (2008). Genetic variability in nicotinic acetylcholine receptors and nicotine addiction: converging evidence from human and animal research. *Behavioural Brain Research, 193*(1), 1–16.

Portugal, G. S., & Gould, T. J. (2009). Nicotine withdrawal disrupts new contextual learning. *Pharmacology Biochemistry and Behavior, 92*(1), 117–123.

Portugal, G. S., Kenney, J. W., & Gould, T. J. (2008). β2 subunit containing acetylcholine receptors mediate nicotine withdrawal deficits in the acquisition of contextual fear conditioning. *Neurobiology of Learning and Memory, 89*(2), 106–113.

Portugal, G. S., Wilkinson, D. S., Kenney, J. W., Sullivan, C., & Gould, T. J. (2012). Strain-dependent effects of acute, chronic, and withdrawal from chronic nicotine on fear conditioning. *Behavior Genetics, 42*(1), 133–150.

Portugal, G. S., Wilkinson, D. S., Turner, J. R., Blendy, J. A., & Gould, T. J. (2012). Developmental effects of acute, chronic, and withdrawal from chronic nicotine on fear conditioning. *Neurobiology of Learning and Memory, 97*(4), 482–494.

Rai, M. F., Hashimoto, S., Johnson, E. E., Janiszak, K. L., Fitzgerald, J., Heber-Katz, E., … Sandell, L. J. (2012). Heritability of articular cartilage regeneration and its association with ear wound healing in mice. *Arthritis & Rheumatism, 64*(7), 2300–2310.

Raybuck, J. D., & Gould, T. J. (2009). Nicotine withdrawal-induced deficits in trace fear conditioning in C57BL/6 mice–a role for high-affinity β2 subunit-containing nicotinic acetylcholine receptors. *European Journal of Neuroscience, 29*(2), 377–387.

Raybuck, J. D., Portugal, G. S., Lerman, C., & Gould, T. J. (2008). Varenicline ameliorates nicotine withdrawal-induced learning deficits in C57BL/6 mice. *Behavioral Neuroscience, 122*(5), 1166.

Rukstalis, M., Jepson, C., Patterson, F., & Lerman, C. (2005). Increases in hyperactive–impulsive symptoms predict relapse among smokers in nicotine replacement therapy. *Journal of Substance Abuse Treatment, 28*(4), 297–304.

Rush, R., Kuryatov, A., Nelson, M. E., & Lindstrom, J. (2002). First and second transmembrane segments of α3, α4, β2, and β4 nicotinic acetylcholine receptor subunits influence the efficacy and potency of nicotine. *Molecular Pharmacology, 61*(6), 1416–1422.

Sabol, S. Z., Nelson, M. L., Fisher, C., Gunzerath, L., Brody, C. L., Hu, S., … Hamer, D. H. (1999). A genetic association for cigarette smoking behavior. *Health Psychology, 18*(1), 7.

Salas, R., Main, A., Gangitano, D., & De Biasi, M. (2007). Decreased withdrawal symptoms but normal tolerance to nicotine in mice null for the α7 nicotinic acetylcholine receptor subunit. *Neuropharmacology, 53*(7), 863–869.

Scerri, C., Stewart, C. A., Breen, K. C., & Balfour, D. J. (2006). The effects of chronic nicotine on spatial learning and bromodeoxyuridine incorporation into the dentate gyrus of the rat. *Psychopharmacology, 184*(3–4), 540–546.

Schwartz, R. D., & Kellar, K. J. (1983). Nicotinic cholinergic receptor binding sites in the brain: regulation in vivo. *Science, 220*(4593), 214–216.

Seguela, P., Wadiche, J., Dineley-Miller, K., Dani, J. A., & Patrick, J. W. (1993). Molecular cloning, functional properties, and distribution of rat brain alpha 7: a nicotinic cation channel highly permeable to calcium. *The Journal of Neuroscience, 13*(2), 596–604.

Sharifzadeh, M., Sharifzadeh, K., Naghdi, N., Ghahremani, M. H., & Roghani, A. (2005). Posttraining intrahippocampal infusion of a protein kinase AII inhibitor impairs spatial memory retention in rats. *Journal of Neuroscience Research, 79*(3), 392–400.

Snyder, F. R., Davis, F. C., & Henningfield, J. E. (1989). The tobacco withdrawal syndrome: performance decrements assessed on a computerized test battery. *Drug and Alcohol Dependence, 23*(3), 259–266.

Socci, D. J., Sanberg, P. R., & Arendash, G. W. (1995). Nicotine enhances Morris water maze performance of young and aged rats. *Neurobiology of Aging, 16*(5), 857–860.

Spear, L. (2000). The adolescent brain and age-related behavioral manifestations. *Neuroscience and Biobehavioral Reviews, 24*(4), 417–463.

Steinberg, L. (2010). A behavioral scientist looks at the science of adolescent brain development. *Brain and Cognition, 72*(1), 160–164.

del Toro, E. D., Juiz, J. M., Peng, X., Lindstrom, J., & Criado, M. (1994). Immunocytochemical localization of the α7 subunit of the nicotinic acetylcholine receptor in the rat central nervous system. *Journal of Comparative Neurology, 349*(3), 325–342.

Trauth, J., Seidler, F., McCook, E., & Slotkin, T. (1999). Adolescent nicotine exposure causes persistent upregulation of nicotinic cholinergic receptors in rat brain regions. *Brain Research, 851*(1–2), 9–19.

Trauth, J., Seidler, F., & Slotkin, T. (2000). An animal model of adolescent nicotine exposure: effects on gene expression and macromolecular constituents in rat brain regions. *Brain Research, 867*(1–2), 29–39.

Wehner, J. M., Keller, J. J., Keller, A. B., Picciotto, M. R., Paylor, R., Booker, T. K., … Balogh, S. A. (2004). Role of neuronal nicotinic receptors in the effects of nicotine and ethanol on contextual fear conditioning. *Neuroscience, 129*(1), 11–24.

Welsby, P. J., Rowan, M., & Anwyl, R. (2007). Beta-amyloid blocks high frequency stimulation induced LTP but not nicotine enhanced LTP. *Neuropharmacology, 53*, 188–195.

Welsby, P. J., Rowan, M. J., & Anwyl, R. (2009). Intracellular mechanisms underlying the nicotinic enhancement of LTP in the rat dentate gyrus. *European Journal of Neuroscience, 29*(1), 65–75.

Wilkinson, D. S., & Gould, T. J. (2013). Withdrawal from chronic nicotine and subsequent sensitivity to nicotine challenge on contextual learning. *Behavioural Brain Research, 250*, 58–61.

Wilkinson, D. S., Turner, J. R., Blendy, J. A., & Gould, T. J. (2013). Genetic background influences the effects of withdrawal from chronic nicotine on learning and high-affinity nicotinic acetylcholine receptor binding in the dorsal and ventral hippocampus. *Psychopharmacology, 225*(1), 201–208.

Willoughby, T., Good, M., Adachi, P., Hamza, C., & Tavernier, R. (2013). Examining the link between adolescent brain development and risk taking from a social developmental perspective. *Brain and Cognition, 83*(3), 315–323.

Enhanced Tobacco Use Vulnerability in Adolescents, Females, and Persons With Diabetes

J.A. Pipkin, T. Ontiveros, L.M. Carcoba, L.E. O'Dell

The University of Texas at El Paso, El Paso, TX, United States

INTRODUCTION

Tobacco use is the number one cause of preventable deaths in the United States, and the health-care costs of tobacco use have been estimated at over $150 billion dollars per year. Epidemiological studies have advanced our understanding of which populations are most vulnerable to tobacco use, and suggest that the efficacy of smoking cessation strategies varies across different groups of people. It is presently unclear why certain populations are more vulnerable to tobacco use and are less responsive to cessation approaches. Thus, much work is needed to understand the factors that contribute to tobacco use in different populations. This understanding will ultimately lead to more effective specialized medications that target the critical factors that modulate tobacco use in different subpopulations. Thus, work in this area has the potential to help reduce health disparities produced by tobacco use.

For the past several years, work in our laboratory has studied the underlying mechanisms that promote tobacco use among certain groups that display enhanced vulnerability to smoking behavior. Along with other laboratories, animal models have been applied to provide studies that will deepen our understanding of the underlying factors that promote tobacco

Negative Affective States and Cognitive Impairments in Nicotine Dependence
http://dx.doi.org/10.1016/B978-0-12-802574-1.00005-3

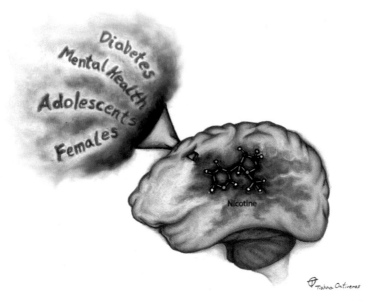

FIGURE 5.1   This image represents certain populations that are more susceptible to the effects of nicotine in the brain. As a result, there are some demographic populations that are more vulnerable to tobacco use than the general population.

use. This chapter is intended to provide a summary of the work that has advanced our current understanding of the role of nicotine reward and withdrawal in modulating tobacco use among vulnerable populations, including adolescents, females, and individuals with diabetes. We also discuss tobacco use vulnerability among persons suffering from anxiety disorders and alcoholism. Although there are many ethnic groups and social factors to consider, we focus on subgroups for which animal models have been applied. Fig. 5.1 depicts different populations that are discussed here that display enhanced susceptibility to tobacco use.

NICOTINE REWARD AND WITHDRAWAL

Tobacco use is motivated by at least two processes involving the positive rewarding effects of nicotine and avoiding the negative consequences of withdrawal from this drug. Fig. 5.2 depicts tobacco use as a balance between experiencing the positive rewarding effects of nicotine and avoiding the negative consequences of withdrawal from chronic exposure to nicotine. Initially, tobacco use is largely motivated by the positive rewarding effects of nicotine that promote continued use. Nicotine also possesses short-term negative effects that may limit initial use or discourage future experimentation with tobacco products. The most common rodent models

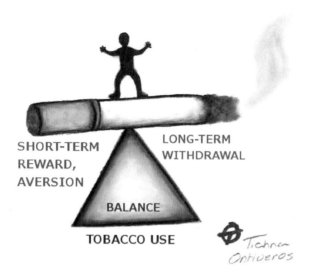

FIGURE 5.2   Tobacco use is depicted as a balance between experiencing the short-term rewarding effects of nicotine and avoiding the long-term effects of nicotine withdrawal that are believed to promote continued tobacco use and relapse. Importantly, nicotine also produces short-term aversive effects that may limit nicotine use.

used to study the rewarding effects of nicotine involve operant responses for nicotine and classical conditioning between the drug and environmental cues (O'Dell & Khroyan, 2009). For example, nicotine intravenous self-administration (IVSA) has been established in humans, primates, dogs, and rodents (Corrigall & Coen, 1989; Goldberg, Spealman, Goldberg, & Goldberg, 1981; Henningfield, Miyasato, & Jasinski, 1985; Risner & Goldberg, 1982). IVSA involves operant learning, whereby the reinforcing properties of a drug are assessed as the ability of a drug to increase the probability of a behavioral response, such as a licking, nose poke response, or pressing a lever (Weeks, 1962). The conditioned place preference (CPP) procedure involves classical conditioning, where the drug serves as the unconditioned stimulus and the environmental context serves as the conditioned stimulus. During conditioning, the rats are given an injection of nicotine, and the animals are confined to a compartment with distinct environmental cues. On intervening days, rats are given a vehicle injection and are confined to an alternate compartment. After conditioning, the rats are allowed to explore the two compartments in a drug-free state. CPP is operationally defined as an increase in time spent in the drug-paired side versus the neutral location (Shaham, Shalev, Lu, de Wit, & Stewart, 2003). It is unlikely that nicotine reinforcement is the sole motivational factor for continued tobacco use and relapse. In fact, some authors have argued that the positive reinforcing effects of tobacco may be more closely related to the ability of this drug to enhance the reinforcing value of other drugs or environmental factors, such as social interaction (Conrad, Flay, & Hill, 1992; Flay, Phil, Hu, & Richardson, 1998).

Chronic exposure to tobacco leads to nicotine dependence and withdrawal during abstinence from smoking. The withdrawal syndrome includes physical symptoms and negative affective states such as intense craving, anxiety, and depression. The emergence of these subjective effects is closely associated with the severity of dependence and the likelihood of smoking relapse (Hughes, 2007; Piper, Cook, Schlam, Jorenby, & Baker, 2011; Ríos-Bedoya, Snedecor, Pomerleau, & Pomerleau, 2008; West, Ussher, Evans, & Rashid, 2006). In rodents, a common method of inducing nicotine dependence is via surgical implantation of osmotic pumps that continuously deliver nicotine for a minimum of at least 5–7 days (Damaj, Kao, & Martin, 2003; O'Dell et al., 2004; Malin & Goyarzu, 2009). Withdrawal is induced following the removal of the nicotine pump (spontaneous withdrawal) or administration of a nicotinic receptor antagonist (precipitated withdrawal). In either method, nicotine withdrawal produces a behavioral profile involving physical signs, including writhes, gasps, shakes, tremors, teeth chattering, chewing, and ptosis (Hamilton, Berger, Perry, & Grunberg, 2009; Hamilton, Perry, Berger, & Grunberg, 2010; Malin et al., 1992; Skjei & Markou, 2003). Nicotine withdrawal has also been shown to produce an increase in negative affective states, as evidenced in place aversion studies where rodents avoid a compartment that was previously paired with nicotine withdrawal (Bruijnzeel, 2012; O'Dell & Khroyan, 2009). The nature of the negative affective state produced by nicotine withdrawal is believed to involve the induction of stress systems, as evidenced by an increase in time spent in the closed arms of an elevated plus maze (Damaj et al., 2003; Irvine, Cheeta, & File, 2001; Pellow, Chopin, File, & Briley, 1985). It has been suggested that drug addiction reflects opponent processes that undergo a dynamic shift in motivational systems from positive to negative reinforcement processes that promote compulsive drug use (Koob & Le Moal, 2001).

ADOLESCENTS

There is growing concern for the marked recent rise in cigarette smoking among adolescents, particularly because it facilitates tobacco dependence during adulthood. As a result, adolescents who smoke are at an increased risk of developing diseases caused by the long-term tobacco use.

Nicotine reward: Clinical reports have not directly compared the rewarding effects of nicotine in adolescent and adult smokers. However, there is evidence suggesting that adults that initiated smoking during adolescence report more pleasant effects and fewer unpleasant effects (dizziness and sickness) following their first smoking episode as compared to adults that initiated smoking in adulthood (Eissenberg & Balster, 2000; Pomerleau,

Pomerleau, Namenek, & Marks, 1999). There is also a myriad of risk factors that promote the initiation of tobacco use during adolescence, including enhanced risk-taking, peer pressure, and weight concerns (Henningfield, Hatsukami, Zeller, & Peters, 2011; Hussaini, Nicholson, Shera, Stettler, & Kinsman, 2011; Nizami, Sobani, Raza, Baloch, & Khan, 2011).

Rodent studies have shown that nicotine reward is enhanced during the adolescent period of development (postnatal day 28–45; Spear, 2000). For example, adolescent rodents display greater nicotine CPP as compared to adults across a wide range of experimental protocols, nicotine doses, and routes of administration (Belluzzi, Lee, Oliff, & Leslie, 2004; Kota, Martin, Robinson, & Damaj, 2007; Shram, Funk, Li, & Lê, 2006; Shram & Lê, 2010; Torres, Natividad, Tejeda, Van Weelden, & O'Dell, 2009; Torres, Tejeda, Natividad, & O'Dell, 2008; Vastola, Douglas, Varlinskaya, & Spear, 2002). Studies using IV and oral SA procedures have shown that nicotine intake is higher in adolescent versus adult rats (Chen, Matta, & Sharp, 2007; Levin, Rezvani, Montoya, Rose, & Swartzwelder, 2003; Levin et al., 2007; 2011; Natividad, Tejeda, Torres, & O'Dell, 2010; Nesil, Kanit, Collins, & Pogun, 2011) and mice (Adriani, Macrì, Pacifici, & Laviola, 2002). Importantly, nicotine also possesses short-term aversive effects that are lower during adolescence. Specifically, adolescent rats display reduced place aversion to an environment (O'Dell, Torres, Natividad, & Tejeda, 2007) and taste aversion to a solution (Shram et al., 2006) that was paired with a high nicotine dose as compared to adults. These data suggest that enhanced nicotine reward and reduced aversive effects may facilitate experimentation with and continued use of tobacco products in young persons.

Nicotine withdrawal: Following chronic tobacco use, clinical studies have revealed that young smokers exhibit milder symptoms of nicotine withdrawal than adults (Smith, Cavallo, Dahl, et al., 2008). Also, withdrawal symptoms on the quit day are not related to relapse behavior in adolescent smokers (Smith, Cavallo, McFetridge, Liss, & Krishnan-Sarin, 2008). Furthermore, treatments that focus on alleviating withdrawal, such as nicotine replacement therapy (NRT), do not improve abstinence rates in adolescent smokers (Bailey et al., 2012; Grimshaw & Stanton, 2006; Hanson, Allen, Jensen, & Hatsukami, 2003). Studies comparing the effectiveness of various tobacco cessation medications report abstinence rates in the range 19.0–36.5% in adults and 4.5–20.6% in adolescents (Bailey et al., 2012; Hudmon, Suchanek, Corelli, & Prokhorov, 2010). However, there are reports showing that young smokers display robust cue-elicited craving despite occasional cigarette use (Carpenter et al., 2014). Thus, the possibility exists that treatments that target withdrawal may not be as effective at reducing tobacco use in adolescents given that they experience less negative states during nicotine withdrawal.

Rodent studies have shown that the behavioral effects of nicotine withdrawal are lower during adolescence. Following chronic nicotine exposure, administration of the nicotinic receptor antagonist mecamylamine precipitates fewer physical signs of withdrawal in adolescent versus adult rats (O'Dell et al., 2004; Shram, Siu, Li, Tyndale, & Lê, 2008) and mice (Kota, Martin, & Damaj, 2008). Nicotine withdrawal also produces an increase in brain reward thresholds in adult rats that is lower in adolescents (O'Dell et al., 2006). Adult rats also display place aversion to a compartment previously paired with nicotine withdrawal, and this effect is lower in adolescents (O'Dell et al., 2007). Nicotine withdrawal also elicits anxiety-like behavior in adult rodents that is lower in adolescents (Kota et al., 2007; Torres, Gentil, Natividad, Carcoba, & O'Dell, 2013; Wilmouth & Spear, 2006). These findings suggest that nicotine withdrawal is lower during the adolescent period of development.

To summarize, it appears that vulnerability to tobacco use in adolescents is driven by two factors: (1) the positive rewarding effects of nicotine are greater, and (2) the negative aversive effects of nicotine withdrawal are reduced. Thus, an inadequate balance between the strong positive rewarding effects of nicotine that are unopposed by minimal negative effects during withdrawal enhances the motivation to use tobacco products during adolescence. The strong rewarding effects of nicotine are depicted in Fig. 5.3 as a large "on" switch in the brain of a young person that is more susceptible to tobacco use. For more detailed information on

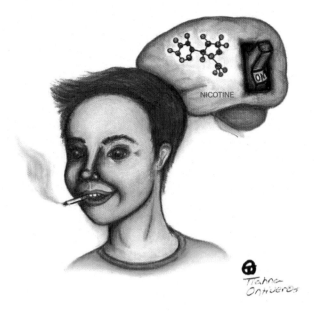

FIGURE 5.3 This image depicts an adolescent engaged in smoking behavior. It is postulated that adolescents experience enhanced rewarding effects of nicotine and weaker symptoms of nicotine withdrawal as compared to adults. Thus, we postulate that the strong rewarding effects of nicotine largely motivate tobacco use in young persons.

the factors that promote tobacco use in adolescents, the reader is referred to the following review papers (Lydon, Wilson, Child, & Geier, 2014; O'Dell, 2009; 2011; Tyas & Pederson, 1998).

FEMALES

There is also growing concern that women are more susceptible to tobacco use and the long-term negative health consequences of smoking as compared to men. Indeed, female smoking behavior is believed to be a major factor that promotes health disparities among women. Despite this well-recognized problem, there is a knowledge gap regarding the factors that promote tobacco use in women.

Nicotine reward: Clinical reports have suggested that women are more sensitive to the rewarding effects of nicotine (Carroll, Lynch, Roth, Morgan, & Cosgrove, 2004; Roth, Cosgrove, & Carroll, 2004). Females display a higher prevalence of smoking and lower quit rates as compared to males (Perkins, Donny, & Caggiula, 1999; Zilberman, Hochgraf, & Andrade, 2003). Self-reports of positive mood effects following cigarette use are also higher in female relative to male smokers (Perkins et al., 2006). Additionally, female smokers display enhanced responding for smoking-related cues compared to males (Perkins et al., 1999).

Preclinical studies have shown that females display more robust CPP produced by nicotine compared to male rats (Torres et al., 2009) and mice (Kota et al., 2008). Female rats also display greater nicotine intake on a demanding schedule of IVSA and following presentation of conditioned stimuli compared to males (Chaudhri et al., 2005). However, another study found that female and male rats display similar levels of nicotine intake as well as extinction and reinstatement of nicotine-seeking behavior following administration of the pharmacological stressor yohimbine (Feltenstein, Ghee, & See, 2012). The authors of the latter report suggested that their lack of sex differences is likely related to their use of lower reinforcement requirements as compared to previous reports.

Nicotine withdrawal: Few clinical studies have directly compared sex differences in nicotine withdrawal. However, it may be suggested that females experience greater nicotine withdrawal during abstinence, given that women consume more tobacco products, exhibit lower quit rates, and are less likely to benefit from NRT than men (Cepeda-Benito, Reynoso, & Erath, 2004; Hammond, 2009; Perkins & Scott, 2008; Piper et al., 2010; Schnoll, Patterson, & Lerman, 2007). Female smokers also experience reduced relief from withdrawal and lower abstinence rates with NRT relative to males (Pomerleau, Tate, Lumley, & Pomerleau, 1994). During abstinence from smoking, women report greater levels of anxiety, depression, and stress (Perkins & Scott, 2008; Schnoll et al., 2007; Xu et al., 2008) and higher levels of cortisol (a biological marker of stress in humans) compared to men (Hogle & Curtin, 2006). Women also report more often than men that the anxiety-reducing effects of cigarettes are the main reason for continued smoking and relapse (Perkins & Scott, 2008; Perkins, Giedgowd, Karelitz, Conklin, & Lerman, 2012; Piper et al., 2010).

Preclinical work in our laboratory has revealed that female rats display larger increases in anxiety-like behavior, corticosterone levels, and changes in the expression of stress-associated genes in the nucleus accumbens than males (Torres et al., 2013). Subsequent studies revealed that the latter effects are absent in ovariectomized females, suggesting that the stress produced by withdrawal is modulated via ovarian hormones (Torres, Pipkin, Ferree, Carcoba, & O'Dell, 2015). Consistent with this, female rats display higher plasma corticosterone levels during nicotine withdrawal as compared to males (Gentile et al., 2011; Skwara, Karwoski, Czambel, Rubin, & Rhodes, 2012). Female mice also display more anxiety-like behavior during nicotine withdrawal than males (Kota et al., 2007; 2008).

To summarize, it is suggested that enhanced vulnerability to tobacco use in females is driven by stronger positive effects of nicotine and more intense stress produced by withdrawal from this drug compared to males. Fig. 5.4 depicts a female that is more susceptible to tobacco use given the strong positive effects of nicotine and intense stress produced by withdrawal from this drug. As a result, both positive rewarding effects and intense negative affective states produced by withdrawal promote continued use and relapse in females. For more information on the factors that

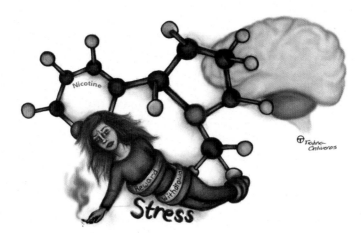

FIGURE 5.4   This image depicts a female engaged in smoking behavior. It is postulated that females experience both strong rewarding effects of nicotine and aversive effects of withdrawal from this drug. Specifically, females experience intense stress during withdrawal that we postulate plays a major role in promoting tobacco use and relapse.

promote tobacco use in females, the reader is referred to the following review papers (Becker, Perry, & Westenbroek, 2012; Carroll & Anker, 2010; O'Dell and Torres, 2014; Torres & O'Dell, 2016).

PERSONS WITH DIABETES

Tobacco products are appealing for persons with diabetes for several reasons, including control of appetite, management of stress, and to improve cognitive processes that may be compromised by chronic diabetes. As the disease progresses, persons with diabetes need to learn how to apply various pharmacological tools in an optimal manner to manage different negative health consequences, as such hunger, anxiety, and cognitive strain (Holt, Cockram, Flyvbjerg, & Goldstein, 2010). The ability of nicotine to cope with these health effects may increase vulnerability to experiment with and ultimately use tobacco. Fig. 5.5 depicts smoking behavior in a diabetic individual that is more susceptible to tobacco use.

Nicotine reward: Clinical evidence suggests that persons with diabetes may be more vulnerable to tobacco use. One way to assess tobacco use vulnerability is to compare smoking rates in the general population with smoking rates in persons with diabetes. Indeed, smoking rates in adolescent males with Type 1 diabetes are significantly higher than in healthy controls (47% versus 38%; Scaramuzza et al., 2010). Few studies have directly compared smoking rates in adults with and without diabetes. A recent examination of cigarette smoking trends from 2001 to 2010 revealed

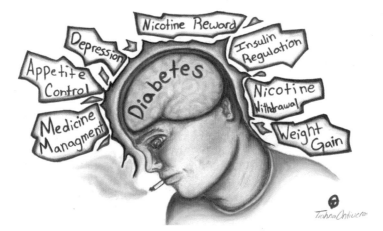

FIGURE 5.5   This image depicts a person with diabetes engaged in smoking behavior. Persons with diabetes face a milieu of physical and emotional states that are often managed with tobacco use. It is postulated that a stronger rewarding effect of nicotine is one important factor that promotes tobacco use in persons with diabetes.

that smoking rates are generally similar in persons with and without diabetes (Fan et al., 2013). However, it is important to note that the latter survey also found that the decline in smoking rates over this period is lower in persons with diabetes, indicating a sustained use of tobacco in persons with diabetes. Bishop et al. (2009) also found that persons with Type 1 diabetes report higher rates of current smoking (12.3%) compared to nondiabetic people (8.6%).

Preclinical studies have revealed that diabetic rats display higher nicotine IVSA compared to healthy controls (O'Dell et al., 2014). A subsequent study revealed that insulin resistance, produced by a high fat diet (HFD) regimen, enhances CPP produced by nicotine (Richardson, Pipkin, O'Dell, & Nazarian, 2014). Interestingly, nicotine CPP was absent in rats that were placed on an HFD regimen but did not display insulin resistance. Thus, the rewarding effects of nicotine were uniquely exacerbated in rats that received the HFD and also displayed insulin resistance, suggesting an enhancement in nicotine reward via a disruption of insulin signaling. Taken together, our findings suggest that the rewarding effects of nicotine are enhanced in diabetic rats due to insulin resistance and lack of insulin signaling rather than the effects of the diet and increased body weight per se. We acknowledge another report showing that mice placed on an HFD regimen do not display nicotine CPP (Blendy et al., 2005). The discrepancy in these reports may be related to metabolic differences between rats and mice and/or different doses of nicotine and routes of administration that were used.

Nicotine withdrawal: Persons with diabetes display lower smoking cessation rates as compared to smokers without diabetes (Gill, Morgan, & MacFarlane, 2005). Interestingly, the latter study also showed that 34–50% of persons with diabetes have never heard of NRT or pharmacological therapies or consider these interventions to be unsafe given their diabetes status. Persons with diabetes also report poorer health outcomes and display lower readiness to quit smoking as compared to nondiabetic persons (Solberg, Desai, O'Connor, Bishop, & Devlin, 2004). Diabetic persons who smoke also display higher levels of stress, negative affect, and depressive clinical symptoms as compared to nonsmokers (Haire-Joshu, Heady, Thomas, Schechtman, & Fisher, 1994; Spangler, Summerson, Bell, & Konen, 2001). Thus, one might expect that persons with diabetes may experience greater anxiety, stress, and depression following smoking cessation that may promote relapse behavior in this population.

To our knowledge, no one has assessed nicotine withdrawal in an animal model of diabetes. Thus, additional studies are needed to better understand the complex mechanisms by which diabetes enhances vulnerability to tobacco use. For additional information on the factors that promote tobacco use in persons with diabetes, the reader is referred to the following review papers (Eliasson, 2003; O'Dell & Nazarian, 2016; Tonstad, 2009).

OTHER POPULATIONS TO CONSIDER

There are other groups to consider that are more susceptible to tobacco use than the general population. Indeed, the propensity for tobacco use in persons with schizophrenia, posttraumatic stress disorder, and depression are reviewed in other chapters of this book. One important factor to consider is the comorbid use of tobacco with other drugs of abuse, such as alcohol. Although tobacco is used to elevate mood and improve cognitive functioning, the comorbid use of drugs complicates the treatment of mental health problems that often coexist with substance addiction, as depicted in Fig. 5.6.

Nicotine reward: Alcohol is the most common substance that is co-abused with tobacco and the vast majority of alcohol-dependent persons use tobacco regularly. Individuals with alcohol use disorder are three to four times more likely than the general population to smoke regularly (Grant, Hasin, Chou, Stinson, & Dawson, 2004). Nicotine administration has been shown to increase alcohol consumption in humans (Barrett, Tichauer, Leyton, & Pihl, 2006). Alcohol administration has also been shown to enhance the rewarding effects of nicotine, as assessed by self-reports of smoking

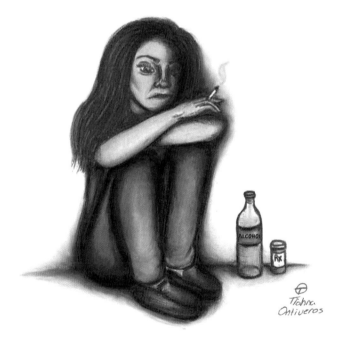

FIGURE 5.6 This image depicts comorbid tobacco and alcohol abuse in persons with mental health issues. Tobacco is often used as a coping strategy to deal with a variety of emotional and cognitive impairments that are alleviated by nicotine. It is postulated that alcohol promotes the rewarding effects of nicotine and withdrawal from this drug.

satisfaction (Glaudtier, Clements, White, Taylor, & Stolerman, 1996; Rose et al., 2004) and feelings of pleasure (Piasecki et al., 2011).

Preclinical studies have shown that nicotine enhances alcohol intake and reinstates alcohol-seeking behavior following extinction in rats (Clark, Lindgren, Brooks, Watson, & Little, 2001; Lê et al., 2000; 2003). Chronic nicotine exposure has also been shown to increase compulsive alcohol intake in rats (Leào et al., 2015; Potthof et al., 1983; Smith, Horan, Gaskin, & Amit, 1999). Direct infusions of nicotine into the basal forebrain also increase alcohol consumption in mice (Sharma, Sahota, & Thakkar, 2014). However, there are reports showing that nicotine decreases alcohol consumption (Dyr, Koros, Bienkowsky, & Kostowki, 1999; Nadal & Samson, 1999; Sharpe & Samson, 2002) and has no effect on CPP produced by alcohol (Gubner, Cunningham, & Phillips, 2015). These discrepancies in the literature may be due to an array of factors such as dose, length of exposure, and the route of administration that is used.

Nicotine withdrawal: Clinical reports have shown that nicotine withdrawal potentiates alcohol craving (Palfai, Monti, Ostafin, & Hutchison, 2000). Alcohol consumption has also been shown promote relapse in individuals that are in the process of quitting smoking (Borland, 1990). Furthermore, in abstinent smokers, NRT has been shown to enhance the subjective rewarding effects of alcohol (Kouri, McCarthy, Faust, & Lukas, 2004).

Preclinical reports have shown that simultaneous withdrawal from alcohol and nicotine produces physical symptoms that are more severe and last longer than withdrawal from either drug alone (Perez, Quijano-Cardé, & De Biasi, 2015). The latter report also revealed that nicotine administration reduces withdrawal symptoms produced by the removal of chronic alcohol. Interestingly, nicotine administration to adolescent (but not adult) mice increases withdrawal signs produced alcohol withdrawal (Riley, Zalud, & Diaz-Granados, 2010). This finding is clinically relevant given that smoking and alcohol use are initiated during the adolescent period. Together, these data suggest alcohol and nicotine interact in a manner that promotes dependence on these abused substances.

CONCLUSION AND CLINICAL IMPLICATIONS

In conclusion, there are clearly certain demographic populations that are more vulnerable to tobacco use. It is recognized that there are a host of social and biological factors that promote tobacco use among the populations discussed here, and more research is needed to better understand the underlying mechanisms that promote tobacco use in these vulnerable groups.

The information presented in this chapter offers many clinical implications to consider. The preclinical research suggests that different vulnerable populations possess a unique profile in which tobacco use is enhanced relative to the general population. In some cases, the factors that promote tobacco use among certain groups overlap. As one example, the rewarding effects of nicotine are greater in adolescent, female, and diabetic rats, suggesting that strong rewarding effects of nicotine is an important factor that promotes tobacco use in these populations. On the other hand, adolescent rats display reduced physical and affective properties of nicotine withdrawal, as compared to females that display intense stress during withdrawal. Taken together, these data suggest that the most effective treatment strategies in certain groups will need to target the unique factors that promote tobacco use in each demographic population. Unfortunately, there is a critical knowledge gap regarding the biological mechanisms that promote enhanced vulnerability to tobacco use in vulnerable populations. A deeper understanding of the brain substrates that enhance vulnerability to tobacco use will guide the development of specialized and more effective cessation treatments for unique populations.

Another clinical implication of the work discussed here is that physicians need to assess the demographic and health background of their patients, as depicted in Fig. 5.7. In this way, health-care professionals will be better equipped to prescribe specialized medications according to the background of the patient. Lastly, it is also important to educate populations that may be more susceptible to tobacco use. This information is vital

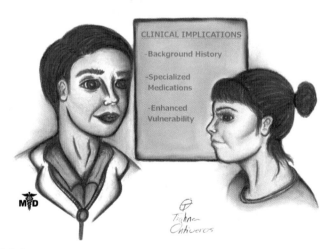

FIGURE 5.7   This image depicts the clinical implications of enhanced tobacco use in certain vulnerable populations. We suggest that the most effective smoking cessation medications will target the specific factors that promote tobacco use in certain demographic groups. This will require that physicians understand the background of their patients and that they apply specialized medications to different patient populations. Education approaches may also be used to inform certain persons about their greater vulnerability to tobacco use as compared to the general population.

to reducing health disparities, especially given that the tobacco industry targets demographic groups (such as young females) that are vulnerable to tobacco use. Thus, educational approaches may help to foster a healthier and tobacco-free lifestyle in vulnerable populations.

Acknowledgments

The authors are grateful for the grant support provided by the American Diabetes Association (7-12-BS-135) and the National Institute on Drug Abuse (R01-DA021274, R24-DA029989, and R25-DA033613). The authors have no relevant conflict of interest to disclose.

References

Adriani, W., Macrì, S., Pacifici, R., & Laviola, G. (2002). Peculiar vulnerability to nicotine oral self-administration in mice during early adolescence. *Neuropsychopharmacology: Official Publication of the American College of Neuropsychopharmacology, 27*, 212–224.

Bailey, S. R., Crew, E. E., Riske, E. C., Ammerman, S., Robinson, T. N., & Killen, J. D. (2012). Efficacy and tolerability of pharmacotherapies to aid smoking cessation in adolescents. *Paediatric Drugs, 14*(2), 91–108.

Barrett, S., Tichauer, M., Leyton, M., & Pihl, R. (2006). Nicotine increases alcohol self-administration in non-dependent male smokers. *Drug and Alcohol Dependence, 81*(2), 197–204.

Becker, J. B., Perry, A. N., & Westenbroek, C. (2012). Sex differences in the neural mechanisms mediating addiction: a new synthesis and hypothesis. *Biology of Sex Differences, 3*(1), 14.

Belluzzi, J. D., Lee, A. G., Oliff, H. S., & Leslie, F. M. (2004). Age-dependent effects of nicotine on locomotor activity and conditioned place preference in rats. *Psychopharmacology, 174*(3), 389–395.

Bishop, F. K., Maahs, D. M., Snell-Bergeon, J. K., Ogden, L. G., Kinney, G. L., & Rewers, M. (2009). Lifestyle risk factors for atherosclerosis in adults with type 1 diabetes. *Diabetes & Vascular Disease Research: Official Journal of the International Society of Diabetes and Vascular Disease, 6*(4), 269–275.

Blendy, J. A., Strasser, A., Walters, C. L., Perkins, K. A., Patterson, F., Berkowitz, R., et al. (2005). Reduced nicotine reward in obesity: cross-comparison in human and mouse. *Psychopharmacology, 180*(2), 306–315.

Borland, R. (1990). Slip-ups and relapse in attempts to quit smoking. *Addictive Behaviors, 15*(3), 235–245.

Bruijnzeel, A. W. (2012). Tobacco addiction and the dysregulation of brain stress systems. *Neuroscience and Biobehavioral Reviews, 36*(5), 1418–1441.

Carpenter, M. J., Saladin, M. E., Larowe, S. D., Mcclure, E. A., Simonian, S., Upadhyaya, H. P., et al. (2014). Craving, cue reactivity, and stimulus control among early-stage young smokers: effects of smoking intensity and gender. *Nicotine & Tobacco Research, 16*(2), 208–215.

Carroll, M. E., & Anker, J. J. (2010). Sex differences and ovarian hormones in animal models of drug dependence. *Hormones and Behavior, 58*(1), 44–56.

Carroll, M. E., Lynch, W. J., Roth, M. E., Morgan, A. D., & Cosgrove, K. P. (2004). Sex and estrogen influence drug abuse. *Trends in Pharmacological Sciences, 25*(5), 273–279.

Cepeda-Benito, A., Reynoso, J., & Erath, S. (2004). Meta-analysis of the efficacy of nicotine replacement therapy for smoking cessation: differences between men and women. *Journal of Consulting and Clinical Psychology, 72*(4), 712–722.

Chaudhri, N., Caggiula, A., Donny, E., Booth, S., Gharib, M., Craven, L., et al. (2005). Sex differences in the contribution of nicotine and nonpharmacological stimuli to nicotine self-administration in rats. *Psychopharmacology, 180*(2), 258–266.

Chen, H., Matta, S. G., & Sharp, B. M. (2007). Acquisition of nicotine self-administration in adolescent rats given prolonged access to the drug. *Neuropsychopharmacology: Official Publication of the American College of Neuropsychopharmacology, 32*, 700–709.

Clark, A., Lindgren, S., Brooks, S. P., Watson, W. P., & Little, H. J. (2001). Chronic infusion of nicotine can increase operant self-administration of alcohol. *Neuropharmacology, 41*(1), 108–117.

Conrad, K. M., Flay, B. R., & Hill, D. (1992). Why children start smoking cigarettes: predictors of onset. *British Journal of Addiction, 87*(12), 1711–1724.

Corrigall, W. A., & Coen, K. M. (1989). Nicotine maintains robust self-administration in rats on a limited-access schedule. *Psychopharmacology, 99*(4), 473–478.

Damaj, M. I., Kao, W., & Martin, B. R. (2003). Characterization of spontaneous and precipitated nicotine withdrawal in the mouse. *Pharmacological Reviews, 307*(2), 526–534.

Dyr, W., Koros, E., Bienkowsky, P., & Kostowki, W. (1999). Involvement of nicotinic acetylcholine receptors in the regulation of alcohol drinking in wistar rats. *Alcohol & Alcoholism, 34*(1), 43–47.

Eissenberg, T., & Balster, R. L. (2000). Initial tobacco use episodes in children and adolescents: current knowledge, future direction. *Drug and Alcohol Dependence, 59*(1), 41–60.

Eliasson, B. (2003). Cigarette smoking and diabetes. *Progress in Cardiovascular Diseases, 45*(5), 405–413.

Eliasson, B., Attvall, S., Taskinen, M. R., & Smith, U. (1997). Smoking cessation improves insulin sensitivity in healthy middle-aged men. *European Journal of Clinical Investigation, 27*, 450–456.

Fan, A. Z., Rock, V., Zhang, X., Li, Y., Elam-Evans, L., & Lina, B. (2013). Trends in cigarette smoking rates and quit attempts among adults with and without diagnosed diabetes: findings from 2001 to 2010 behavioral risk factors surveillance system. *Preventing Chronic Disease, 10*, E160.

Feltenstein, M., Ghee, S., & See, R. (2012). Nicotine self-administration and reinstatement of nicotine-seeking in male and female rats. *Drug and Alcohol Dependence, 121*, 240–246.

Flay, B. R., Phil, D., Hu, F. B., & Richardson, J. (1998). Psychosocial predictors of different stages of cigarette smoking among high school students. *Preventive Medicine, 27*(5B), A9–A18.

Gentile, N. E., Andrekanic, J. D., Karwoski, T. E., Czambel, R. K., Rubin, R. T., & Rhodes, M. E. (2011). Sexually diergic hypothalamic-pituitary-adrenal (HPA) responses to single-dose nicotine, continuous nicotine infusion, and nicotine withdrawal by mecamylamine in rats. *Brain Research Bulletin, 85*(3–4), 145–152.

Gill, G. V., Morgan, C., & MacFarlane, I. A. (2005). Awareness and use of smoking cessation treatments among diabetic patients. *Diabetic Medicine, 22I*(5), 658–660.

Glaudtier, S., Clements, K., White, J., Taylor, C., & Stolerman, I. (1996). Alcohol and the reward value of cigarette smoking. *Behavioral Pharmacology, 7*(2).

Goldberg, S. R., Spealman, R. D., Goldberg, S., & Goldberg, D. M. (1981). Persistent behavior at high rates maintained by intravenous self-administration of nicotine. *Science, 214*(4520), 573–575.

Grant, B. F., Hasin, D. S., Chou, S., Stinson, F. S., & Dawson, D. A. (2004). Nicotine dependence and psychiatric disorders in the United States: results from the National Epidemiologic Survey on alcohol and related conditions. *Archives of General Psychiatry, 61*(11), 1107–1115.

Grimshaw, G., & Stanton, A. (2006). Tobacco cessation interventions for young people. *Cochrane Database of Systematic Reviews*, 1–60.

Gubner, N., Cunningham, C., & Phillips, T. (2015). Nicotine enhances the locomotor stimulating but not the conditioned rewarding effect of ethanol in DBA/2J mice. *Alcoholism: Clinical and Experimental Research, 39*(1), 64–72.

Haire-Joshu, D., Heady, S., Thomas, L., Schechtman, K., & Fisher, E. B. J. (1994). Depressive symptomatology and smoking among persons with diabetes. *Research in Nursing & Health, 17*, 273–282.

Hamilton, K. R., Berger, S. S., Perry, M. E., & Grunberg, N. E. (2009). Behavioral effects of nicotine withdrawal in adult male and female rats. *Pharmacology Biochemistry and Behavior, 92*(1), 51–59.

Hamilton, K. R., Perry, M. E., Berger, S. S., & Grunberg, N. E. (2010). Behavioral effects of nicotine withdrawal differ by genetic strain in male and female adolescent rats. *Nicotine & Tobacco Research, 12*(12), 1236–1245.

Hammond, S. K. (2009). Global patterns of nicotine and tobacco consumption. *Nicotine Psychopharmacology, 192*, 3–28.

Hanson, K., Allen, S., Jensen, S., & Hatsukami, D. (2003). Treatment of adolescent smokers with the nicotine patch. *Nicotine & Tobacco Research, 5*(4), 515–526.

Henningfield, J. E., Hatsukami, D. K., Zeller, M., & Peters, E. (2011). Conference on abuse liability and appeal of tobacco products: conclusions and recommendations. *Drug and Alcohol Dependence, 116*(1), 1–7.

Henningfield, J. E., Miyasato, K., & Jasinski, D. R. (1985). Abuse liability and pharmacodynamics characteristic of intravenous and inhaled nicotine. *The Journal of Pharmacology and Experimental Therapeutics, 234*(1), 1–12.

Hogle, J., & Curtin, J. (2006). Sex differences in negative affective response during nicotine withdrawal. *Psychophysiology, 43*(4), 344–356.

Holt, R. I., Cockram, C., Flyvbjerg, A., & Goldstein, B. J. (2010). In R. I. Holt, C. Cockram, A. Flyvbjerg, & B. J. Goldstein (Eds.), *Textbook of diabetes* (4th ed.). Wiley-Blackwell.

Hudmon, K., Suchanek, R., Corelli, L., & Prokhorov, A. V. (2010). Current approaches to pharmacotherapy for smoking cessation. *Therapeutic Advances in Respiratory Disease,* 35–47.

Hughes, J. R. (2007). Effects of abstinence from tobacco: valid symptoms and time course. *Nicotine & Tobacco Research, 9*(3), 315–327.

Hussaini, A. E., Nicholson, L. M., Shera, D., Stettler, N., & Kinsman, S. (2011). Adolescent obesity as a risk factor for high-level nicotine addiction in young women. *Journal of Adolescent Health, 49*(5), 511–517.

Irvine, E. E., Cheeta, S., & File, S. E. (2001). Tolerance to nicotine's effects in the elevated plus-maze and increased anxiety during withdrawal. *Pharmacology Biochemistry and Behavior, 68*(2), 319–325.

Koob, G., & Le Moal, M. (2001). Drug addiction, dysregulation of reward, and allostasis. *Neuropsychopharmacology: Official Publication of the American College of Neuropsychopharmacology, 24*(2), 97–129.

Kota, D., Martin, B. R., & Damaj, M. I. (2008). Age-dependent differences in nicotine reward and withdrawal in female mice. *Psychopharmacology, 198*(2), 201–210.

Kota, D., Martin, B. R., Robinson, S. E., & Damaj, M. I. (2007). Nicotine dependence and reward differ between adolescent and adult male mice. *The Journal of Pharmacology and Experimental Therapeutics, 322*(1), 399–407.

Kouri, E. M., McCarthy, E. M., Faust, A. H., & Lukas, S. E. (2004). Pretreatment with transdermal nicotine enhances some of ethanol's acute effects in men. *Drug and Alcohol Dependence, 75*(1), 55–65.

Leào, R., Cruz, F., Vendruscolo, L., Guglielmo, G., Logrip, M., Planeta, C., et al. (2015). Chronic nicotine activates stress/reward-related brain regions and facilitates the transition to compulsive alcohol drinking. *Journal of Neuroscience, 35*(15), 6241–6253.

Lê, A. D., Corrigall, W. A., Watchus, J., Harding, S., Juzytsch, W., & Li, T.-K. (2000). Involvement of nicotinic receptors in alcohol self-administration. *Alcoholism: Clinical and Experimental Research, 24*(2), 155–163.

Levin, E. D., Lawrence, S. S., Petro, A., Horton, K., Rezvani, A. H., Seidler, F. J., et al. (2007). Adolescent vs. adult-onset nicotine self-administration in male rats: duration of effect and differential nicotinic receptor correlates. *Neurotoxicology and Teratology, 29*(4), 458–465.

Levin, E. D., Rezvani, A. H., Montoya, D., Rose, J. E., & Swartzwelder, H. S. (2003). Adolescent-onset nicotine self-administration modeled in female rats. *Psychopharmacology, 169*(2), 141–149.

Levin, E. D., Slade, S., Wells, C., Cauley, M., Petro, A., Vendittelli, A., et al. (2011). Threshold of adulthood for the onset of nicotine self-administration in male and female rats. *Behavioural Brain Research, 225*(2), 473–481.

Lê, A. D., Wang, A., Harding, S., Juzytsch, W., & Shaham, Y. (2003). Nicotine increases alcohol self-administration and reinstates alcohol seeking in rats. *Psychopharmacology, 168*(1–2), 216–221.

Lydon, D. M., Wilson, S. J., Child, A., & Geier, C. F. (2014). Adolescent brain maturation and smoking: what we know and where we're headed. *Neuroscience and Biobehavioral Reviews, 45*, 323–342.

Malin, D. H., & Goyarzu, P. (2009). Rodent models of nicotine withdrawal syndrome. *Handbook of Experimental Pharmacology, 192*, 401–434.

Malin, D. H., Lake, J. R., Newlin-Maultsby, P., Roberts, L. K., Lanier, J. G., Carter, V. A., et al. (1992). Rodent model of nicotine abstinence syndrome. *Pharmacology Biochemistry and Behavior, 43*(3), 779–784.

Nadal, R., & Samson, H. H. (1999). Operant ethanol self-administration after nicotine treatment and withdrawal. *Alcohol, 17*(2), 139–147.

Natividad, L. A., Tejeda, H. A., Torres, O. V., & O'Dell, L. E. (2010). Nicotine withdrawal produces a decrease in extracellular levels of dopamine in the nucleus accumbens that is lower in adolescent versus adult male rats. *Synapse, 64*(2), 136–145.

Nesil, T., Kanit, L., Collins, A. C., & Pogun, S. (2011). Individual differences in oral nicotine intake in rats. *Neuropharmacology, 61*(1–2), 189–201.

Nizami, S., Sobani, Z., Raza, E., Baloch, N., & Khan, J. A. (2011). Causes of smoking in Pakistan: an analysis of social factors. *The Journal of the Pakistan Medical Association, 61*(2), 198–201.

O'Dell, L. E., BruijnzelL, A. W., Ghozland, S., Markou, A., & Koob, G. F. (2004). Nicotine withdrawal in adolescent and adult rats. *Annals of the New York Academy of Sciences, 1021*(1), 167–174.

O'Dell, L. E., Natividad, L. A., Pipkin, J. A., Roman, F., Torres, I., Jurado, J., et al. (2014). Enhanced nicotine self-administration and suppressed dopaminergic systems in a rat model of diabetes. *Addiction Biology, 19*, 1006–1019.

O'Dell, L. E., & Torres, O. V. (2014). A mechanistic hypothesis of the factors that enhance vulnerability to nicotine use in females. *Neuropharmacology, 76*(1), 566–580.

O'Dell, L. E. (2009). A psychobiological framework of the substrates that mediate nicotine use during adolescence. *Neuropharmacology, 52*(1), 263–278.

O'Dell, L. E. (2011). NICO-TEEN: neural substrates that mediate adolescent tobacco abuse. *Neuropsychopharmacology: Official Publication of the American College of Neuropsychopharmacology, 36*(1), 356–357.

O'Dell, L., Bruijnzeel, A., Smith, R., Parsons, L., Merves, M., Goldberger, B., et al. (2006). Diminished nicotine withdrawal in adolescent rats: implications for vulnerability to addiction. *Psychopharmacology, 186*(4), 612–619.

O'Dell, L. E., & Khroyan, T. V. (2009). Rodent models of nicotine reward: what do they tell us about tobacco abuse in humans? *Pharmacology Biochemistry and Behavior, 91*(4), 481–488.

O'Dell, L. E., & Nazarian, A. (2016). Enhanced vulnerability to tobacco use in persons with diabetes: a behavioral and neurobiological framework. *Progress in Neuro-Psychopharmacology and Biological Psychiatry, 65*, 288–296.

O'Dell, L. E., Torres, O. V., Natividad, L. A., & Tejeda, H. A. (2007). Adolescent nicotine exposure produces less affective measures of withdrawal relative to adult nicotine exposure in male rats. *Neurotoxicology and Teratology, 29*(1), 17–22.

Palfai, T. P., Monti, P. M., Ostafin, B., & Hutchison, K. (2000). Effects of nicotine deprivation on alcohol-related information processing and drinking behavior. *Journal of Abnormal Psychology, 109*(1), 96–105.

Pellow, S., Chopin, P., File, S. E., & Briley, M. (1985). Validation of open: closed arm entries in an elevated plus-maze as a measure of anxiety in the rat. *Journal of Neuroscience Methods, 14*(3), 149–167.

Perez, E., Quijano-Cardé, N., & De Biasi, M. (2015). Nicotinic mechanisms modulate ethanol withdrawal and modify time course and symptoms severity of simultaneous withdrawal from alcohol and nicotine. *Neuropsychopharmacology: Official Publication of the American College of Neuropsychopharmacology, 40*(10), 2327–2336.

Perkins, K. A., Donny, E., & Caggiula, A. R. (1999). Sex differences in nicotine effects and self-administration: review of human and animal evidence. *Nicotine & Tobacco Research, 1*(4), 301–315.

Perkins, K. A., Doyle, T., Ciccocioppo, M., Conklin, C., Sayette, M., & Caggiula, A. (2006). Sex differences in the influence of nicotine dose instructions on the reinforcing and self-reported rewarding effects of smoking. *Psychopharmacology, 184*(3–4), 600–607.

Perkins, K. A., Giedgowd, G. E., Karelitz, J. L., Conklin, C. A., & Lerman, C. (2012). Smoking in response to negative mood in men versus women as a function of distress tolerance. *Nicotine & Tobacco Research, 14*(12), 1418–1425.

Perkins, K. A., & Scott, J., Levine, M., D'amico, D., Miller, A., Broge, M. (2008). Sex differences in long-term smoking cessation rates due to nicotine patch. *Nicotine & Tobacco Research, 10*(7), 1245–1251.

Piasecki, T. , & Jahng, S., Wood, P., Robertson, B., Epler, A., Cronk, N., et al. (2011). The subjective effects of alcohol–tobacco co-use: an ecological momentary assessment investigation. *Journal of Abnormal Psychology, 120*(3), 557–571.

Piper, M. E., Cook, J. W., Schlam, T. R., Jorenby, D. E., & Baker, T. B., Cronk, N. (2011). Anxiety diagnoses in smoker seeking cessation treatment: relations with tobacco dependence, withdrawal, outcome and response to treatment. *Addiction, 106*(2), 418–427.

Piper, M. E., Cook, J. W., Schlam, T. R., Jorenby, D. E., & Smith, S. S., Bolt, D. M., et al. (2010). Gender, race, and education differences in abstinence rates among participants in two randomized smoking cessation trials. *Nicotine & Tobacco Research, 12*(6), 647–657.

Piper, M. E., Cook, J. W., Schlam, T. R., Jorenby, D. E., Smith, S. S., Bolt, D. M., et al. (2010). Gender, race, and education differences in abstinence rates among participants in two randomized smoking cessation trials. *Nicotine & Tobacco Research, 12*(6), 647–657.

Pomerleau, C. S., Pomerleau, O. F., & Namenek, R. J., & Marks, J. L. (1999). Initial exposure to nicotine in college-age women smokers and never-smokers. *Journal of Addictive Diseases, 18*(3), 13–19.

Pomerleau, C., Tate, J., Lumley, M., & Pomerleau, O. (1994). Gender differences in prospectively versus retrospectively assessed smoking withdrawal symptoms. *Journal of Substance Abuse, 6*(4), 433–440.

Potthoff, A. D., Ellison, G., Lumley, M., & Nelson, L. (1983). Ethanol intake increases during continuous administration of amphetamine and nicotine, but not several other drugs. *Pharmacology Biochemistry and Behavior, 18*(4), 489–493.

Richardson, J. R., Pipkin, J. A., & O'Dell, L. E., & Nazarian, A. (2014). Insulin resistant rats display enhanced rewarding effects of nicotine. *Drug and Alcohol Dependence, 140*(4), 205–207.

Riley, H. H., Zalud, A. W., O'Dell, L. E., & Diaz-Granados, J. L. (2010). The influence of a chronic adolescent nicotine exposure on ethanol withdrawal severity during adulthood in C3H mice. *Alcohol, 44*(1), 81–87.

Ríos-Bedoya, C. F., Snedecor, S. M., & Pomerleau, C. S., & Pomerleau, O. F. (2008). Association of withdrawal with nicotine dependence as measured by the fagerstrom test for nicotine dependence (FTND). *Addictive Behaviors, 33*(8), 1086–1089.

Risner, M. E., Snedecor, S. M., Pomerleau, C. S., & Goldberg, S. R. (1982). A comparison of nicotine and cocaine self-administration in the dog: fixed-ratio and progressive-ratio schedules of intravenous drug infusion. *The Journal of Pharmacology and Experimental Therapeutics, 224*(2), 319–326.

Rose, J. , & Brauer, L. , Behm, F., Cramblett, M., Calkins, K., & Lawhon, D. (2004). Psychopharmacological interactions between nicotine and ethanol. *Nicotine & Tobacco Research, 6*(1), 133–144.

Roth, M. E., Cosgrove, K. P., Behm, F., Cramblett, M., Calkins, K., & Carroll, M. E. (2004). Sex differences in the vulnerability to drug abuse: a review of preclinical studies. *Neuroscience and Biobehavioral Reviews, 28*(6), 533–546.

Scaramuzza, A. , De Palma, A. , & Mameli, C. , Spiri, D., Santoro, L., & Zuccotti, G. V. (2010). Adolescents with type 1 diabetes and risky behaviour. *Acta Paediatrics, 99*(8), 1237–1241.

Schnoll, R., Patterson, F., Mameli, C., Spiri, D., Santoro, L., & Lerman, C. (2007). Treating tobacco dependence in women. *Journal of Women's Health, 16*(8), 1211–1218.

Shaham, Y., Shalev, U., & Lu, L., de Wit, H., & Stewart, J. (2003). The reinstatement model of drug relapse: history, methodology and major findings. *Psychopharmacology, 168*(1–2), 3–20.

Sharma, R., Sahota, P., Lu, L., de Wit, H., & Thakkar, M. (2014). Nicotine administration in the cholinergic basal forebrain increases alcohol consumption in C57BL/6J mice. *Alcoholism: Clinical and Experimental Research, 38*(5), 1315–1320.

Sharpe, A. L., Sahota, P., & Samson, H. H. (2002). Repeated nicotine injections decrease operant ethanol self-administration. *Alcohol, 28*(1), 1–7.

Shram, M. J., & Funk, D. , Li, Z., & Lê, A. D. (2006). Periadolescent and adult rats respond differently in tests measuring the rewarding and aversive effects of nicotine. *Psychopharmacology, 186*(2), 201–208.

Shram, M. J., Funk, D., Li, Z., & Lê, A. D. (2010). Adolescent male Wistar rats are more responsive than adult rats to the conditioned rewarding effects of intravenously administered nicotine in the place conditioning procedure. *Behavioural Brain Research, 206*(2), 240–244.

Shram, M. , & Siu, E. , Li, Z., Tyndale, R., & Lê, A. (2008). Interactions between age and the aversive effects of nicotine withdrawal under mecamylamine-precipitated and spontaneous conditions in male Wistar rats. *Psychopharmacology, 198*(2), 181–190.

Skjei, K. L., Siu, E., Li, Z., Tyndale, R., & Markou, A. (2003). Effects of repeated withdrawal episodes, nicotine dose, and duration of nicotine exposure on the severity and duration of nicotine withdrawal in rats. *Pyschopharmacology, 168*(3), 280–292.

Skwara, A. J., & Karwoski, T. E., Czambel, R. K., Rubin, R. T., & Rhodes, M. E. (2012). Influence of environmental enrichment on hypothalamic-pituitary-adrenal (HPA) responses to single-dose nicotine, continuous nicotine by osmotic mini-pumps, and nicotine withdrawal by mecamylamine in male and female rats. *Behavioural Brain Research, 234*(1), 1–10.

Smith, A. E., Cavallo, D. A., Dahl, T. , Wu, R. , & George, T. P., & Krishnan-Sarin, S. (2008). Effects of acute tobacco abstinence in adolescent smokers compared with nonsmokers. *Journal of Adolescent Health, 43*(1), 46–54.

Smith, A. E., Cavallo, D. A., McFetridge, A., Liss, T., George, T. P., & Krishnan-Sarin, S. (2008). Preliminary examination of tobacco withdrawal in adolescent smokers during smoking cessation treatment. *Nicotine & Tobacco Research, 10*(7), 1253–1259.

Smith, B. R., Horan, J. T., Gaskin, S., Liss, T., & Amit, Z. (1999). Exposure to nicotine enhances acquisition of ethanol drinking by laboratory rats in a limited access paradigm. *Psychopharmacology, 142*(7), 408–412.

Solberg, L. I., Desai, J. R., O'Connor, P. J., & Bishop, D. B., & Devlin, H. M. (2004). Diabetic patients who smoke: are they different? *Annals of Family Medicine, 2*(1), 26–32.

Spangler, J. G., Summerson, J. H., Bell, R. A., Bishop, D. B., & Konen, J. C. (2001). Smoking status and psychosocial variables in type 1 diabetes mellitus. *Addictive Behaviors, 26*(1), 21–29.

Spear, L. P., Summerson, J. H., Bell, R. A., & Konen, J. C. (2000). The adolescent brain and age-related behavioral manifestations. *Neuroscience and Biobehavioral Reviews, 24*(4), 417–463.

Tonstad, S. (2009). Cigarette smoking, smoking cessation, and diabetes. *Diabetes Research and Clinical Practice, 85*(1), 4–13.

Torres, O. V., Gentil, L. G., Natividad, L. A., Carcoba, L. M., & O'Dell, L. E. (2013). Behavioral, biochemical, and molecular indices of stress are enhanced in female versus male rats experiencing nicotine withdrawal. *Frontiers in Psychiatry, 4*(1), 38.

Torres, O. V., Natividad, L. A., Tejeda, H. A., Van Weelden, S. A., & O'Dell, L. E. (2009). Female rats display dose-dependent differences to the rewarding and aversive effects of nicotine in an age-, hormone-, and sex-dependent manner. *Psychopharmacology, 206*(2), 303–312.

Torres, O. V., & O'Dell, L. E. (February 4, 2016). Stress is a principal factor that promotes tobacco use in females. *Progress in Neuro-Psychopharmacology and Biological Psychiatry, 65,* 260–268.

Torres, O. V., & Pipkin, J. A., Ferree, P., Carcoba, L. M., & O'Dell, L. E. (2015). Nicotine withdrawal increases stress-associated genes in the nucleus accumbens of female rats in a hormone-dependent manner. *Nicotine & Tobacco Research, 17*(4), 422–430.

Torres, O. V., Tejeda, H. A., Natividad, L. A., Carcoba, L. M., & O'Dell, L. E. (2008). Enhanced vulnerability to the rewarding effects of nicotine during the adolescent period of development. *Pharmacology Biochemistry and Behavior, 90*(4), 658–663.

Tyas, S. L., Tejeda, H. A., Natividad, L. A., & Pederson, L. L. (1998). Psychosocial factors related to adolescent smoking: a critical review of the literature. *Tobacco Control, 7*(4), 409–420.

Vastola, B. J., & Douglas, L. A., Varlinskaya, E. I., & Spear, L. P. (2002). Nicotine-induced conditioned place preference in adolescent and adult rats. *Physiology & Behavior, 77*(1), 107–114.

Weeks, J. R., Douglas, L. A., Varlinskaya, E. I., & Spear, L. P. (1962). Experimental morphine addiction: method for automatic intravenous injections in unrestrained rats. *Science, 138*(3537), 143–144.

West, R. , Ussher, M., Evans, M., & Rashid, M. (2006). Assessing DSM-IV nicotine withdrawal symptoms: a comparison and evaluation of five different scales. *Pyschopharmacology, 184*(3–4), 619–627.

Wilmouth, C. E., Ussher, M., Evans, M., & Spear, L. P. (2006). Withdrawal from chronic nicotine in adolescent and adult rats. *Pharmacology Biochemistry and Behavior, 85*(3), 648–657.

Xu, J. , & Azizian, A. , Monterosso, J., Domier, C., Brody, A., London, E., et al. (2008). Gender effects on mood and cigarette craving during early abstinence and resumption of smoking. *Nicotine & Tobacco Research, 10*(11), 1653–1661.

Zilberman, M. L., Hochgraf, P. B., & Andrade, A. G. (2003). Gender difference in treatment-seeking Brazilian drug-dependent individuals. *Substance Abuse, 24*(1), 17–23.

Detrimental Effects of Prenatal Exposure to Tobacco Smoke and Nicotine

T. Schneider

University of Central Lancashire, Preston, United Kingdom

INTRODUCTION

Tobacco smoking during pregnancy is associated with a plethora of detrimental effects in offspring, including spontaneous abortions (George, Granath, Johansson, Anneren, & Cnattingius, 2006), preterm birth and stillbirth (Ion & Bernal, 2015), fetal growth retardation and low birth weight (Eskenazi, Prehn, & Christianson, 1995; Salihu, Aliyu, & Kirby, 2005), and sudden infant death syndrome (SIDS) (Rajs, Rasten-Almqvist, Falck, Eksborg, & Andersson, 1997), as well as neurobehavioral aberrations like attention deficit hyperactivity disorder (ADHD), conduct disorder, and substance abuse (D'Onofrio et al., 2008; Goldschmidt, Cornelius, & Day, 2012; Lindblad & Hjern, 2010; Roberts et al., 2005; Thapar et al., 2003). Smoking reduction during pregnancy can ameliorate these aberrations (Blatt, Moore, Chen, Van Hook, & DeFranco, 2015; Lindley, Becker, Gray, & Herman, 2000).

Despite the clear evidence of the harmful effects of cigarette smoking on offspring, approximately 15–20% of all women still smoke during pregnancy, even if the majority of them declare the desire to quit (Murin, Rafii, & Bilello, 2011; Smedberg, Lupattelli, Mardby, & Nordeng, 2014; Swamy, Reddick, Brouwer, Pollak, & Myers, 2011; Tong et al., 2013). Both human and nonhuman animal studies have shown that it is the highly addictive nature of nicotine that makes smoking cessation so difficult (Buchhalter, Fant, & Henningfield, 2008; Okuyemi, Ahluwalia, & Harris,

Negative Affective States and Cognitive Impairments in Nicotine Dependence
http://dx.doi.org/10.1016/B978-0-12-802574-1.00006-5

2000). Indeed, only 20–30% of pregnant tobacco smokers succeed in quitting, with half of them relapsing shortly after parturition (Ashford, Hahn, Hall, Rayens, & Noland, 2009; Harmer & Memon, 2013), which results in significant childhood exposure to tobacco smoke with serious health consequences (Al-Sayed & Ibrahim, 2014). Chances of quitting smoking tobacco are lower in mothers with lower social status, a smoking partner, a higher degree of addiction (Harmer & Memon, 2013), and a history of psychiatric and conduct problems (Park et al., 2009; Prusakowski, Shofer, Rhodes, & Mills, 2011).

Active maternal smoking is just one pathway of fetal exposure to nicotine. Others include exposure of pregnant women to environmental tobacco smoke (ETS), and maternal use of smokeless tobacco products or nicotine replacement therapy (NRT) (Mannino, Moorman, Kingsley, Rose, & Repace, 2001; Oncken et al., 2008; Slotkin, 2008). Although smoking rates among women living in the developed world are declining (Cnattingius, 2004), a lot of women in the third world have started to use tobacco due to rapid cultural and financial changes (Ng et al., 2014). This is accompanied by high environmental tobacco exposure, especially at home (Nichter et al., 2010), which can lead to a similar range of detrimental effects as smoking by mothers (DiFranza, Aligne, & Weitzman, 2004; George et al., 2006; Rogers, 2008).

There is no doubt that prenatal tobacco smoke and nicotine exposure leads to adverse health, behavioral, and cognitive effects in children whose mothers either smoked cigarettes or were exposed to environmental tobacco during pregnancy; however, lifestyle, socioeconomic status, genetic factors, and complex chemical assembly in tobacco smoke make it difficult to show direct causality in humans. This causality has been established in nonhuman animal studies, showing widespread deleterious effects of prenatal exposure to nicotine and tobacco products. The objective of this chapter is to provide an overview of prenatal nicotine and tobacco smoke exposure and its impact on somatic and neurobehavioral aberrations in offspring with special emphasis on preclinical data.

FUNCTIONAL ROLE OF NICOTINIC ACETYLCHOLINE RECEPTORS IN THE DEVELOPING NERVOUS SYSTEM

Activation of nicotinic acetylcholine receptors (nAChRs) by acetylcholine (ACh) during the prenatal period plays a vital role in cell survival, neuronal pathfinding, the formation of motor and sensory circuits (Abreu-Villaca, Filgueiras, & Manhaes, 2011; Feller, 2002; Myers et al., 2005; Papke & Heinemann, 1991), as well as in the development of catecholaminergic systems (Azam, Chen, & Leslie, 2007; Exley, Clements, Hartung, McIntosh, & Cragg, 2008; O'Leary, Loughlin, Chen, & Leslie, 2008) important for the regulation of motivation, attention, cognition, and mood in the mature brain (Brennan & Arnsten, 2008; Nestler & Carlezon, 2006).

In women who smoke, use NRT, or are exposed to ETS during pregnancy, nicotine crosses the placenta (Lambers & Clark, 1996; Schulte-Hobein, Schwartz-Bickenbach, Abt, Plum, & Nau, 1992) and can change developmental trajectories controlled by the ACh system through activation of nAChRs. For example, prenatal exposure to nicotine decreases the number of cells in the brain during the fetal and early neonatal periods (Shingo & Kito, 2005; Slotkin, Cho, & Whitmore, 1987), enhances a switch from cellular proliferation to differentiation (Navarro, Seidler, Eylers, et al., 1989; Navarro, Seidler, Schwartz, et al., 1989), increases expression of nAChR binding sites in the fetus (Falk, Nordberg, Seiger, Kjaeldgaard, & Hellstrom-Lindahl, 2005; Tizabi & Perry, 2000; Van de Kamp & Collins, 1994), and is associated with a plethora of adverse cardiovascular, respiratory, endocrine, metabolic, and neurobehavioral outcomes (Bruin, Gerstein, & Holloway, 2010; Winzer-Serhan, 2008). Mechanisms of those adverse effects have been mimicked and tested in nonhuman animal models.

SOMATIC EFFECTS OF PRENATAL EXPOSURE TO TOBACCO SMOKE AND NICOTINE

Cardiovascular Outcomes

Prenatal exposure to tobacco smoke is a well-established factor that dose-dependently increases the risk for SIDS (Fleming & Blair, 2007). The etiology of SIDS involves a dysregulation of neural control of cardiorespiratory processes and aberrant responses to hypoxia (Prandota, 2004). Rats treated prenatally with nicotine exhibit increased spontaneous apnea in the first 2 days of life (Huang, Brown, Costy-Bennett, Luo, & Fregosi, 2004) and increased vulnerability to death from hypoxic challenge (Fewell, Smith, & Ng, 2001; Slotkin, Lappi, McCook, Lorber, & Seidler, 1995). There are several mechanisms that might be responsible for those changes. First, prenatal nicotine alters the activity of cardiorespiratory neurons in the brainstem during both normal breathing and episodes of hypoxia (Huang et al., 2004; Kamendi et al., 2006). Prenatal nicotine, through increased cholinergic activation of the vagal nerve, results in increased heart rates during normal respiration (Neff, Wang, Baxi, Evans, & Mendelowitz, 2003), but also in the excitation of those cardio-inhibitory neurons, through cholinergic enhancement of glutamate release during hypoxic episodes, leading to increased risk of hypoxia-induced mortality (Evans, Wang, Neff, & Mendelowitz, 2005; Huang et al., 2007). Second, the aberrant response to hypoxia following prenatal nicotine exposure might be mediated by changes in central and peripheral adrenergic systems (Slotkin et al., 1995), critical for regulation of neonatal respiration (Viemari, 2008), and dysregulated in SIDS (Leiter & Bohm, 2007). For example, prenatal nicotine exposure decreases the baseline activity of noradrenergic neurons but sensitizes them to hypoxia-induced activation (Slotkin et al., 1995), resulting in excessive release of central norepinephrine, which inhibits the ventilatory response by activation of brainstem alpha-2-adrenergic receptors. At the same time, prenatal nicotine exposure diminishes hypoxia-induced release of norepinephrine from adrenal chromaffin cells (Buttigieg et al., 2008; Slotkin et al., 1995). Both processes can contribute to the increased incidence of SIDS in the offspring of mothers who smoked during pregnancy.

Hypertension is yet another consequence associated with *in utero* exposure to tobacco smoking in humans (Beratis, Panagoulias, & Varvarigou, 1996). Nonhuman animal studies suggest that this effect may be mediated by nicotine alone. Indeed, fetal and neonatal nicotine exposure in rats results in increased blood pressure during adulthood (Gao et al., 2008) linked to endothelial dysfunctions (Xiao, Huang, Lawrence, Yang, & Zhang, 2007), changes in renal structure and function (Mao et al., 2009), and/or changes in the composition and amount of perivascular adipose tissue impairing the contractile response of blood vessels (Gao et al., 2005).

Prenatal nicotine exposure also leads to stress-induced cardiac defects in the offspring, including increased myocardial infarct size and decreased postischemic recovery of the left ventricle function (Lawrence et al., 2008), and a higher incidence of arrhythmias in response to stress (Feng et al., 2010). Taken together, nonhuman animal studies demonstrate that developmental nicotine exposure may play a key role in cardiovascular defects following prenatal exposure to tobacco smoke in humans.

Metabolic Outcomes

There is a link between maternal tobacco smoking and subsequent obesity and type 2 diabetes in children even after adjustment for a wide range of confounding factors, including birth weight, socioeconomic status, and maternal diet (Cupul-Uicab, Skjaerven, Haug, Melve, et al., 2012; Cupul-Uicab, Skjaerven, Haug, Travlos, et al., 2012; Power & Jefferis, 2002; Syme et al., 2010; Wideroe, Vik, Jacobsen, & Bakketeig, 2003). In rats, maternal nicotine exposure during pregnancy and lactation results in increased body weight (Newman, Shytle, & Sanberg, 1999; Somm et al., 2008), altered perivascular adipose tissue composition and function (Gao et al., 2008), and impaired glucose homeostasis (Holloway et al., 2005), in the offspring. Rats treated perinatally with nicotine have significantly upregulated levels of proopiomelanocortin messenger RNA (mRNA) in the arcuate nucleus of the hypothalamus (Huang & Winzer-Serhan, 2007), a precursor for the anorexic peptide alpha-melanocortin-stimulating hormone and a regulator of appetite (Butler, 2006), suggesting nicotine-induced changes in hypothalamic mechanisms of satiety.

Nicotine exposure during pregnancy and lactation can also result in endocrine and metabolic changes in rats resembling disturbed glucose metabolism observed in type 2 diabetes in humans (Holloway et al., 2005). Type 2 diabetes results from a progressive reduction in the ability of the pancreas to produce sufficient insulin to maintain normal glucose homeostasis (Marchetti, Del Prato, Lupi, & Del Guerra, 2006), via a reduced number of insulin-secreting cells and/or abnormal insulin secretion from the beta cells, accompanied by a reduced sensitivity to insulin action (Butler et al., 2003). In rats, fetal and neonatal exposure to nicotine increases beta cell apoptosis and decreases pancreatic islet cell capacity, leading to glucose and insulin intolerance, hyperinsulinemia, and increased body weight during adulthood (Bruin et al., 2010; Bruin, Gerstein, Morrison, & Holloway, 2008; Somm et al., 2008). Even second-generation offspring of dams exposed to nicotine during pregnancy show elevated blood pressure, increased fasting serum insulin, and an enhanced insulin response to an oral glucose challenge (Holloway, Cuu, Morrison, Gerstein, & Tarnopolsky, 2007).

Respiratory Outcomes

Maternal smoking during pregnancy is associated with diminished lung function and increased risk of wheezing and asthma in children (Burke et al., 2012; Maritz & Harding, 2011), and exacerbated airflow limitations induced by smoking in chronic obstructive pulmonary disease (Upton, Smith, McConnachie, Hart, & Watt, 2004). In rodents, pre- and perinatal exposure to nicotine has a negative impact on lung development and post-natal lung function (Campos, Bravo, & Eugenin, 2009; Maritz, 2008). For example, nicotine impairs alveolarization in the lungs, decreases internal lung surface for gas exchange, accelerates aging of the lungs, and induces emphysema in rats exposed to nicotine perinatally (Maritz & Windvogel, 2003); however, these changes are transient and disappear by adulthood (Petre et al., 2011).

Fertility Outcomes

An association between prenatal exposure to tobacco smoke and decreased quality of semen in men and fecundity in women has been suggested by epidemiological studies (Hakonsen, Ernst, & Ramlau-Hansen, 2014). Nonhuman animal data suggest that nicotine exposure may be critical in the development of adverse reproductive effects in the offspring of women who smoked during pregnancy. Nicotine exposure during prenatal and neonatal development results in reduced fertility, dysregulation of ovarian steroidogenesis, altered follicle dynamics, increased ovarian cell apoptosis, and decreased ovarian angiogenesis in female offspring (Holloway, Kellenberger, & Petrik, 2006; Petrik et al., 2009). The results for male offspring are less profound, with some transient defects noted in the histopathology of testes in peripubertal, but not adult, animals (Lagunov et al., 2011), and with no functional aberrations during either developmental period. This is consistent with a study in dizygotic twins, which reported that *in utero* exposure to tobacco smoke reduced fecundity in the female, but not male, twin (Jensen et al., 2006).

LONG-TERM NEUROBEHAVIORAL EFFECTS OF PRENATAL EXPOSURE TO TOBACCO SMOKE AND NICOTINE

Human Studies

Children of mothers who smoked during pregnancy display more externalizing behaviors (eg, aggressive and overactive) (Orlebeke, Knol, & Verhulst, 1997, 1999); deficits in learning, memory, and sustained attention; increased impulsivity, as measured by performance on a response inhibition task and a continuous performance task; and lower scores on overall cognitive function (Cho, Frijters, Zhang, Miller, & Gruen, 2013; Fried & Watkinson, 2001; Jacobsen, Slotkin, Mencl, Frost, & Pugh, 2007; Kristjansson, Fried, & Watkinson, 1989; McCartney, Fried, & Watkinson, 1994), with increased risk for psychiatric disorders, including ADHD, conduct disorders, and substance abuse (Latimer et al., 2012; Linnet et al., 2003; Milberger, Biederman, Faraone, & Jones, 1998; Roberts et al., 2005; Weissman, Warner, Wickramaratne, & Kandel, 1999). Early changes in catecholaminergic signaling induced by prenatal exposure to nicotine might be responsible for some of those psychiatric aberrations (Thapar et al., 2003; Weissman et al., 1999) and for an increased risk of addiction, especially tobacco smoking, during adolescence (Buka, Shenassa, & Niaura, 2003; Porath & Fried, 2005). Interestingly, adolescent smokers whose mothers smoked cigarettes during pregnancy experience more severe memory deficits during nicotine withdrawal, which can make quitting more difficult for them (Jacobsen, Slotkin, Westerveld, Mencl, & Pugh, 2006). Vulnerability to externalizing psychopathology in children is increased even by maternal exposure to secondhand smoke (Gatzke-Kopp & Beauchaine, 2007).

Although there seems to be overwhelming evidence for a deleterious effect of *in utero* exposure to tobacco smoking on behavior and cognition later in life and on increased risk for childhood-onset psychiatric disorders, it is difficult to separate these effects from other confounding environmental and genetic factors (D'Onofrio et al., 2008; Thapar, Cooper, Eyre, & Langley, 2013; Thapar et al., 2009). Indeed, when data are corrected for confounding factors such as age of the mother, socioeconomic status, or mother's education and IQ, the relationship between prenatal exposure to tobacco smoking and cognitive performance in children is drastically reduced or disappears (Lambe, Hultman, Torrang, Maccabe, & Cnattingius, 2006; Lassen & Oei, 1998); however, some studies reported a significant relationship between tobacco smoking during pregnancy and cognitive problems in children even after correcting for those confounding factors (Naeye & Peters, 1984).

It has also been suggested that mothers who continue to smoke during pregnancy can try to self-medicate their own psychological and behavioral problems, which can have a heritable genetic base that can be transferred to their children (Breslau, Kilbey, & Andreski, 1991; Munafo, Heron, & Araya, 2008; Wakschlag et al., 2003). For example, it has been suggested that common genetic vulnerability factors may exist for both maternal tobacco smoking and offspring ADHD that may explain the increased rate of ADHD among children of smokers (Maher, Marazita, Ferrell, & Vanyukov, 2002; Munafo & Johnstone, 2008). Indeed, both hyperactivity-impulsivity and oppositional behaviors are significantly associated with polymorphisms of the dopamine transporter in the children of pregnant smokers (Kahn, Khoury, Nichols, & Lanphear, 2003; Neuman et al., 2007). Therefore, maternal smoking during pregnancy might be an independent risk factor for ADHD that can also increase the risk of developing ADHD in those with a genetic predisposition. Similarly, reduced academic achievement and impaired intellectual abilities in children whose mothers smoked during pregnancy can be partially explained, as mentioned above, by maternal age, education, intelligence, or socioeconomic status (Lambe et al., 2006; Naeye & Peters, 1984), which can affect the home environment and parenting style. Nonetheless, quitting smoking during pregnancy proves beneficial for perceptual performance as well as quantitative and verbal skills in young children (Sexton, Fox, & Hebel, 1990).

The long-term significance of lower birth weight, yet another detrimental effect of prenatal exposure to tobacco smoke and nicotine (Eskenazi et al., 1995), on neurobehavioral aberrations is still unclear; however, studies in humans have found associations between low birth weight and long-term cognitive deficits (Gianni et al., 2007; Hack, 2006; Taylor, Klein, Drotar, Schluchter, & Hack, 2006) and behavioral disorders, including ADHD (Hayes & Sharif, 2009). Therefore, lower birth weight in children whose mothers smoked during pregnancy might be a risk factor for a number of neurobehavioral and cognitive aberrations, but tobacco smoke and nicotine exposure trigger the process. Importantly, the direct impact of prenatal nicotine exposure on birth weight remains significant after controlling for maternal genetic influences (Thapar et al., 2009). The relative impact of genetic and environmental factors on the neurobehavioral and cognitive aberrations in children prenatally exposed to tobacco smoke and nicotine can be disentangled in nonhuman animal models.

Preclinical Studies

The long-term consequences of fetal and neonatal exposure to nicotine on the central nervous system have been extensively studied in numerous nonhuman animal models (reviewed in Dwyer, McQuown, & Leslie, 2009; Pauly & Slotkin, 2008; Winzer-Serhan, 2008). Prenatal nicotine exposure in rodents leads to persistent alterations in cholinergic (Gold, Keller, & Perry, 2009) and catecholaminergic neurotransmitter systems (Oliff & Gallardo, 1999), with serious negative behavioral consequences. For example, chronic prenatal exposure to nicotine in rats leads to increased high-affinity nicotine binding in fetal and neonatal brains (Navarro, Seidler, Eylers, et al., 1989; Tizabi & Perry, 2000; Tizabi, Russell, Nespor, Perry, & Grunberg, 2000), which disappears or changes, in some regions, into a decreased high-affinity binding by adolescence (Chen, Parker, Matta, & Sharp, 2005). Prenatal nicotine exposure also elevates brain levels of dopamine, norepinephrine, and their metabolites during the late prenatal and early postnatal periods (Onal et al., 2004; Ribary & Lichtensteiger, 1989). Although those levels return to baseline by adulthood (Ribary & Lichtensteiger, 1989), changes in cholinergic regulation of catecholamine signaling at the synaptic level persist throughout all developmental stages, leading to, for example, decreased nicotine-induced dopamine release in the nucleus accumbens in adolescent rats (Kane, Fu, Matta, & Sharp, 2004). This might have important implications as the monoamine systems regulate the neural circuitries underlying motivation, attention, cognition, and mood (Brennan & Arnsten, 2008; Lammel, Lim, & Malenka, 2014; Nestler & Carlezon, 2006). Nicotine-induced alterations in these circuits may not manifest until their full maturation during adolescence, which clearly emerges as a key period for increased behavioral problems and initiation of substance abuse (Paus, Keshavan, & Giedd, 2008), and for the onset of anxiety disorders, bipolar disorder, depression, eating disorders, psychosis, and substance abuse (Rutherford, Mayes, & Potenza, 2010; Wermter et al., 2010) in humans.

Prenatal exposure to nicotine seems to trigger similar behavioral aberrations in rodents as compared to humans. For example, gestational nicotine exposure leads to hyperactivity in both rats and mice (Pauly, Sparks, Hauser, & Pauly, 2004; Paz, Barsness, Martenson, Tanner, & Allan, 2007; Tizabi, Popke, Rahman, Nespor, & Grunberg, 1997; Tizabi et al., 2000; Vaglenova, Birru, Pandiella, & Breese, 2004); however, these findings are not entirely consistent since some studies found either no difference in locomotor activity in adult rats (Schneider et al., 2011) or hypoactivity in preweaning animals prenatally exposed to nicotine, which was most likely stress related and disappeared after continued exposure to the testing environment (LeSage, Gustaf, Dufek, & Pentel, 2006). Rats prenatally exposed to nicotine show also enhanced locomotor responses to a nicotine challenge on postnatal day 14 (males only) (Shacka, Fennell, & Robinson, 1997) and increased cocaine-induced locomotor sensitization (Franke, Belluzzi, & Leslie, 2007), which corresponds to certain aspects of drug addiction (Steketee & Kalivas, 2011); decreased cocaine-induced stereotypy in adolescence; less initial motivation for a food reward, but increased motivation for and total intake of cocaine (Franke, Park, Belluzzi, & Leslie, 2008; Paz et al., 2007); increased nicotine self-administration in adolescent female rats following a withdrawal period (Levin et al., 2006); and increased consumption of nicotine in a free-choice two-bottle test in adolescent males (Schneider, Bizarro, Asherson, & Stolerman, 2012). Interestingly, prenatal nicotine exposure in rats enhanced dopamine receptor D5 (DRD5) mRNA expression in the striatum (Schneider et al., 2011), and changes in DRD5 have been linked to ADHD (Johansson et al., 2008; Li, Sham, Owen, & He, 2006) and to lower performance scores on the Test of Variables of Attention continuous performance test in ADHD patients and their parents (Manor et al., 2004).

Prenatal exposure to nicotine also leads to increased anxiety in rodents (Sobrian, Marr, & Ressman, 2003; Vaglenova et al., 2004), somatosensory deficits (Abou-Donia et al., 2006), several cognitive impairments, including attention and memory deficits (Levin, Briggs, Christopher, & Rose, 1993; Levin, Wilkerson, Jones, Christopher, & Briggs, 1996; Schneider et al., 2012, 2011; Sorenson, Raskin, & Suh, 1991), and impairments in the acquisition and retention of avoidance behavior (Genedani, Bernardi, & Bertolini, 1983; Vaglenova et al., 2008). However, these findings are again not entirely consistent since some studies found decreased anxiety, although that was linked to increased risk-taking or novelty-seeking behavior (Schneider et al., 2012), and no decrement in avoidance behavior or spatial learning in rodents prenatally exposed to nicotine (Bertolini, Bernardi, & Genedani, 1982; Levin et al., 1993, 1996; Paulson et al., 1994). Potential interference between increased anxiety in novel environments and cognitive performance in rodents prenatally exposed to nicotine requires further studies, especially since many of the cognitive aberrations in nicotine-exposed animals are limited to the early acquisition phase of learning and memory tests (Levin et al., 1993, 1996). Some of the reported neurobehavioral outcomes of prenatal exposure to nicotine are gender specific, with overall greater impact in males (Pauly et al., 2004; Peters & Tang, 1982; Vaglenova et al., 2008).

Prenatal nicotine exposure is also related to developmental delays and maturational deficits in rodents (Ajarem & Ahmad, 1998; Bertolini et al., 1982; Schneider, Bizarro, Asherson, & Stolerman, 2010; Vaglenova et al., 2008), providing compelling evidence that nicotine can be the single most important factor triggering the negative effects of tobacco smoking on neurodevelopment.

Despite some disparities in the cognitive and locomotor test results described above, impairments in attention, memory, and learning reported in rodents exposed to nicotine *in utero* are consistent with the cognitive deficits found in psychiatric disorders such as ADHD. Our own data from rats prenatally exposed to nicotine support epidemiological studies showing increased levels of ADHD-related behaviors among those whose mothers smoked during pregnancy (Milberger et al., 1998; Thapar et al., 2003; Weissman et al., 1999). Our results also stress the importance of a developmental stage of animals during testing and of using measures of cognitive dimensions that can be more directly linked to comparable aspects of cognitive performance, attentional problems, and impulsivity observed in human studies. The Five Choice Serial Reaction Time Test (5-CSRTT), in which reaction time, response accuracy, omission errors, and anticipatory responses are thought to reflect processes related to attention and impulsivity in human studies using continuous performance tests (Winstanley, Eagle, & Robbins, 2006), might be a good example of such a test. In our model, rats prenatally exposed to nicotine show both increased inattentiveness and impulsivity in the 5-CSRTT in adulthood (Schneider et al., 2011), but only increased impulsivity in adolescence (Schneider et al., 2012), which suggests a developmental change in the expression of cognitive aberrations in rats prenatally exposed to nicotine and resembles human data showing significant increase in anticipatory responses (ie, impulsivity) in children with ADHD (Bedard et al., 2003; Wada, Yamashita, Matsuishi, Ohtani, & Kato, 2000) and in adolescents whose mothers smoked during pregnancy, but not attentional problems in vigilance tests (Fried & Watkinson, 2001; Kristjansson et al., 1989). Similarly, we found an increased consumption of nicotine in adolescent, but not adult, rats prenatally exposed to nicotine (Schneider et al., 2012), which again stresses the importance of developmental aspects in the effects of prenatal exposure to nicotine. Interestingly, we found no difference in a standard locomotor activity test either in adolescent or adult rats in our model (Schneider et al., 2012, 2011), but when we modified the procedure and exposed adolescent rats to the same environment over 9 consecutive days, a clear hyperactivity was seen in rats prenatally exposed to nicotine (Schneider et al., 2012). This is in line with human data showing that overactivity in ADHD is more pronounced under constant (habituated) and unstimulating conditions and that it normalizes in novel or stimulating environments (Antrop, Roeyers, Van Oost, & Buysse, 2000; Sagvolden, Aase, Zeiner, & Berger, 1998). Therefore, preclinical studies in rodents prenatally exposed to nicotine challenge suggestions that the observed association between ADHD and maternal smoking in pregnancy is mediated entirely by genetic effects (D'Onofrio et al., 2008; Thapar et al., 2009).

CONCLUSIONS

There is clear evidence from both human epidemiological studies and preclinical models that exposure to tobacco smoke in utero is harmful for the fetus and leads to a wide variety of negative reproductive, somatic, and neurobehavioral effects in the offspring. Nonhuman animal studies confirmed that nicotine alone may be a key chemical responsible for many of the long-term effects in the offspring of mothers that smoked during pregnancy, including type 2 diabetes, obesity, hypertension, impaired fertility, cardiorespiratory dysfunctions, as well as neurobehavioral aberrations like ADHD, conduct disorder, and substance abuse.

References

Abou-Donia, M. B., Khan, W. A., Dechkovskaia, A. M., Goldstein, L. B., Bullman, S. L., & Abdel-Rahman, A. (2006). In utero exposure to nicotine and chlorpyrifos alone, and in combination produces persistent sensorimotor deficits and Purkinje neuron loss in the cerebellum of adult offspring rats. *Archives of Toxicology, 80,* 620–631.

Abreu-Villaca, Y., Filgueiras, C. C., & Manhaes, A. C. (2011). Developmental aspects of the cholinergic system. *Behavioural Brain Research, 221,* 367–378.

Ajarem, J. S., & Ahmad, M. (1998). Prenatal nicotine exposure modifies behavior of mice through early development. *Pharmacology, Biochemistry, and Behavior, 59,* 313–318.

Al-Sayed, E. M., & Ibrahim, K. S. (2014). Second-hand tobacco smoke and children. *Toxicology and Industrial Health, 30,* 635–644.

Antrop, I., Roeyers, H., Van Oost, P., & Buysse, A. (2000). Stimulation seeking and hyperactivity in children with ADHD. Attention deficit hyperactivity disorder. *Journal of Child Psychology and Psychiatry, and Allied Disciplines, 41,* 225–231.

Ashford, K. B., Hahn, E., Hall, L., Rayens, M. K., & Noland, M. (2009). Postpartum smoking relapse and secondhand smoke. *Public Health Reports, 124,* 515–526.

Azam, L., Chen, Y., & Leslie, F. M. (2007). Developmental regulation of nicotinic acetylcholine receptors within midbrain dopamine neurons. *Neuroscience, 144,* 1347–1360.

Bedard, A. C., Ickowicz, A., Logan, G. D., Hogg-Johnson, S., Schachar, R., & Tannock, R. (2003). Selective inhibition in children with attention-deficit hyperactivity disorder off and on stimulant medication. *Journal of Abnormal Child Psychology, 31,* 315–327.

Beratis, N. G., Panagoulias, D., & Varvarigou, A. (1996). Increased blood pressure in neonates and infants whose mothers smoked during pregnancy. *The Journal of Pediatrics, 128,* 806–812.

Bertolini, A., Bernardi, M., & Genedani, S. (1982). Effects of prenatal exposure to cigarette smoke and nicotine on pregnancy, offspring development and avoidance behavior in rats. *Neurobehavioral Toxicology and Teratology, 4,* 545–548.

Blatt, K., Moore, E., Chen, A., Van Hook, J., & DeFranco, E. A. (2015). Association of reported trimester-specific smoking cessation with fetal growth restriction. *Obstetrics and Gynecology, 125,* 1452–1459.

Brennan, A. R., & Arnsten, A. F. (2008). Neuronal mechanisms underlying attention deficit hyperactivity disorder: the influence of arousal on prefrontal cortical function. *Annals of the New York Academy of Sciences, 1129,* 236–245.

Breslau, N., Kilbey, M., & Andreski, P. (1991). Nicotine dependence, major depression, and anxiety in young adults. *Archives of General Psychiatry, 48,* 1069–1074.

Bruin, J. E., Gerstein, H. C., & Holloway, A. C. (2010). Long-term consequences of fetal and neonatal nicotine exposure: a critical review. *Toxicological Sciences: An Official Journal of the Society of Toxicology, 116,* 364–374.

Bruin, J. E., Gerstein, H. C., Morrison, K. M., & Holloway, A. C. (2008). Increased pancreatic beta-cell apoptosis following fetal and neonatal exposure to nicotine is mediated via the mitochondria. *Toxicological Sciences: An Official Journal of the Society of Toxicology, 103*, 362–370.

Buchhalter, A. R., Fant, R. V., & Henningfield, J. E. (2008). Novel pharmacological approaches for treating tobacco dependence and withdrawal: current status. *Drugs, 68*, 1067–1088.

Buka, S. L., Shenassa, E. D., & Niaura, R. (2003). Elevated risk of tobacco dependence among offspring of mothers who smoked during pregnancy: a 30-year prospective study. *The American Journal of Psychiatry, 160*, 1978–1984.

Burke, H., Leonardi-Bee, J., Hashim, A., Pine-Abata, H., Chen, Y., Cook, D. G., et al. (2012). Prenatal and passive smoke exposure and incidence of asthma and wheeze: systematic review and meta-analysis. *Pediatrics, 129*, 735–744.

Butler, A. A. (2006). The melanocortin system and energy balance. *Peptides, 27*, 281–290.

Butler, A. E., Janson, J., Bonner-Weir, S., Ritzel, R., Rizza, R. A., & Butler, P. C. (2003). Beta-cell deficit and increased beta-cell apoptosis in humans with type 2 diabetes. *Diabetes, 52*, 102–110.

Buttigieg, J., Brown, S., Zhang, M., Lowe, M., Holloway, A. C., & Nurse, C. A. (2008). Chronic nicotine in utero selectively suppresses hypoxic sensitivity in neonatal rat adrenal chromaffin cells. *FASEB Journal: Official Publication of the Federation of American Societies for Experimental Biology, 22*, 1317–1326.

Campos, M., Bravo, E., & Eugenin, J. (2009). Respiratory dysfunctions induced by prenatal nicotine exposure. *Clinical and Experimental Pharmacology and Physiology, 36*, 1205–1217.

Chen, H., Parker, S. L., Matta, S. G., & Sharp, B. M. (2005). Gestational nicotine exposure reduces nicotinic cholinergic receptor (nAChR) expression in dopaminergic brain regions of adolescent rats. *The European Journal of Neuroscience, 22*, 380–388.

Cho, K., Frijters, J. C., Zhang, H., Miller, L. L., & Gruen, J. R. (2013). Prenatal exposure to nicotine and impaired reading performance. *The Journal of Pediatrics, 162*, 713–718 e712.

Cnattingius, S. (2004). The epidemiology of smoking during pregnancy: smoking prevalence, maternal characteristics, and pregnancy outcomes. *Nicotine and Tobacco Research: Official Journal of the Society for Research on Nicotine and Tobacco, 6*(Suppl. 2), S125–S140.

Cupul-Uicab, L. A., Skjaerven, R., Haug, K., Melve, K. K., Engel, S. M., & Longnecker, M. P. (2012a). In utero exposure to maternal tobacco smoke and subsequent obesity, hypertension, and gestational diabetes among women in the MoBa cohort. *Environmental Health Perspectives, 120*, 355–360.

Cupul-Uicab, L. A., Skjaerven, R., Haug, K., Travlos, G. S., Wilson, R. E., Eggesbo, M., et al. (2012b). Exposure to tobacco smoke in utero and subsequent plasma lipids, ApoB, and CRP among adult women in the MoBa cohort. *Environmental Health Perspectives, 120*, 1532–1537.

DiFranza, J. R., Aligne, C. A., & Weitzman, M. (2004). Prenatal and postnatal environmental tobacco smoke exposure and children's health. *Pediatrics, 113*, 1007–1015.

D'Onofrio, B. M., Van Hulle, C. A., Waldman, I. D., Rodgers, J. L., Harden, K. P., Rathouz, P. J., et al. (2008). Smoking during pregnancy and offspring externalizing problems: an exploration of genetic and environmental confounds. *Development and Psychopathology, 20*, 139–164.

Dwyer, J. B., McQuown, S. C., & Leslie, F. M. (2009). The dynamic effects of nicotine on the developing brain. *Pharmacology and Therapeutics, 122*, 125–139.

Eskenazi, B., Prehn, A. W., & Christianson, R. E. (1995). Passive and active maternal smoking as measured by serum cotinine: the effect on birthweight. *American Journal of Public Health, 85*, 395–398.

Evans, C., Wang, J., Neff, R., & Mendelowitz, D. (2005). Hypoxia recruits a respiratory-related excitatory pathway to brainstem premotor cardiac vagal neurons in animals exposed to prenatal nicotine. *Neuroscience, 133*, 1073–1079.

Exley, R., Clements, M. A., Hartung, H., McIntosh, J. M., & Cragg, S. J. (2008). Alpha6-containing nicotinic acetylcholine receptors dominate the nicotine control of dopamine neurotransmission in nucleus accumbens. *Neuropsychopharmacology: Official Publication of the American College of Neuropsychopharmacology, 33*, 2158–2166.

Falk, L., Nordberg, A., Seiger, A., Kjaeldgaard, A., & Hellstrom-Lindahl, E. (2005). Smoking during early pregnancy affects the expression pattern of both nicotinic and muscarinic acetylcholine receptors in human first trimester brainstem and cerebellum. *Neuroscience, 132*, 389–397.

Feller, M. B. (2002). The role of nAChR-mediated spontaneous retinal activity in visual system development. *Journal of Neurobiology, 53*, 556–567.

Feng, Y., Caiping, M., Li, C., Can, R., Feichao, X., Li, Z., et al. (2010). Fetal and offspring arrhythmia following exposure to nicotine during pregnancy. *Journal of Applied Toxicology: JAT, 30*, 53–58.

Fewell, J. E., Smith, F. G., & Ng, V. K. (2001). Prenatal exposure to nicotine impairs protective responses of rat pups to hypoxia in an age-dependent manner. *Respiratory Physiology, 127*, 61–73.

Fleming, P., & Blair, P. S. (2007). Sudden infant death syndrome and parental smoking. *Early Human Development, 83*, 721–725.

Franke, R. M., Belluzzi, J. D., & Leslie, F. M. (2007). Gestational exposure to nicotine and monoamine oxidase inhibitors influences cocaine-induced locomotion in adolescent rats. *Psychopharmacology, 195*, 117–124.

Franke, R. M., Park, M., Belluzzi, J. D., & Leslie, F. M. (2008). Prenatal nicotine exposure changes natural and drug-induced reinforcement in adolescent male rats. *The European Journal of Neuroscience, 27*, 2952–2961.

Fried, P. A., & Watkinson, B. (2001). Differential effects on facets of attention in adolescents prenatally exposed to cigarettes and marihuana. *Neurotoxicology and Teratology, 23*, 421–430.

Gao, Y. J., Holloway, A. C., Su, L. Y., Takemori, K., Lu, C., & Lee, R. M. (2008). Effects of fetal and neonatal exposure to nicotine on blood pressure and perivascular adipose tissue function in adult life. *European Journal of Pharmacology, 590*, 264–268.

Gao, Y. J., Holloway, A. C., Zeng, Z. H., Lim, G. E., Petrik, J. J., Foster, W. G., et al. (2005). Prenatal exposure to nicotine causes postnatal obesity and altered perivascular adipose tissue function. *Obesity Research, 13*, 687–692.

Gatzke-Kopp, L. M., & Beauchaine, T. P. (2007). Direct and passive prenatal nicotine exposure and the development of externalizing psychopathology. *Child Psychiatry and Human Development, 38*, 255–269.

Genedani, S., Bernardi, M., & Bertolini, A. (1983). Sex-linked differences in avoidance learning in the offspring of rats treated with nicotine during pregnancy. *Psychopharmacology, 80*, 93–95.

George, L., Granath, F., Johansson, A. L., Anneren, G., & Cnattingius, S. (2006). Environmental tobacco smoke and risk of spontaneous abortion. *Epidemiology, 17*, 500–505.

Gianni, M. L., Picciolini, O., Vegni, C., Gardon, L., Fumagalli, M., & Mosca, F. (2007). Twelve-month neurofunctional assessment and cognitive performance at 36 months of age in extremely low birth weight infants. *Pediatrics, 120*, 1012–1019.

Gold, A. B., Keller, A. B., & Perry, D. C. (2009). Prenatal exposure of rats to nicotine causes persistent alterations of nicotinic cholinergic receptors. *Brain Research, 1250*, 88–100.

Goldschmidt, L., Cornelius, M. D., & Day, N. L. (2012). Prenatal cigarette smoke exposure and early initiation of multiple substance use. *Nicotine and Tobacco Research: Official Journal of the Society for Research on Nicotine and Tobacco, 14*, 694–702.

Hack, M. (2006). Young adult outcomes of very-low-birth-weight children. *Seminars in Fetal and Neonatal Medicine, 11*, 127–137.

Hakonsen, L. B., Ernst, A., & Ramlau-Hansen, C. H. (2014). Maternal cigarette smoking during pregnancy and reproductive health in children: a review of epidemiological studies. *Asian Journal of Andrology, 16*, 39–49.

Harmer, C., & Memon, A. (2013). Factors associated with smoking relapse in the postpartum period: an analysis of the child health surveillance system data in Southeast England. *Nicotine and Tobacco Research: Official Journal of the Society for Research on Nicotine and Tobacco, 15*, 904–909.

Hayes, B., & Sharif, F. (2009). Behavioural and emotional outcome of very low birth weight infants–literature review. *The Journal of Maternal-fetal and Neonatal Medicine: the Official Journal of the European Association of Perinatal Medicine, the Federation of Asia and Oceania Perinatal Societies, the International Society of Perinatal Obstetricians, 22*, 849–856.

Holloway, A. C., Cuu, D. Q., Morrison, K. M., Gerstein, H. C., & Tarnopolsky, M. A. (2007). Transgenerational effects of fetal and neonatal exposure to nicotine. *Endocrine, 31*, 254–259.

Holloway, A. C., Kellenberger, L. D., & Petrik, J. J. (2006). Fetal and neonatal exposure to nicotine disrupts ovarian function and fertility in adult female rats. *Endocrine, 30*, 213–216.

Holloway, A. C., Lim, G. E., Petrik, J. J., Foster, W. G., Morrison, K. M., & Gerstein, H. C. (2005). Fetal and neonatal exposure to nicotine in Wistar rats results in increased beta cell apoptosis at birth and postnatal endocrine and metabolic changes associated with type 2 diabetes. *Diabetologia, 48*, 2661–2666.

Huang, L. Z., & Winzer-Serhan, U. H. (2007). Nicotine regulates mRNA expression of feeding peptides in the arcuate nucleus in neonatal rat pups. *Developmental Neurobiology, 67*, 363–377.

Huang, Y. H., Brown, A. R., Costy-Bennett, S., Luo, Z., & Fregosi, R. F. (2004). Influence of prenatal nicotine exposure on postnatal development of breathing pattern. *Respiratory Physiology and Neurobiology, 143*, 1–8.

Huang, Z. G., Griffioen, K. J., Wang, X., Dergacheva, O., Kamendi, H., Gorini, C., et al. (2007). Nicotinic receptor activation occludes purinergic control of central cardiorespiratory network responses to hypoxia/hypercapnia. *Journal of Neurophysiology, 98*, 2429–2438.

Ion, R., & Bernal, A. L. (2015). Smoking and preterm birth. *Reproductive Sciences, 22*(8), 918–926.

Jacobsen, L. K., Slotkin, T. A., Mencl, W. E., Frost, S. J., & Pugh, K. R. (2007). Gender-specific effects of prenatal and adolescent exposure to tobacco smoke on auditory and visual attention. *Neuropsychopharmacology: Official Publication of the American College of Neuropsychopharmacology, 32*, 2453–2464.

Jacobsen, L. K., Slotkin, T. A., Westerveld, M., Mencl, W. E., & Pugh, K. R. (2006). Visuospatial memory deficits emerging during nicotine withdrawal in adolescents with prenatal exposure to active maternal smoking. *Neuropsychopharmacology: Official Publication of the American College of Neuropsychopharmacology, 31*, 1550–1561.

Jensen, T. K., Joffe, M., Scheike, T., Skytthe, A., Gaist, D., Petersen, I., et al. (2006). Early exposure to smoking and future fecundity among Danish twins. *International Journal of Andrology, 29*, 603–613.

Johansson, S., Halleland, H., Halmoy, A., Jacobsen, K. K., Landaas, E. T., Dramsdahl, M., et al. (2008). Genetic analyses of dopamine related genes in adult ADHD patients suggest an association with the DRD5-microsatellite repeat, but not with DRD4 or SLC6A3 VNTRs. *American Journal of Medical Genetics Part B: Neuropsychiatric Genetics, 147B*, 1470–1475.

Kahn, R. S., Khoury, J., Nichols, W. C., & Lanphear, B. P. (2003). Role of dopamine transporter genotype and maternal prenatal smoking in childhood hyperactive-impulsive, inattentive, and oppositional behaviors. *The Journal of Pediatrics, 143*, 104–110.

Kamendi, H., Stephens, C., Dergacheva, O., Wang, X., Huang, Z. G., Bouairi, E., et al. (2006). Prenatal nicotine exposure alters the nicotinic receptor subtypes that modulate excitation of parasympathetic cardiac neurons in the nucleus ambiguus from primarily alpha3beta2 and/or alpha6betaX to alpha3beta4. *Neuropharmacology, 51*, 60–66.

Kane, V. B., Fu, Y., Matta, S. G., & Sharp, B. M. (2004). Gestational nicotine exposure attenuates nicotine-stimulated dopamine release in the nucleus accumbens shell of adolescent Lewis rats. *The Journal of Pharmacology and Experimental Therapeutics, 308*, 521–528.

Kristjansson, E. A., Fried, P. A., & Watkinson, B. (1989). Maternal smoking during pregnancy affects children's vigilance performance. *Drug and Alcohol Dependence, 24*, 11–19.

Lagunov, A., Anzar, M., Sadeu, J. C., Khan, M. I., Bruin, J. E., Woynillowicz, A. K., et al. (2011). Effect of in utero and lactational nicotine exposure on the male reproductive tract in peripubertal and adult rats. *Reproductive Toxicology, 31*, 418–423.

Lambe, M., Hultman, C., Torrang, A., Maccabe, J., & Cnattingius, S. (2006). Maternal smoking during pregnancy and school performance at age 15. *Epidemiology, 17*, 524–530.

Lambers, D. S., & Clark, K. E. (1996). The maternal and fetal physiologic effects of nicotine. *Seminars in Perinatology, 20*, 115–126.

Lammel, S., Lim, B. K., & Malenka, R. C. (2014). Reward and aversion in a heterogeneous midbrain dopamine system. *Neuropharmacology, 76*(Pt B), 351–359.

Lassen, K., & Oei, T. P. (1998). Effects of maternal cigarette smoking during pregnancy on long-term physical and cognitive parameters of child development. *Addictive Behaviors, 23*, 635–653.

Latimer, K., Wilson, P., Kemp, J., Thompson, L., Sim, F., Gillberg, C., et al. (2012). Disruptive behaviour disorders: a systematic review of environmental antenatal and early years risk factors. *Child: Care, Health and Development, 38*, 611–628.

Lawrence, J., Xiao, D., Xue, Q., Rejali, M., Yang, S., & Zhang, L. (2008). Prenatal nicotine exposure increases heart susceptibility to ischemia/reperfusion injury in adult offspring. *The Journal of Pharmacology and Experimental Therapeutics, 324*, 331–341.

Leiter, J. C., & Bohm, I. (2007). Mechanisms of pathogenesis in the sudden infant death syndrome. *Respiratory Physiology and Neurobiology, 159*, 127–138.

LeSage, M. G., Gustaf, E., Dufek, M. B., & Pentel, P. R. (2006). Effects of maternal intravenous nicotine administration on locomotor behavior in pre-weanling rats. *Pharmacology, Biochemistry, and Behavior, 85*, 575–583.

Levin, E. D., Briggs, S. J., Christopher, N. C., & Rose, J. E. (1993). Prenatal nicotine exposure and cognitive performance in rats. *Neurotoxicology and Teratology, 15*, 251–260.

Levin, E. D., Wilkerson, A., Jones, J. P., Christopher, N. C., & Briggs, S. J. (1996). Prenatal nicotine effects on memory in rats: pharmacological and behavioral challenges. *Brain Research. Developmental Brain Research, 97*, 207–215.

Levin, E. D., Lawrence, S., Petro, A., Horton, K., Seidler, F. J., & Slotkin, T. A. (2006). Increased nicotine self-administration following prenatal exposure in female rats. *Pharmacology, Biochemistry, and Behavior, 85*, 669–674.

Li, D., Sham, P. C., Owen, M. J., & He, L. (2006). Meta-analysis shows significant association between dopamine system genes and attention deficit hyperactivity disorder (ADHD). *Human Molecular Genetics, 15*, 2276–2284.

Lindblad, F., & Hjern, A. (2010). ADHD after fetal exposure to maternal smoking. *Nicotine & Tobacco Research: Official Journal of the Society for Research on Nicotine and Tobacco, 12*, 408–415.

Lindley, A. A., Becker, S., Gray, R. H., & Herman, A. A. (2000). Effect of continuing or stopping smoking during pregnancy on infant birth weight, crown-heel length, head circumference, ponderal index, and brain:body weight ratio. *American Journal of Epidemiology, 152*, 219–225.

Linnet, K. M., Dalsgaard, S., Obel, C., Wisborg, K., Henriksen, T. B., Rodriguez, A., et al. (2003). Maternal lifestyle factors in pregnancy risk of attention deficit hyperactivity disorder and associated behaviors: review of the current evidence. *The American Journal of Psychiatry, 160*, 1028–1040.

Maher, B. S., Marazita, M. L., Ferrell, R. E., & Vanyukov, M. M. (2002). Dopamine system genes and attention deficit hyperactivity disorder: a meta-analysis. *Psychiatric Genetics, 12*, 207–215.

Mannino, D. M., Moorman, J. E., Kingsley, B., Rose, D., & Repace, J. (2001). Health effects related to environmental tobacco smoke exposure in children in the United States: data from the Third National Health and Nutrition Examination Survey. *The Archives of Pediatrics and Adolescent Medicine, 155*, 36–41.

Manor, I., Corbex, M., Eisenberg, J., Gritsenkso, I., Bachner-Melman, R., Tyano, S., et al. (2004). Association of the dopamine D5 receptor with attention deficit hyperactivity disorder (ADHD) and scores on a continuous performance test (TOVA). *American Journal of Medical Genetics Part B: Neuropsychiatric Genetics, 127B,* 73–77.

Mao, C., Wu, J., Xiao, D., Lv, J., Ding, Y., Xu, Z., et al. (2009). The effect of fetal and neonatal nicotine exposure on renal development of AT(1) and AT(2) receptors. *Reproductive Toxicology, 27,* 149–154.

Marchetti, P., Del Prato, S., Lupi, R., & Del Guerra, S. (2006). The pancreatic beta-cell in human Type 2 diabetes. *Nutrition, Metabolism, and Cardiovascular Diseases: NMCD, 16*(Suppl. 1), S3–S6.

Maritz, G. S. (2008). Nicotine and lung development. *Birth Defects Research Part C, Embryo Today: Reviews, 84,* 45–53.

Maritz, G. S., & Harding, R. (2011). Life-long programming implications of exposure to tobacco smoking and nicotine before and soon after birth: evidence for altered lung development. *International Journal of Environmental Research and Public Health [Electronic Resource], 8,* 875–898.

Maritz, G. S., & Windvogel, S. (2003). Chronic maternal nicotine exposure during gestation and lactation and the development of the lung parenchyma in the offspring. Response to nicotine withdrawal. *Pathophysiology, 10,* 69–75.

McCartney, J. S., Fried, P. A., & Watkinson, B. (1994). Central auditory processing in school-age children prenatally exposed to cigarette smoke. *Neurotoxicology and Teratology, 16,* 269–276.

Milberger, S., Biederman, J., Faraone, S. V., & Jones, J. (1998). Further evidence of an association between maternal smoking during pregnancy and attention deficit hyperactivity disorder: findings from a high-risk sample of siblings. *Journal of Clinical Child and Adolescent Psychology, 27,* 352–358.

Munafo, M. R., Heron, J., & Araya, R. (2008). Smoking patterns during pregnancy and postnatal period and depressive symptoms. *Nicotine and Tobacco Research: Official Journal of the Society for Research on Nicotine and Tobacco, 10,* 1609–1620.

Munafo, M. R., & Johnstone, E. C. (2008). Smoking status moderates the association of the dopamine D4 receptor (DRD4) gene VNTR polymorphism with selective processing of smoking-related cues. *Addiction Biology, 13,* 435–439.

Murin, S., Rafii, R., & Bilello, K. (2011). Smoking and smoking cessation in pregnancy. *Clinics in Chest Medicine, 32,* 75–91 viii.

Myers, C. P., Lewcock, J. W., Hanson, M. G., Gosgnach, S., Aimone, J. B., Gage, F. H., et al. (2005). Cholinergic input is required during embryonic development to mediate proper assembly of spinal locomotor circuits. *Neuron, 46,* 37–49.

Naeye, R. L., & Peters, E. C. (1984). Mental development of children whose mothers smoked during pregnancy. *Obstetrics and Gynecology, 64,* 601–607.

Navarro, H. A., Seidler, F. J., Eylers, J. P., Baker, F. E., Dobbins, S. S., Lappi, S. E., et al. (1989a). Effects of prenatal nicotine exposure on development of central and peripheral cholinergic neurotransmitter systems. Evidence for cholinergic trophic influences in developing brain. *The Journal of Pharmacology and Experimental Therapeutics, 251,* 894–900.

Navarro, H. A., Seidler, F. J., Schwartz, R. D., Baker, F. E., Dobbins, S. S., & Slotkin, T. A. (1989b). Prenatal exposure to nicotine impairs nervous system development at a dose which does not affect viability or growth. *Brain Research Bulletin, 23,* 187–192.

Neff, R. A., Wang, J., Baxi, S., Evans, C., & Mendelowitz, D. (2003). Respiratory sinus arrhythmia: endogenous activation of nicotinic receptors mediates respiratory modulation of brainstem cardioinhibitory parasympathetic neurons. *Circulation Research, 93,* 565–572.

Nestler, E. J., & Carlezon, W. A., Jr. (2006). The mesolimbic dopamine reward circuit in depression. *Biological Psychiatry, 59,* 1151–1159.

Neuman, R. J., Lobos, E., Reich, W., Henderson, C. A., Sun, L. W., & Todd, R. D. (2007). Prenatal smoking exposure and dopaminergic genotypes interact to cause a severe ADHD subtype. *Biological Psychiatry, 61,* 1320–1328.

Newman, M. B., Shytle, R. D., & Sanberg, P. R. (1999). Locomotor behavioral effects of prenatal and postnatal nicotine exposure in rat offspring. *Behavioural Pharmacology, 10,* 699–706.

Ng, M., Freeman, M. K., Fleming, T. D., Robinson, M., Dwyer-Lindgren, L., Thomson, B., et al. (2014). Smoking prevalence and cigarette consumption in 187 countries, 1980–2012. *JAMA: the Journal of the American Medical Association, 311*, 183–192.

Nichter, M., Greaves, L., Bloch, M., Paglia, M., Scarinci, I., Tolosa, J. E., et al. (2010). Tobacco use and secondhand smoke exposure during pregnancy in low- and middle-income countries: the need for social and cultural research. *Acta Obstetricia et Gynecologica Scandinavica, 89*, 465–477.

Okuyemi, K. S., Ahluwalia, J. S., & Harris, K. J. (2000). Pharmacotherapy of smoking cessation. *Archives of Family Medicine, 9*, 270–281.

O'Leary, K. T., Loughlin, S. E., Chen, Y., & Leslie, F. M. (2008). Nicotinic acetylcholine receptor subunit mRNA expression in adult and developing rat medullary catecholamine neurons. *The Journal of Comparative Neurology, 510*, 655–672.

Oliff, H. S., & Gallardo, K. A. (1999). The effect of nicotine on developing brain catecholamine systems. *Frontiers in Bioscience, 4*, D883–D897.

Onal, A., Uysal, A., Ulker, S., Delen, Y., Yurtseven, M. E., & Evinc, A. (2004). Alterations of brain tissue in fetal rats exposed to nicotine in utero: possible involvement of nitric oxide and catecholamines. *Neurotoxicology and Teratology, 26*, 103–112.

Oncken, C., Dornelas, E., Greene, J., Sankey, H., Glasmann, A., Feinn, R., et al. (2008). Nicotine gum for pregnant smokers: a randomized controlled trial. *Obstetrics and Gynecology, 112*, 859–867.

Orlebeke, J. F., Knol, D. L., & Verhulst, F. C. (1997). Increase in child behavior problems resulting from maternal smoking during pregnancy. *Archives of Environmental Health, 52*, 317–321.

Orlebeke, J. F., Knol, D. L., & Verhulst, F. C. (1999). Child behavior problems increased by maternal smoking during pregnancy. *Archives of Environmental Health, 54*, 15–19.

Papke, R. L., & Heinemann, S. F. (1991). The role of the beta 4-subunit in determining the kinetic properties of rat neuronal nicotinic acetylcholine alpha 3-receptors. *Journal of Physiology, 440*, 95–112.

Park, E. R., Chang, Y., Quinn, V., Regan, S., Cohen, L., Viguera, A., et al. (2009). The association of depressive, anxiety, and stress symptoms and postpartum relapse to smoking: a longitudinal study. *Nicotine and Tobacco Research: Official Journal of the Society for Research on Nicotine and Tobacco, 11*, 707–714.

Paulson, R. B., Shanfeld, J., Vorhees, C. V., Cole, J., Sweazy, A., & Paulson, J. O. (1994). Behavioral effects of smokeless tobacco on the neonate and young Sprague Dawley rat. *Teratology, 49*, 293–305.

Pauly, J. R., & Slotkin, T. A. (2008). Maternal tobacco smoking, nicotine replacement and neurobehavioural development. *Acta Paediatrica, 97*, 1331–1337.

Pauly, J. R., Sparks, J. A., Hauser, K. F., & Pauly, T. H. (2004). In utero nicotine exposure causes persistent, gender-dependant changes in locomotor activity and sensitivity to nicotine in C57Bl/6 mice. *International Journal of Developmental Neuroscience: the Official Journal of the International Society for Developmental Neuroscience, 22*, 329–337.

Paus, T., Keshavan, M., & Giedd, J. N. (2008). Why do many psychiatric disorders emerge during adolescence? *Nature Reviews. Neuroscience, 9*, 947–957.

Paz, R., Barsness, B., Martenson, T., Tanner, D., & Allan, A. M. (2007). Behavioral teratogenicity induced by nonforced maternal nicotine consumption. *Neuropsychopharmacology: Official Publication of the American College of Neuropsychopharmacology, 32*, 693–699.

Peters, D. A., & Tang, S. (1982). Sex-dependent biological changes following prenatal nicotine exposure in the rat. *Pharmacology, Biochemistry, and Behavior, 17*, 1077–1082.

Petre, M. A., Petrik, J., Ellis, R., Inman, M. D., Holloway, A. C., & Labiris, N. R. (2011). Fetal and neonatal exposure to nicotine disrupts postnatal lung development in rats: role of VEGF and its receptors. *International Journal of Toxicology, 30*, 244–252.

Petrik, J. J., Gerstein, H. C., Cesta, C. E., Kellenberger, L. D., Alfaidy, N., & Holloway, A. C. (2009). Effects of rosiglitazone on ovarian function and fertility in animals with reduced fertility following fetal and neonatal exposure to nicotine. *Endocrine, 36*, 281–290.

Porath, A. J., & Fried, P. A. (2005). Effects of prenatal cigarette and marijuana exposure on drug use among offspring. *Neurotoxicology and Teratology, 27*, 267–277.

Power, C., & Jefferis, B. J. (2002). Fetal environment and subsequent obesity: a study of maternal smoking. *International Journal of Epidemiology, 31*, 413–419.

Prandota, J. (2004). Possible pathomechanisms of sudden infant death syndrome: key role of chronic hypoxia, infection/inflammation states, cytokine irregularities, and metabolic trauma in genetically predisposed infants. *American Journal of Therapeutics, 11*, 517–546.

Prusakowski, M. K., Shofer, F. S., Rhodes, K. V., & Mills, A. M. (2011). Effect of depression and psychosocial stressors on cessation self-efficacy in mothers who smoke. *Maternal and Child Health Journal, 15*, 620–626.

Rajs, J., Rasten-Almqvist, P., Falck, G., Eksborg, S., & Andersson, B. S. (1997). Sudden infant death syndrome: postmortem findings of nicotine and cotinine in pericardial fluid of infants in relation to morphological changes and position at death. *Pediatric Pathology and Laboratory Medicine, 17*, 83–97.

Ribary, U., & Lichtensteiger, W. (1989). Effects of acute and chronic prenatal nicotine treatment on central catecholamine systems of male and female rat fetuses and offspring. *The Journal of Pharmacology and Experimental Therapeutics, 248*, 786–792.

Roberts, K. H., Munafo, M. R., Rodriguez, D., Drury, M., Murphy, M. F., Neale, R. E., et al. (2005). Longitudinal analysis of the effect of prenatal nicotine exposure on subsequent smoking behavior of offspring. *Nicotine and Tobacco Research: Official Journal of the Society for Research on Nicotine and Tobacco, 7*, 801–808.

Rogers, J. M. (2008). Tobacco and pregnancy: overview of exposures and effects. *Birth Defects Research Part C, Embryo Today: Reviews, 84*, 1–15.

Rutherford, H. J., Mayes, L. C., & Potenza, M. N. (2010). Neurobiology of adolescent substance use disorders: implications for prevention and treatment. *Child and Adolescent Psychiatric Clinics of North America, 19*, 479–492.

Sagvolden, T., Aase, H., Zeiner, P., & Berger, D. (1998). Altered reinforcement mechanisms in attention-deficit/hyperactivity disorder. *Behavioural Brain Research, 94*, 61–71.

Salihu, H. M., Aliyu, M. H., & Kirby, R. S. (2005). In utero nicotine exposure and fetal growth inhibition among twins. *American Journal of Perinatology, 22*, 421–427.

Schneider, T., Bizarro, L., Asherson, P. J., & Stolerman, I. P. (2010). Gestational exposure to nicotine in drinking water: teratogenic effects and methodological issues. *Behavioural Pharmacology, 21*, 206–216.

Schneider, T., Bizarro, L., Asherson, P. J., & Stolerman, I. P. (2012). Hyperactivity, increased nicotine consumption and impaired performance in the five-choice serial reaction time task in adolescent rats prenatally exposed to nicotine. *Psychopharmacology, 223*, 401–415.

Schneider, T., Ilott, N., Brolese, G., Bizarro, L., Asherson, P. J., & Stolerman, I. P. (2011). Prenatal exposure to nicotine impairs performance of the 5-choice serial reaction time task in adult rats. *Neuropsychopharmacology: Official Publication of the American College of Neuropsychopharmacology, 36*, 1114–1125.

Schulte-Hobein, B., Schwartz-Bickenbach, D., Abt, S., Plum, C., & Nau, H. (1992). Cigarette smoke exposure and development of infants throughout the first year of life: influence of passive smoking and nursing on cotinine levels in breast milk and infant's urine. *Acta Paediatrica, 81*, 550–557.

Sexton, M., Fox, N. L., & Hebel, J. R. (1990). Prenatal exposure to tobacco: II. Effects on cognitive functioning at age three. *International Journal of Epidemiology, 19*, 72–77.

Shacka, J. J., Fennell, O. B., & Robinson, S. E. (1997). Prenatal nicotine sex-dependently alters agonist-induced locomotion and stereotypy. *Neurotoxicology and Teratology, 19*, 467–476.

Shingo, A. S., & Kito, S. (2005). Effects of nicotine on neurogenesis and plasticity of hippocampal neurons. *Journal of Neural Transmission, 112*, 1475–1478.

Slotkin, T. A. (2008). If nicotine is a developmental neurotoxicant in animal studies, dare we recommend nicotine replacement therapy in pregnant women and adolescents? *Neurotoxicology and Teratology, 30*, 1–19.

Slotkin, T. A., Cho, H., & Whitmore, W. L. (1987). Effects of prenatal nicotine exposure on neuronal development: selective actions on central and peripheral catecholaminergic pathways. *Brain Research Bulletin, 18*, 601–611.

Slotkin, T. A., Lappi, S. E., McCook, E. C., Lorber, B. A., & Seidler, F. J. (1995). Loss of neonatal hypoxia tolerance after prenatal nicotine exposure: implications for sudden infant death syndrome. *Brain Research Bulletin, 38*, 69–75.

Smedberg, J., Lupattelli, A., Mardby, A. C., & Nordeng, H. (2014). Characteristics of women who continue smoking during pregnancy: a cross-sectional study of pregnant women and new mothers in 15 European countries. *BMC Pregnancy and Childbirth, 14*, 213.

Sobrian, S. K., Marr, L., & Ressman, K. (2003). Prenatal cocaine and/or nicotine exposure produces depression and anxiety in aging rats. *Progress in Neuro-psychopharmacology and Biological Psychiatry, 27*, 501–518.

Somm, E., Schwitzgebel, V. M., Vauthay, D. M., Camm, E. J., Chen, C. Y., Giacobino, J. P., et al. (2008). Prenatal nicotine exposure alters early pancreatic islet and adipose tissue development with consequences on the control of body weight and glucose metabolism later in life. *Endocrinology, 149*, 6289–6299.

Sorenson, C. A., Raskin, L. A., & Suh, Y. (1991). The effects of prenatal nicotine on radial-arm maze performance in rats. *Pharmacology, Biochemistry, and Behavior, 40*, 991–993.

Steketee, J. D., & Kalivas, P. W. (2011). Drug wanting: behavioral sensitization and relapse to drug-seeking behavior. *Pharmacological Reviews, 63*, 348–365.

Swamy, G. K., Reddick, K. L., Brouwer, R. J., Pollak, K. I., & Myers, E. R. (2011). Smoking prevalence in early pregnancy: comparison of self-report and anonymous urine cotinine testing. *The Journal of Maternal-fetal and Neonatal Medicine: the Official Journal of the European Association of Perinatal Medicine, the Federation of Asia and Oceania Perinatal Societies, the International Society of Perinatal Obstetricians, 24*, 86–90.

Syme, C., Abrahamowicz, M., Mahboubi, A., Leonard, G. T., Perron, M., Richer, L., et al. (2010). Prenatal exposure to maternal cigarette smoking and accumulation of intra-abdominal fat during adolescence. *Obesity, 18*, 1021–1025.

Taylor, H. G., Klein, N., Drotar, D., Schluchter, M., & Hack, M. (2006). Consequences and risks of <1000-g birth weight for neuropsychological skills, achievement, and adaptive functioning. *Journal of Developmental and Behavioral Pediatrics: JDBP, 27*, 459–469.

Thapar, A., Cooper, M., Eyre, O., & Langley, K. (2013). What have we learnt about the causes of ADHD? *Journal of Child Psychology and Psychiatry, and Allied Disciplines, 54*, 3–16.

Thapar, A., Fowler, T., Rice, F., Scourfield, J., van den Bree, M., Thomas, H., et al. (2003). Maternal smoking during pregnancy and attention deficit hyperactivity disorder symptoms in offspring. *The American Journal of Psychiatry, 160*, 1985–1989.

Thapar, A., Rice, F., Hay, D., Boivin, J., Langley, K., van den Bree, M., et al. (2009). Prenatal smoking might not cause attention-deficit/hyperactivity disorder: evidence from a novel design. *Biological Psychiatry, 66*, 722–727.

Tizabi, Y., & Perry, D. C. (2000). Prenatal nicotine exposure is associated with an increase in [125I]epibatidine binding in discrete cortical regions in rats. *Pharmacology, Biochemistry, and Behavior, 67*, 319–323.

Tizabi, Y., Popke, E. J., Rahman, M. A., Nespor, S. M., & Grunberg, N. E. (1997). Hyperactivity induced by prenatal nicotine exposure is associated with an increase in cortical nicotinic receptors. *Pharmacology, Biochemistry, and Behavior, 58*, 141–146.

Tizabi, Y., Russell, L. T., Nespor, S. M., Perry, D. C., & Grunberg, N. E. (2000). Prenatal nicotine exposure: effects on locomotor activity and central [125I]alpha-BT binding in rats. *Pharmacology, Biochemistry, and Behavior, 66*, 495–500.

Tong, V. T., Dietz, P. M., Morrow, B., D'Angelo, D. V., Farr, S. L., Rockhill, K. M., et al. (2013). Trends in smoking before, during, and after pregnancy–pregnancy risk assessment monitoring system, United States, 40 sites, 2000–2010. *MMWR. Surveillance Summaries: Morbidity and Mortality Weekly Report. Surveillance Summaries/CDC, 62*, 1–19.

Upton, M. N., Smith, G. D., McConnachie, A., Hart, C. L., & Watt, G. C. (2004). Maternal and personal cigarette smoking synergize to increase airflow limitation in adults. *American Journal of Respiratory and Critical Care Medicine, 169*, 479–487.

Vaglenova, J., Birru, S., Pandiella, N. M., & Breese, C. R. (2004). An assessment of the long-term developmental and behavioral teratogenicity of prenatal nicotine exposure. *Behavioural Brain Research, 150*, 159–170.

Vaglenova, J., Parameshwaran, K., Suppiramaniam, V., Breese, C. R., Pandiella, N., & Birru, S. (2008). Long-lasting teratogenic effects of nicotine on cognition: gender specificity and role of AMPA receptor function. *Neurobiology of Learning and Memory, 90*, 527–536.

Van de Kamp, J. L., & Collins, A. C. (1994). Prenatal nicotine alters nicotinic receptor development in the mouse brain. *Pharmacology, Biochemistry, and Behavior, 47*, 889–900.

Viemari, J. C. (2008). Noradrenergic modulation of the respiratory neural network. *Respiratory Physiology and Neurobiology, 164*, 123–130.

Wada, N., Yamashita, Y., Matsuishi, T., Ohtani, Y., & Kato, H. (2000). The test of variables of attention (TOVA) is useful in the diagnosis of Japanese male children with attention deficit hyperactivity disorder. *Brain and Development, 22*, 378–382.

Wakschlag, L. S., Pickett, K. E., Middlecamp, M. K., Walton, L. L., Tenzer, P., & Leventhal, B. L. (2003). Pregnant smokers who quit, pregnant smokers who don't: does history of problem behavior make a difference? *Social Science and Medicine, 56*, 2449–2460.

Weissman, M. M., Warner, V., Wickramaratne, P. J., & Kandel, D. B. (1999). Maternal smoking during pregnancy and psychopathology in offspring followed to adulthood. *Journal of the American Academy of Child and Adolescent Psychiatry, 38*, 892–899.

Wermter, A. K., Laucht, M., Schimmelmann, B. G., Banaschewski, T., Sonuga-Barke, E. J., Rietschel, M., et al. (2010). From nature versus nurture, via nature and nurture, to gene x environment interaction in mental disorders. *European Child and Adolescent Psychiatry, 19*, 199–210.

Wideroe, M., Vik, T., Jacobsen, G., & Bakketeig, L. S. (2003). Does maternal smoking during pregnancy cause childhood overweight? *Paediatric and Perinatal Epidemiology, 17*, 171–179.

Winstanley, C. A., Eagle, D. M., & Robbins, T. W. (2006). Behavioral models of impulsivity in relation to ADHD: translation between clinical and preclinical studies. *Clinical Psychology Review, 26*, 379–395.

Winzer-Serhan, U. H. (2008). Long-term consequences of maternal smoking and developmental chronic nicotine exposure. *Frontiers in Bioscience, 13*, 636–649.

Xiao, D., Huang, X., Lawrence, J., Yang, S., & Zhang, L. (2007). Fetal and neonatal nicotine exposure differentially regulates vascular contractility in adult male and female offspring. *The Journal of Pharmacology and Experimental Therapeutics, 320*, 654–661.

Contribution of Translational Genetic Research to Our Understanding of Nicotine Dependence

F.S. Hall[1], Y. Arime[2], Y. Saber[1], I. Sora[3]

[1]University of Toledo, Toledo, OH, United States; [2]Dokkyo Medical University School of Medicine, Mibu, Japan; [3]Kobe University Graduate School of Medicine, Chuo-ku, Kobe, Japan

HUMAN GENETICS: WHAT SHOULD WE SEEK TO MODEL IN ANIMAL STUDIES?

Nicotine dependence liability has a substantial genetic component (Broms et al., 2006; Morley et al., 2007), much of which is associated with general drug dependence liability (Uhl, Drgon, Johnson, Li, et al., 2008), but a portion of which appears to be specific for nicotine dependence. The history of the genetic study of addiction has an initial pre-genomic phase and a post-genomic phase (Hall, Drgonova, Jain, & Uhl, 2013). In the pre-genomic phase, the genes considered to be important for studies of addiction were nominated solely based upon *a priori* neurobiological considerations, eg, the targets of drugs of abuse, neurotransmitter receptors, and transporters. In the case of nicotine dependence, this led to a focus on nicotinic receptor genes. This emphasis has persisted into the post-genomic era of addiction research despite substantial evidence from genome-wide association studies (GWAS) that a substantial portion of genes involved in addiction liability are from other gene classes (Uhl, Drgon, Johnson, Fatusin, et al., 2008). GWAS studies have shown that cell adhesion molecules, in particular, are substantially overrepresented in GWAS for addiction liability, nicotine dependence, and smoking cessation

Negative Affective States and Cognitive Impairments in Nicotine Dependence
http://dx.doi.org/10.1016/B978-0-12-802574-1.00007-7

success (Lind et al., 2010; Uhl et al., 2010, 2007, Uhl, Liu, et al., 2008c). Furthermore, each the genetic loci identified in these studies contributes to only a small proportion of the overall genetic liability for nicotine dependence and nicotine cessation. On this basis, cumulative risk scores representing the collective influence of multiple genes have been used in smoking cessation trials (Rose, Behm, Drgon, Johnson, & Uhl, 2010).

Despite the implications of this post-genomic work, a great deal of genetic research has continued to focus on nicotinic receptor variants in part because, unlike what is generally observed for other classes of abused substances (Hall, 2016), there is a good deal of evidence for the involvement of genetic variation in nicotinic system genes in nicotine dependence ((eg, Saccone et al., 2009; Thorgeirsson et al., 2010), and for review, see Bierut (2009)). Negative findings are certainly found as well (Gelernter et al., 2015; Hubacek, Lanska, & Adamkova, 2014), even for genes for which there are many highly replicated associations with measures of nicotine dependence, such as variants in the α5-α3-β4 gene cluster (see Bierut (2009) for a full description of these studies). Many reasons have been suggested to account for this situation, but certainly one factor is that the effect size for each individual gene locus is likely to be quite small. Consequently, the collected influence of all nicotinic receptor-system gene variants has been suggested to account for less than 10% of the total phenotypic variance in nicotine dependence (Saccone et al., 2009), consistent with a polygenic and heterogeneous genetic architecture. This means that there are likely to be many negative findings, even for real effects.

Additionally, when the collected findings are analyzed, researchers have tended to lump all genetic studies of nicotine dependence together, even though particular associations are much more likely to involve specific phenotypes (sometimes conceived as intermediate phenotypes or endophenotypes). Indeed, the examination of a limited set of phenotypes has been suggested to have impeded identification of the genetic basis of nicotine dependence (Loukola et al., 2014), and the observation of a significant association is dependent upon the particular phenotype examined (Rice et al., 2012). Those authors found more specific associations for particular nicotine dependence phenotypes, although none as strong as that observed for menthol preference (Uhl, Walther, Behm, & Rose, 2011), which appears to be a highly unusual case. Of particular interest—given some of the chapters in this book examining the role of cognitive deficits in nicotine dependence—one locus in the Rice et al., (2012) study was quite near a linkage locus for Attention Deficit Hyperactivity Disorder (ADHD) (Romanos et al., 2008). As another example of this issue, in a study of variation in the α5 and α3 nicotinic receptor subunits (CHRNA5 and CHRNA3, respectively), Bousman, Rivard, Haese, Ambrosone, and Hyland (2012) found significant associations with cigarettes per day (CPD), but not time to first cigarette or the composite heavy smoking index, nor was there any association with nicotine cessation. In one final example, Broms et al., (2012) examined the association of multiple α5-α3-β4 gene cluster variants with multiple dependence phenotypes, DSM diagnostic criteria, and comorbid conditions. Significant associations were found for some markers with some of the phenotypes, but there was substantial independence of these associations for particular dependence phenotypes. Data of this kind would seem to reinforce both the polygenic and heterogeneous nature of the genetics of nicotine dependence: multiple loci within each gene appear to be associated with different nicotine dependence phenotypes, each accounting for a very small percentage of the overall variance. Indeed, Broms et al., (2012) noted that their findings were in accordance with the findings of Thorgeirsson et al., (2008) in which variation in a particular CHRNA3 locus accounted for only 1% of the variance in CPD, or one CPD.

These findings raise the rather important issue of what would be the most meaningful phenotypes to study in human association studies (which also has reverse translational implications for animal studies). The most commonly used measures address quantity of tobacco consumption, some indirect measure of motivation or overall diagnostic status; none of the commonly used measures directly address the psychological reasons for smoking, eg, what effects are produced by cigarettes that maintain the behavior. This has come about partially because the emphasis in clinical studies has been on highly dependent individuals for whom these reasons may be long lost in the past, so current drug use is driven by conditioning and habit. Habit, conditioning, and craving are certainly important factors in nicotine dependence; however, if questioned after nicotine cessation failure, smokers will often give much more specific psychological explanations for their smoking. Studies have begun to address genetic contributions to more specific phenotypes. For example, a study using the risk score approach (Belsky et al., 2013), intended to reflect the collective genetic risk of drug dependence, based upon the findings of several meta-analyses of GWAS for cigarettes smoked per day (Consortium 2010; Liu et al., 2010; Thorgeirsson et al., 2010), examined associations with several phenotypes. This genetic risk score was unrelated to smoking initiation, but it was related to several measures of the transition to heavier smoking and nicotine dependence. Most importantly for the present discussion, this risk score was associated with smoking to alleviate stress. Based upon much of the discussion in the rest of this book, it would seem likely that one such composite score might be sought that reflected genetic contributions to stress-alleviation, another to reduction in negative affect, another to alleviation of attentional deficits, and so forth. It would not necessarily be expected that such scores be completely independent, as suggested by the pleiotropic effects described by Broms et al., (2012). GWAS for smoking cessation, via several different treatment approaches, share substantial overlap, but they have much less overlap with GWAS for nicotine dependence (Drgon, Johnson, et al., 2009, Drgon, Montoya, et al., 2009b).

The current state of nicotine dependence studies in humans suggests several potential problems for animal studies. Since the genetic architecture of nicotine dependence, like dependence on other substances, appears to reflect the highly polygenic and heterogeneous contributions of numerous genes, it might be thought that one-by-one manipulation of individual genes in animal models might not be sufficient to produce differences in dependence phenotypes. However, the sorts of manipulations (most often gene knockouts) used in mice likely produce much larger consequences on gene function than human variants. Although this may be a problem for the comparison to human variants, it can still confirm the importance of those genes in responses to nicotine or nicotine dependence. In any case, as we shall see, mutant strains created on the basis of nomination from human genetic studies, including those from more recent GWAS (Uhl, Drgonova, & Hall, 2014), have generally been shown to have altered nicotine responses or nicotine dependence phenotypes. Moreover, in agreement with the foregoing argument, many of the effects of particular gene mutations tend to produce rather specific phenotypic effects.

GENETIC STUDIES OF POSITIVE REINFORCEMENT IN MICE

Many approaches have contributed to the understanding of the genetic basis of nicotine dependence using mouse models, although the involvement of specific genes has been primarily elucidated using targeted gene mutations. These studies have implicated multiple nicotinic receptor subunits (nAChRs) in the behavioral effects of nicotine. The distribution of nAChRs is quite complex (as an example, see the description of these receptor combinations in the habenula and interpeduncular nucleus in Grady et al., (2009)), but fits with the known functions of the regions in which they are found. The emphasis in these studies has been upon the positive reinforcing effects of nicotine, and upon the neurocircuitry involved in drug reinforcement and drug seeking. Intravenous (IV) self-administration (SA) of nicotine is reduced or eliminated in β_2 nicotinic receptor subunit KO (β_2 KO) mice (Orejarena et al., 2012; Pons et al., 2008), as is nicotine conditioned place preference (CPP) (Mineur et al., 2009; Walters, Brown, Changeux, Martin, & Damaj, 2006) and oral nicotine consumption to some extent (Levin et al., 2009). Nicotine SA in β_2 KO mice is rescued by viral-mediated re-expression of β_2 nAChRs in the ventral tegmental area (VTA), which also restore nicotine- and varenicline-induced elevations in DA release in the nucleus accumbens (NAc) (Reperant et al., 2010), as well as some other behavioral and neural responses to nicotine (Mineur et al., 2009). In the VTA, β_2 nAChRs are expressed on both DAergic and GABAergic neurons, and reinforcing actions of nicotine are mediated by the concerted activity of DA and GABA neurons via β_2 nAChRs (Tolu et al., 2013). Deletions of other nAChR genes also affect the positive reinforcing effects of nicotine and related functions, including α_7 nicotinic receptor subunit KO (α7 KO) (Besson et al., 2012; Levin et al., 2009), α_5 nicotinic receptor subunit KO (α5 KO) (Morel et al., 2014), α_4 nicotinic receptor subunit KO (α4 KO) (Pons et al., 2008), and α_6 nicotinic receptor subunit KO (α6 KO) mice (Pons et al., 2008). Although a spatially based intracranial (IC) SA procedure found that α4 KO, but not α6 KO, mice have reduced IC nicotine SA in the VTA and nicotine-induced DA neuron burst-firing (Exley et al., 2011), both mutations affected DA release in the NAc. Nicotine selectively activates DA neurons in the posterior VTA (Exley et al., 2011), which is eliminated in α4 KO mice and potentiated in a mutant strain with genetically enhanced α4 activity. Although complete α4 KO does not affect nicotine IV SA or CPP (Cahir, Pillidge, Drago, & Lawrence, 2011), conditional α_4 deletion in DA neurons eliminates nicotine CPP (McGranahan, Patzlaff, Grady, Heinemann, & Booker, 2011). This finding may suggest that different α_4^* nAChR populations have different roles in nicotine reinforcement.

KO studies have been criticized because they have largely examined only the mechanisms underlying the acute effects of nicotine and consequently may not say much about genetic variants underlying nicotine dependence, and do not reflect the sort of genetic variation seen in humans. Other studies may address the consequences of the sort of variation seen in humans. Insertion of an α_4 nAChR S248F mutation into mice that induces greater sensitivity to low-dose nicotine also increases nicotine IV SA at low doses (Cahir et al., 2011). Similarly, genetic insertion of a naturally occurring mouse T529A *Chrna4* polymorphism increases nicotine CPP and oral nicotine consumption (Wilking, Hesterberg, Crouch, Homanics, & Stitzel, 2010). Some gene mutations indirectly influence nAChR expression, such as the protein kinase Cϵ KO that reduces oral nicotine consumption and CPP, α6, and β3 subunit expression in striatum and VTA, and nicotine-stimulated DA release (Lee & Messing, 2011).

Studies of other drugs of abuse (Hall et al., 2002; Sora et al., 2001) suggest that some genetic mechanisms separately affect ascending or descending portions of dose–response relationships (Uhl et al., 2002, 2014). Such effects broaden or contract effective reinforcing dose ranges, which would be particularly important for nicotine given its notoriously narrow dose range for many behavioral and physiological effects. One of the best examples of this type of effect is found in α5 KO mice, in which there is a widening of the effective dose range for nicotine SA (Fowler, Lu, Johnson, Marks, & Kenny, 2011) and CPP (Jackson et al., 2010) because of reduced aversive effects of high nicotine doses. These effects involve α_5 nAChRs in the medial habenula (Fowler et al., 2011), as viral-mediated gene rescue in the medial habenula reverses the effects of α5 KO. Additionally, DA neuron-specific rescue of WT α5 nAChR expression rescues the effect of α5 KO on nicotine IV SA, which is not observed with a partial loss of function human α5 gene variant associated with nicotine dependence (Morel et al., 2014). Studies in mutant mice with several gain of function nAChR variants (for review, see Drenan and Lester (2012)) have contributed to this overall picture as well. Although some of these mutants are not viable, others enhance nicotinic stimulation of DA neurons and behavior associated with DA function (Cohen et al., 2012), including mutants with increased activity at $α_6^*$ nAChRs (Cohen et al., 2012) and $α_4^*$ nAChRs (Drenan et al., 2010).

Most of the studies discussed thus far in this chapter have demonstrated effects of genetic mutations on acute (or subacute) effects of nicotine, the presumption being that differences in acute nicotine responses influence subsequent chronic effects. Numerous other non-nicotinic genes have also been studied, primarily those already known to be involved in reinforcement circuitry. Deletion of the genes for the μ opioid receptor (MOP KO), δ opioid receptor (DOP KO), β-endorphin, or preproenkephalin (PPE KO) eliminate or reduce nicotine CPP (Berrendero, Kieffer, & Maldonado, 2002, 2005, 2012; Trigo, Zimmer, & Maldonado, 2009). The effects of MOP KO are not surprising as MOP KO has broad effects on drug reinforcement (Hall & Uhl, 2006), but MOP KO also reduces other acute and chronic nicotine effects (Berrendero et al., 2002). Although neither DOP KO nor preprodynorphin (PPD) KO affect a variety of acute and chronic nicotine effects (Berrendero et al., 2012; Galeote, Berrendero, Bura, Zimmer, & Maldonado, 2009), PPD KO increases nicotine SA for low nicotine doses (Galeote et al., 2009). Other gene mutants have also been shown to affect positive reinforcement. Full consideration of this topic is beyond the scope of the present chapter (see Marks (2013) for a fuller consideration), but this brief survey shows that many of these findings are consistent with human genetic studies, particularly for nAChRs. However, the variance associated with these genes in human studies comprises only a small percentage of the overall variance associated with nicotine dependence, focusing primarily on those identified based on *a priori* considerations, leaving the question of where to look to account for the rest of the variance. As summarized in more detail elsewhere in this book, self-medication and negative reinforcement mechanisms have been suggested to have a greater role in drug dependence (Koob, 2015), including perhaps its genetic basis.

MOUSE MODELS OF NEGATIVE REINFORCEMENT

Negative reinforcement might occur in nicotine-dependent individuals by acting upon premorbid deficits or by acting to reverse deficits that emerge during nicotine withdrawal (Hiroi & Scott, 2009; Markou, Kosten, & Koob, 1998). Nicotine withdrawal certainly produces undesirable effects, including changes in mood, cognition, and weight gain. These effects play a role in smoking relapse (Patterson et al., 2010), but that does not necessarily address the question of whether the original conditioning resulted from effects of nicotine on a premorbid state or upon effects resulting from nicotine withdrawal. These need not be mutually exclusive of course, as withdrawal effects are likely to be more pronounced in individuals with premorbid impairments.

There is certainly evidence for a genetic component to the development of nicotine dependence and tolerance, as can be seen in differences in the rate and magnitude of tolerance and withdrawal development across rodent strains (Jackson, Walters, Miles, Martin, & Damaj, 2009b; Marks, Romm, Gaffney, & Collins, 1986; Marks, Stitzel, & Collins, 1986). Work with KO mice demonstrates different rates of acute desensitization depending on subunit composition of nAChRs (Grady, Wageman, Patzlaff, & Marks, 2012), which may influence the development of tolerance and consequent withdrawal. Indeed, many genetic mutations in nAChRs that affect acute nicotine responses also influence the development of tolerance and withdrawal, including in $\alpha 7$ KO (Jackson, Martin, Changeux, & Damaj, 2008; Salas, Main, Gangitano, & De Biasi, 2007; Stoker, Olivier, & Markou, 2012), $\alpha 2$ KO (Salas, Sturm, Boulter, & De Biasi, 2009), and $\alpha 5$ KO (Jackson et al., 2008; Salas et al., 2009) mice. Salas et al. (2009) associated this with the high expression of these receptors in the habenula/interpeduncular nucleus and the ability of IC mecamylamine injections to precipitate withdrawal. By contrast, $\beta 2$ KO does not affect somatic withdrawal, but it alters affective withdrawal signs, including precipitated-withdrawal conditioned aversion and spontaneous withdrawal-induced anxiety (Jackson et al., 2008). Other nicotine tolerance studies have addressed phenotypes with more limited application to human drug dependence, such as elimination of tolerance to hyperthermic and hypolocomotor effects of nicotine in $\alpha 4$ KO mice, and enhancements in mutant mice harboring α_4 nAChR L9A mutation, which renders them hypersensitive to nicotine (Tapper, McKinney, Marks, & Lester, 2007).

Many of the non-nicotinic gene mutants shown to affect positive reinforcement also affect nicotine tolerance and withdrawal, including MOR KO and PPE KO (Berrendero et al., 2002, 2005), CB2 KO (Navarrete et al., 2013), and HINT1 KO (Jackson, Wang, Barbier, Damaj, & Chen, 2013) mice. Withdrawal-induced somatic responses, anxiety, elevations in corticosterone, FOS activation, and reductions in BDNF-positive cells are all reduced in GABA$_B$ KO mice (Varani, Moutinho, Bettler, & Balerio, 2012; Varani, Pedron, Bettler, & Balerio, 2014), although some acute responses to nicotine are also affected. On the other hand, preprohypocretin KO has only been shown to affect withdrawal (Plaza-Zabala, Flores, Maldonado, & Berrendero, 2012). The majority of these studies have examined only somatic signs of dependence. There is some evidence for divergence of effects on somatic and affective withdrawal (Jackson et al., 2008).

A broader consideration of nicotine withdrawal effects, and those that might be involved in self-medication, is certainly warranted. The affective and cognitive deficits induced by nicotine withdrawal in humans that are relevant to negative reinforcement are discussed in more detail elsewhere in this book [see also Hall et al., (2015)], but they will be summarized briefly here. Nicotine withdrawal impairs attention and reaction time (Gross, Jarvik, & Rosenblatt, 1993; Hughes, Keenan, & Yellin, 1989; Keenan, Hatsukami, & Anton, 1989), working memory (Carlson et al., 2009; Sweet et al., 2010), and other aspects of cognition ((George et al., 2002; Hatsukami, Fletcher, Morgan, Keenan, & Amble, 1989); see also Heishman, Taylor, and Henningfield (1994) for review). These deficits are improved by smoking or nicotine replacement (Atzori, Lemmonds, Kotler, Durcan, & Boyle, 2008; Kollins, McClernon, & Epstein, 2009; Loughead et al., 2010; Myers, Taylor, Moolchan, & Heishman, 2008; Sacco et al., 2005; Snyder & Henningfield, 1989), and smokers that experience greater cognitive impairments during withdrawal are more likely to suffer relapse (Patterson et al., 2010). As regards affect, the irritability and other affective symptoms of withdrawal are well-known, and can be ameliorated by nicotine (Myers et al., 2008). Affective changes may reflect pre-morbid predisposition, but certainly stress is a commonly reported factor in nicotine cessation failure and has been shown to increase motivation for nicotine in abstinent smokers (Colamussi, Bovbjerg, & Erblich, 2007), and it is central to some negative reinforcement theories (Koob, 2015).

There is substantial comorbidity between smoking and psychiatric diagnoses [(Lawrence, Mitrou, & Zubrick, 2009), see also chapters elsewhere in this book]. Indeed, psychological and neurobiological attributes that predispose individuals to nicotine addiction might also predispose them to these other disorders (Paterson & Markou, 2007). Pro-addiction phenotypes, as well as nicotine use in the presence of active symptoms, could produce negative reinforcement and self-medication. The concept of self-medication suggests a higher level awareness of the consequences of nicotine use, but negative reinforcement need not involve such awareness. Other studies in genetically modified mice addressing premorbid or post-dependence affective and cognitive symptoms may be laying the groundwork for understanding the genetic basis of these processes in humans.

GENETIC PREDISPOSITION TO AFFECTIVE DEFICITS

The high comorbidity between smoking and affective and anxiety disorders (Beckham et al., 1995; Breslau, Kilbey, & Andreski, 1991; Chen et al., 2012; Dickerson, O'Malley, Canive, Thuras, & Westermeyer, 2009; Glassman et al., 1988; Grabe et al., 2001; Koenen et al., 2005; Roberts, Fuemmeler,

McClernon, & Beckham, 2008; Waxmonsky et al., 2005), in part, is a foundation for self-treatment theories in nicotine dependence (Markou et al., 1998). Indeed, a history of major depression is associated with smoking cessation failure (Covey, Glassman, Stetner, & Becker, 1993; Glassman et al., 1988, 1993), comorbid disorders involve some shared genetic risk (Koenen et al., 2005), and nicotine self-treatment develops (at least in part) after the onset of symptoms (Feldner, Babson, & Zvolensky, 2007). In other instances, whether smoking in comorbid individuals is primarily initiated after the onset of symptoms, in response to prodromal symptomatology, or during withdrawal-induced exacerbation of affective symptoms remains to be seen. In any case, "stress-reducing" and anxiolytic effects of nicotine are commonly reported in smokers, yet such effects are difficult to demonstrate in animal models, in part because of the notoriously narrow effective dose ranges for nicotine effects and because these effects may only occur in predisposed individuals. Supporting this latter view, mice that overexpress the acetylcholinesterase R isoform have increased anxiety that is normalized by long-term nicotine consumption (Salas & De Biasi, 2008).

Genetic mutations in mice that influence affect appear to be at least somewhat different from those that affect positive reinforcement and cognition. Interestingly, $\alpha 7$ KO has no effect in tests of anxiety (Salas et al., 2007), in contrast to its effects on positive reinforcement and cognition (discussed later). Genetic deletions of the β_3 and β_4 nicotinic receptor subunits (in $\beta 3$ KO and $\beta 4$ KO mice) produce differences in tests of anxiety and depression (Booker, Butt, Wehner, Heinemann, & Collins, 2007; Salas, Pieri, Fung, Dani, & De Biasi, 2003; Semenova, Contet, Roberts, & Markou, 2012), and the antidepressant-like effects of nicotine in the forced swim test are eliminated in $\beta 4$ KO mice (Arias, Targowska-Duda, Feuerbach, & Jozwiak, 2015). Differences in anxiety are observed in $\alpha 5$ KO mice, but these effects are sex-dependent, perhaps due to sex hormone–dependent regulation of $\alpha 5$ nAChR gene expression (Gangitano, Salas, Teng, Perez, & De Biasi, 2009). Anhedonia associated with both spontaneous and precipitated nicotine withdrawal, as determined by changes by IC self-stimulation thresholds, is reduced in $\beta 2$ KO mice (Stoker, Marks, & Markou, 2015). Some of these effects may involve some of the same circuitry that influence positive reinforcement, as conditional $\alpha 4$ nAChR deletion in DA neurons eliminates the anxiolytic effects of nicotine (McGranahan et al., 2011). DA also appears to be involved in the nicotine withdrawal conditioned aversion, which is absent in DA D2 receptor KO mice (Grieder et al., 2010). The effects of metabotropic glutamate receptor 5 KO (Stoker, Olivier, & Markou, 2012a) and β-endorphin KO (Trigo et al., 2009) may also suggest that there is an overlap between genes involved in positive and negative reinforcement processes, although there are some differences.

There are many gene mutants that alter affective phenotypes which are not all necessarily going to be relevant to negative reinforcement mechanisms in nicotine dependence of course. A more important demonstration of potential predisposition to nicotine dependence due to negative reinforcement is found in the normalization of anxiety by nicotine in mice that overexpress the R isoform of acetylcholinesterase (Salas & De Biasi, 2008). Future research needs to emphasize this sort of study design, or even better, voluntary nicotine consumption, which has greater translational validity.

GENETIC PREDISPOSITION TO COGNITIVE DEFICITS

Genetic studies find that the contributions of specific nAChRs to cognition and cognitive enhancement by nicotine are quite specific for different cognitive processes, perhaps reflecting the heterogeneity of underlying cognitive impairments in smokers. For instance, α7 KO impairs procedural learning, but it does not appear to affect attentional set-shifting, reversal learning, span capacity, aversively motivated learning, or short-term memory (Young, Meves, Tarantino, Caldwell, & Geyer, 2011), nor contextual learning (Wehner et al., 2004). KO studies suggest that α7 nAChRs are involved in other cognitive processes as well, including spatial learning (Levin et al., 2009), visuospatial episodic memory (Fernandes, Hoyle, Dempster, Schalkwyk, & Collier, 2006), positive reward associative learning (Young et al., 2011), and spatial discrimination (Levin et al., 2009), but not aversive contextual learning (Davis & Gould, 2006; 2007; Davis, Kenney, & Gould, 2007; Wehner et al., 2004; Young et al., 2011), which seems to involve other nAChRs. Interestingly, α7 KO mice are less sensitive to some ethanol-induced cognitive impairments (Wehner et al., 2004), which might suggest that the genetic underpinnings of codependency might be different from single dependencies. As discussed subsequently, β2 nAChRs are involved in contextual and cued fear conditioning; the reversal of ethanol-induced impairments in these processes by nicotine involve β2 nAChRs in the cingulate cortex (Gulick & Gould, 2009). These findings exemplify the complexities of cholinergic roles in cognition. Thus, even when reductions in gene function do not affect cognitive function, other alterations in those genes do so; Paylor et al., (1998) found no effect of α7 KO on spatial learning, but viral-mediated elevation of α7 nAChR expression in the hippocampus enhanced spatial learning (Ren et al., 2007).

β2 nAChRs are involved in cognitive processes somewhat distinct from α7 nAChRs. Old, but not young, β2 KO mice have deficits in fear conditioning and contextual learning (Caldarone, Duman, & Picciotto, 2000; Wehner et al., 2004). Moreover, nicotine-induced enhancement of fear conditioning, passive avoidance, contextual learning, and spatial discrimination are eliminated in β2 KO mice (Davis & Gould, 2007; Levin et al., 2009; Picciotto et al., 1995; Wehner et al., 2004), as are β2 nAChR-mediated signal transduction events (Jackson, Walters, & Damaj, 2009; Kenney, Florian, Portugal, Abel, & Gould, 2010). More importantly, nicotine withdrawal–induced deficits in contextual conditioning and trace cued fear conditioning are eliminated in β2 KO mice (Davis & Gould, 2009; Portugal, Kenney, & Gould, 2008; Raybuck & Gould, 2009), indicating the potential of more specific involvement of β2 nAChRs in certain cognitive aspects of withdrawal. Some of these findings might reflect opponent processes by which acute nicotine-induced enhancements lead to deficits in withdrawal.

Cognitive effects in α7 KO and β2 KO mice are consistent with developmental reductions in glutamatergic synaptic function and altered GABA/glutamate balance in the hippocampus (Lozada et al., 2012a; 2012b), hippocampal deficits in long-term potentiation, and long-term depression (Graw, Freund, Floyd, Dell'Acqua, & Leonard, 2011), and alterations in AMPA/NMDA receptor ratios in the VTA (Gao et al., 2010). In β2 KO and α5 KO mice, nicotinic excitation of cortical pyramidal cells is reduced, but excitatory effects of muscarinic stimulation are enhanced, shifting the balance of nicotinic to muscarinic excitation (Tian, Bailey, De Biasi, Picciotto, & Lambe, 2011). These findings suggest that the broader circuitry involved in learning and memory should be considered in the study of the genetic differences underlying cognitive impairments that might lead to self-medication with nicotine and consequent negative reinforcement produced by alleviation of such impairments. As an example, working memory impairments in human caspase 3 over-expressing mice, reflected by age-independent deficits in span capacity, are reversed by nicotine (Young et al., 2007).

As is the case for cognition generally, many genetic manipulations affect attentional function. Impairments of choice accuracy in the 5-choice serial reaction time task are observed in α5 KO (Bailey, De Biasi, Fletcher, & Lambe, 2010) and α7 KO (Hoyle, Genn, Fernandes, & Stolerman, 2006; Young et al., 2004) mice. In α5 KO mice, these effects are seen at shorter stimulus durations, which increase attentional demand. Nicotine did not improve these deficits, but only a limited dose range was examined in the Bailey et al., (2010) study, and Hoyle et al., (2006) examined nicotine effects only under conditions of high basal performance. Attention-improving effects of nicotine may only be evident when performance is impaired, as was seen by de Bruin, Fransen, Duytschaever, Grantham, and Megens (2006).

Complementing these studies, differences in pre-attentional processes have also been studied. Strain comparisons suggest that some forms of auditory sensory gating are mediated by α7 nAChRs (Mexal et al., 2007; Stevens et al., 1996), effects that can be ameliorated by nicotine or selective α7 nAChR agonists (Feuerbach et al., 2009; Stevens, Kem, Mahnir, & Freedman, 1998). Impairments appear to be specific for particular pre-attentional processes, as pre-pulse inhibition of acoustic startle (PPI) is not affected in α7 KO mice (Paylor et al., 1998; Young et al., 2011). Latent inhibition is unaffected in β2 KO mice (Caldarone et al., 2000), but the effect of nicotine on the N40 component of auditory evoked–related potentials is eliminated (Rudnick, Koehler, Picciotto, & Siegel, 2009). Mechanistic studies support these findings in a general way as effects of prefrontocortical cholinergic transients and consequent glutamatergic transients on cue detection are affected in both α7 KO and β2 KO mice (Parikh, Ji, Decker, & Sarter, 2010).

These studies indicate that certain genetically induced pre-attentional impairments can be ameliorated by nicotine. Observations in dopamine transporter (DAT) KO mice support this view and also provide a potential connection between genetic variation, psychiatric comorbidities, and nicotine dependence. DAT KO mice have been suggested to model aspects of behavioral impairments in ADHD (Arime et al., 2011, 2012; Arime, Kasahara, Hall, Uhl, & Sora, 2012; Arime, Kubo, & Sora, 2011; Yamashita et al., 2006). Deficits in PPI are observed in DAT KO mice (Ralph, Paulus, Fumagalli, Caron, & Geyer, 2001; Yamashita et al., 2006), impairments that are reversed by drugs that treat ADHD (Yamashita et al., 2006), as well as the selective NET blocker nisoxetine (Arime et al., 2012; Yamashita et al., 2006), which has a similar mode of action to atomoxetine. These changes are accompanied by regional and sub-type-specific changes in nAChRs (Weiss, Tzavara, et al., 2007). Of particular relevance to the present discussion, nicotine treatment improves PPI deficits (Uchiumi et al., 2013), hyperactivity (Uchiumi et al., 2013; Weiss, Nosten-Bertrand, McIntosh, Giros, & Martres, 2007), and learning impairments (Weiss, Nosten-Bertrand, et al., 2007a) in DAT KO mice. Moreover, the effects of nicotine were specifically related to α7 nAChRs using the antagonist methyllycaconitine (Uchiumi et al., 2013).

WHERE DO WE GO NEXT?

The studies discussed here demonstrate a progression in the study of the genetic basis of nicotine dependence. In part, this reflects the overall transition in genetics from initial *a priori* hypotheses to those based on broader GWAS findings and a greater understanding of the polygenic and heterogeneous basis of addiction. Moreover, it also reflects a changing consideration of the heterogeneous basis of nicotine dependence, including negative reinforcement as well as positive reinforcement, and self-medication for a variety of cognitive and affective impairments with nicotine. There are both translational and reverse translational implications of this work. Future work in this area will require diverse animal models, genetic and behavioral, to address the diverse affective and cognitive bases of nicotine dependence. A priority will be to recreate genetic mutations related to each aspect of human nicotine dependence in order to understand their specific contributions. At the same time, human genetic studies will need to be refined to address many of the more specific phenotypes addressed in preclinical studies.

Acknowledgments

This work was supported in part by the University of Toledo.

References

Arias, H. R., Targowska-Duda, K. M., Feuerbach, D., & Jozwiak, K. (2015). The antidepressant-like activity of nicotine, but not of 3-furan-2-yl-N-p-tolyl-acrylamide, is regulated by the nicotinic receptor beta4 subunit. *Neurochemistry International, 87,* 110–116.

Arime, Y., Kubo, Y., & Sora, I. (2011). Animal models of attention-deficit/hyperactivity disorder. *Biological & Pharmaceutical Bulletin, 34,* 1373–1376.

Arime, Y., Kasahara, Y., Hall, F. S., Uhl, G. R., & Sora, I. (2012). Cortico-subcortical neuro-modulation involved in the amelioration of prepulse inhibition deficits in dopamine transporter knockout mice. *Neuropsychopharmacology: Official Publication of the American College of Neuropsychopharmacology, 37,* 2522–2530.

Atzori, G., Lemmonds, C. A., Kotler, M. L., Durcan, M. J., & Boyle, J. (2008). Efficacy of a nicotine (4 mg)-containing lozenge on the cognitive impairment of nicotine withdrawal. *Journal of Clinical Psychopharmacology, 28,* 667–674.

Bailey, C. D., De Biasi, M., Fletcher, P. J., & Lambe, E. K. (2010). The nicotinic acetylcholine receptor alpha5 subunit plays a key role in attention circuitry and accuracy. *The Journal of Neuroscience: the Official Journal of the Society for Neuroscience, 30,* 9241–9252.

Beckham, J. C., Roodman, A. A., Shipley, R. H., Hertzberg, M. A., Cunha, G. H., Kudler, H. S., et al. (1995). Smoking in Vietnam combat veterans with posttraumatic-stress-disorder. *Journal of Traumatic Stress, 8,* 461–472.

Belsky, D. W., Moffitt, T. E., Baker, T. B., Biddle, A. K., Evans, J. P., Harrington, H., et al. (2013). Polygenic risk and the developmental progression to heavy, persistent smoking and nicotine dependence: evidence from a 4-decade longitudinal study. *JAMA Psychiatry, 70,* 534–542.

Berrendero, F., Kieffer, B. L., & Maldonado, R. (2002). Attenuation of nicotine-induced antinociception, rewarding effects, and dependence in mu-opioid receptor knock-out mice. *The Journal of Neuroscience: the Official Journal of the Society for Neuroscience, 22,* 10935–10940.

Berrendero, F., Mendizabal, V., Robledo, P., Galeote, L., Bilkei-Gorzo, A., Zimmer, A., et al. (2005). Nicotine-induced antinociception, rewarding effects, and physical dependence are decreased in mice lacking the preproenkephalin gene. *The Journal of Neuroscience: the Official Journal of the Society for Neuroscience, 25,* 1103–1112.

Berrendero, F., Plaza-Zabalala, A., Galeote, L., Flores, A., Bura, S. A., Kieffer, B. L., et al. (2012). Influence of delta-opioid receptors in the behavioral effects of nicotine. *Neuropsychopharmacology: Official Publication of the American College of Neuropsychopharmacology, 37,* 2332–2344.

Besson, M., David, V., Baudonnat, M., Cazala, P., Guilloux, J. P., Reperant, C., et al. (2012). Alpha7-nicotinic receptors modulate nicotine-induced reinforcement and extracellular dopamine outflow in the mesolimbic system in mice. *Psychopharmacology, 220,* 1–14.

Bierut, L. J. (2009). Nicotine dependence and genetic variation in the nicotinic receptors. *Drug and Alcohol Dependence, 104*(Suppl. 1), S64–S69.

Booker, T. K., Butt, C. M., Wehner, J. M., Heinemann, S. F., & Collins, A. C. (2007). Decreased anxiety-like behavior in beta3 nicotinic receptor subunit knockout mice. *Pharmacology, Biochemistry, and Behavior, 87*, 146–157.

Bousman, C. A., Rivard, C., Haese, J. D., Ambrosone, C., & Hyland, A. (2012). Alpha-5 and -3 nicotinic receptor gene variants predict nicotine dependence but not cessation: findings from the COMMIT cohort. *American Journal of Medical Genetics. Part B, Neuropsychiatric Genetics: the Official Publication of the International Society of Psychiatric Genetics, 159B*, 227–235.

Breslau, N., Kilbey, M., & Andreski, P. (1991). Nicotine dependence, major depression, and anxiety in young adults. *Archives of General Psychiatry, 48*, 1069–1074.

Broms, U., Silventoinen, K., Madden, P. A., Heath, A. C., & Kaprio, J. (2006). Genetic architecture of smoking behavior: a study of Finnish adult twins. *Twin Research and Human Genetics: the Official Journal of the International Society for Twin Studies, 9*, 64–72.

Broms, U., Wedenoja, J., Largeau, M. R., Korhonen, T., Pitkaniemi, J., Keskitalo-Vuokko, K., et al. (2012). Analysis of detailed phenotype profiles reveals CHRNA5-CHRNA3-CHRNB4 gene cluster association with several nicotine dependence traits. *Nicotine & Tobacco Research: Official Journal of the Society for Research on Nicotine and Tobacco, 14*, 720–733.

Cahir, E., Pillidge, K., Drago, J., & Lawrence, A. J. (2011). The necessity of alpha4* nicotinic receptors in nicotine-driven behaviors: dissociation between reinforcing and motor effects of nicotine. *Neuropsychopharmacology: Official Publication of the American College of Neuropsychopharmacology, 36*, 1505–1517.

Caldarone, B. J., Duman, C. H., & Picciotto, M. R. (2000). Fear conditioning and latent inhibition in mice lacking the high affinity subclass of nicotinic acetylcholine receptors in the brain. *Neuropharmacology, 39*, 2779–2784.

Carlson, J. M., Gilbert, D. G., Riise, H., Rabinovich, N. E., Sugai, C., & Froeliger, B. (2009). Serotonin transporter genotype and depressive symptoms moderate effects of nicotine on spatial working memory. *Experimental and Clinical Psychopharmacology, 17*, 173–180.

Chen, L. S., Xian, H., Grucza, R. A., Saccone, N. L., Wang, J. C., Johnson, E. O., et al. (2012). Nicotine dependence and comorbid psychiatric disorders: examination of specific genetic variants in the CHRNA5-A3-B4 nicotinic receptor genes. *Drug and Alcohol Dependence, 123*, S42–S51.

Cohen, B. N., Mackey, E. D. W., Grady, S. R., Mckinney, S., Patzlaff, N. E., Wageman, C. R., et al. (2012). Nicotinic cholinergic mechanisms causing elevated dopamine release and abnormal locomotor behavior. *Neuroscience, 200*, 31–41.

Colamussi, L., Bovbjerg, D. H., & Erblich, J. (2007). Stress- and cue-induced cigarette craving: effects of a family history of smoking. *Drug and Alcohol Dependence, 88*, 251–258.

Consortium, TaG. (2010). Genome-wide meta-analyses identify multiple loci associated with smoking behavior. *Nature Genetics, 42*, 441–447.

Covey, L. S., Glassman, A. H., Stetner, F., & Becker, J. (1993). Effect of history of alcoholism or major depression on smoking cessation. *American Journal of Psychiatry, 150*, 1546–1547.

Davis, J. A., & Gould, T. J. (2006). The effects of DHBE and MLA on nicotine-induced enhancement of contextual fear conditioning in C57BL/6 mice. *Psychopharmacology, 184*, 345–352.

Davis, J. A., & Gould, T. J. (2007). Beta 2 subunit-containing nicotinic receptors mediate the enhancing effect of nicotine on trace cued fear conditioning in C57BL/6 mice. *Psychopharmacology, 190*, 343–352.

Davis, J. A., & Gould, T. J. (2009). Hippocampal nAChRs mediate nicotine withdrawal-related learning deficits. *European Neuropsychopharmacology: the Journal of the European College of Neuropsychopharmacology, 19*, 551–561.

Davis, J. A., Kenney, J. W., & Gould, T. J. (2007). Hippocampal alpha4beta2 nicotinic acetylcholine receptor involvement in the enhancing effect of acute nicotine on contextual fear conditioning. *The Journal of Neuroscience: the Official Journal of the Society for Neuroscience, 27*, 10870–10877.

de Bruin, N. M., Fransen, F., Duytschaever, H., Grantham, C., & Megens, A. A. (2006). Attentional performance of (C57BL/6Jx129Sv)F2 mice in the five-choice serial reaction time task. *Physiology & Behavior, 89*, 692–703.

Dickerson, D. L., O'Malley, S. S., Canive, J., Thuras, P., & Westermeyer, J. (2009). Nicotine dependence and psychiatric and substance use comorbidities in a sample of American Indian male veterans. *Drug and Alcohol Dependence, 99*, 169–175.

Drenan, R. M., & Lester, H. A. (2012). Insights into the neurobiology of the nicotinic cholinergic system and nicotine addiction from mice expressing nicotinic receptors harboring gain-of-function mutations. *Pharmacological Reviews, 64*, 869–879.

Drenan, R. M., Grady, S. R., Steele, A. D., McKinney, S., Patzlaff, N. E., McIntosh, J. M., et al. (2010). Cholinergic modulation of locomotion and striatal dopamine release is mediated by alpha 6 alpha 4*Nicotinic acetylcholine receptors. *The Journal of Neuroscience: the Official Journal of the Society for Neuroscience, 30*, 9877–9889.

Drgon, T., Johnson, C., Walther, D., Albino, A. P., Rose, J. E., & Uhl, G. R. (2009). Genome-wide association for smoking cessation success: participants in a trial with adjunctive denicotinized cigarettes. *Molecular Medicine, 15*, 268–274.

Drgon, T., Montoya, I., Johnson, C., Liu, Q. R., Walther, D., Hamer, D., et al. (2009). Genome-wide association for nicotine dependence and smoking cessation success in NIH research volunteers. *Molecular Medicine, 15*, 21–27.

Exley, R., Maubourguet, N., David, V., Eddine, R., Evrard, A., Pons, S., et al. (2011). Distinct contributions of nicotinic acetylcholine receptor subunit alpha4 and subunit alpha6 to the reinforcing effects of nicotine. *Proceedings of the National Academy of Sciences USA, 108*, 7577–7582.

Feldner, M. T., Babson, K. A., & Zvolensky, M. J. (2007). Smoking, traumatic event exposure, and post-traumatic stress: a critical review of the empirical literature. *Clinical Psychology Review, 27*, 14–45.

Fernandes, C., Hoyle, E., Dempster, E., Schalkwyk, L. C., & Collier, D. A. (2006). Performance deficit of alpha7 nicotinic receptor knockout mice in a delayed matching-to-place task suggests a mild impairment of working/episodic-like memory. *Genes, Brain and Behavior, 5*, 433–440.

Feuerbach, D., Lingenhoehl, K., Olpe, H. R., Vassout, A., Gentsch, C., Chaperon, F., et al. (2009). The selective nicotinic acetylcholine receptor alpha7 agonist JN403 is active in animal models of cognition, sensory gating, epilepsy and pain. *Neuropharmacology, 56*, 254–263.

Fowler, C. D., Lu, Q., Johnson, P. M., Marks, M. J., & Kenny, P. J. (2011). Habenular alpha5 nicotinic receptor subunit signalling controls nicotine intake. *Nature, 471*, 597–601.

Galeote, L., Berrendero, F., Bura, S. A., Zimmer, A., & Maldonado, R. (2009). Prodynorphin gene disruption increases the sensitivity to nicotine self-administration in mice. *International Journal of Neuropsychopharmacology, 12*, 615–625.

Gangitano, D., Salas, R., Teng, Y., Perez, E., & De Biasi, M. (2009). Progesterone modulation of alpha 5 nAChR subunits influences anxiety-related behavior during estrus cycle. *Genes, Brain and Behavior, 8*, 398–406.

Gao, M., Jin, Y., Yang, K. C., Zhang, D., Lukas, R. J., & Wu, J. (2010). Mechanisms involved in systemic nicotine-induced glutamatergic synaptic plasticity on dopamine neurons in the ventral tegmental area. *The Journal of Neuroscience: the Official Journal of the Society for Neuroscience, 30*, 13814–13825.

Gelernter, J., Kranzler, H. R., Sherva, R., Almasy, L., Herman, A. I., Koesterer, R., et al. (2015). Genome-wide association study of nicotine dependence in American populations: identification of novel risk loci in both African-Americans and European-Americans. *Biological Psychiatry, 77*, 493–503.

George, T. P., Vessicchio, J. C., Termine, A., Sahady, D. M., Head, C. A., Pepper, W. T., et al. (2002). Effects of smoking abstinence on visuospatial working memory function in schizophrenia. *Neuropsychopharmacology: Official Publication of the American College of Neuropsychopharmacology, 26,* 75–85.

Glassman, A. H., Stetner, F., Walsh, B. T., Raizman, P. S., Fleiss, J. L., Cooper, T. B., et al. (1988). Heavy smokers, smoking cessation, and clonidine. Results of a double-blind, randomized trial. *JAMA, 259,* 2863–2866.

Glassman, A. H., Covey, L. S., Dalack, G. W., Stetner, F., Rivelli, S. K., Fleiss, J., et al. (1993). Smoking cessation, clonidine, and vulnerability to nicotine among dependent smokers. *Clinical Pharmacology and Therapeutics, 54,* 670–679.

Grabe, H. J., Meyer, C., Hapke, U., Rumpf, H. J., Freyberger, H. J., Dilling, H., et al. (2001). Lifetime-comorbidity of obsessive-compulsive disorder and subclinical obsessive-compulsive disorder in northern Germany. *European Archives of Psychiatry and Clinical Neuroscience, 251,* 130–135.

Grady, S. R., Moretti, M., Zoli, M., Marks, M. J., Zanardi, A., Pucci, L., et al. (2009). Rodent Habenulo-interpeduncular pathway expresses a large variety of uncommon nAChR subtypes, but only the alpha 3 beta 4*and alpha 3 beta 3 beta 4*Subtypes mediate acetylcholine release. *The Journal of Neuroscience: The Official Journal of the Society for Neuroscience, 29,* 2272–2282.

Grady, S. R., Wageman, C. R., Patzlaff, N. E., & Marks, M. J. (2012). Low concentrations of nicotine differentially desensitize nicotinic acetylcholine receptors that include alpha 5 or alpha 6 subunits and that mediate synaptosomal neurotransmitter release. *Neuropharmacology, 62,* 1935–1943.

Graw, S., Freund, R., Floyd, K., Dell'Acqua, M., & Leonard, S. (2011). Loss of LTP in alpha 7 neuronal nicotinic receptor (alpha 7*) knockout mice is strain dependent. *Schizophrenia Bulletin, 37,* 34.

Grieder, T. E., Sellings, L. H., Vargas-Perez, H., Ting, A. K. R., Siu, E. C., Tyndale, R. F., et al. (2010). Dopaminergic signaling mediates the motivational response underlying the opponent process to chronic but not acute nicotine. *Neuropsychopharmacology: Official Publication of the American College of Neuropsychopharmacology, 35,* 943–954.

Gross, T. M., Jarvik, M. E., & Rosenblatt, M. R. (1993). Nicotine abstinence produces content-specific Stroop interference. *Psychopharmacology, 110,* 333–336.

Gulick, D., & Gould, T. J. (2009). The hippocampus and cingulate cortex differentially mediate the effects of nicotine on learning versus on ethanol-induced learning deficits through different effects at nicotinic receptors. *Neuropsychopharmacology: Official Publication of the American College of Neuropsychopharmacology, 34,* 2167–2179.

Hall, F. S., & Uhl, G. R. (2006). Transgenic mouse studies reveal substantial roles for opioid receptors in the rewarding effects of several classes of addictive drugs. *Current Psychiatry Reviews, 2,* 27–37.

Hall, F. S., Li, X. F., Sora, I., Xu, F., Caron, M., Lesch, K. P., et al. (2002). Cocaine mechanisms: enhanced cocaine, fluoxetine and nisoxetine place preferences following monoamine transporter deletions. *Neuroscience, 115,* 153–161.

Hall, F. S., Drgonova, J., Jain, S., & Uhl, G. R. (2013). Implications of genome wide association studies for addiction: are our a priori assumptions all wrong? *Pharmacology & Therapeutics, 140,* 267–279.

Hall, F. S., Der-Avakian, A., Gould, T. J., Markou, A., Shoaib, M., & Young, J. W. (2015). Negative affective states and cognitive impairments in nicotine dependence. *Neuroscience and Biobehavioral Reviews, 58,* 168–185.

Hall, F. S. (2016). Reverse translational implications of genome-wide association studies for addiction genetics. In V. R. Preedy (Ed.), *The neuropathology of drug addictions and drug misuse* (pp. 153–164). London: Elsevier.

Hatsukami, D., Fletcher, L., Morgan, S., Keenan, R., & Amble, P. (1989). The effects of varying cigarette deprivation duration on cognitive and performance tasks. *Journal of Substance Abuse, 1,* 407–416.

Heishman, S. J., Taylor, R. C., & Henningfield, J. E. (1994). Nicotine and Smoking: a review of effects on nicotine performance. *Experimental Clinical Psychopharmacology, 2*, 345–395.

Hiroi, N., & Scott, D. (2009). Constitutional mechanisms of vulnerability and resilience to nicotine dependence. *Molecular Psychiatry, 14*, 653–667.

Hoyle, E., Genn, R. F., Fernandes, C., & Stolerman, I. P. (2006). Impaired performance of alpha7 nicotinic receptor knockout mice in the five-choice serial reaction time task. *Psychopharmacology, 189*, 211–223.

Hubacek, J. A., Lanska, V., & Adamkova, V. (2014). Lack of an association between SNPs within the cholinergic receptor genes and smoking behavior in a Czech post-MONICA study. *Genetic Molecular Biology, 37*, 625–630.

Hughes, J. R., Keenan, R. M., & Yellin, A. (1989). Effect of tobacco withdrawal on sustained attention. *Addictive Behaviors, 14*, 577–580.

Jackson, K. J., Martin, B. R., Changeux, J. P., & Damaj, M. I. (2008). Differential role of nicotinic acetylcholine receptor subunits in physical and affective nicotine withdrawal signs. *Pharmacological Reviews, 325*, 302–312.

Jackson, K. J., Walters, C. L., & Damaj, M. I. (2009a). Beta 2 subunit-containing nicotinic receptors mediate acute nicotine-induced activation of calcium/calmodulin-dependent protein kinase II-dependent pathways in vivo. *Pharmacological Reviews, 330*, 541–549.

Jackson, K. J., Walters, C. L., Miles, M. F., Martin, B. R., & Damaj, M. I. (2009b). Characterization of pharmacological and behavioral differences to nicotine in C57Bl/6 and DBA/2 mice. *Neuropharmacology, 57*, 347–355.

Jackson, K. J., Marks, M. J., Vann, R. E., Chen, X., Gamage, T. F., Warner, J. A., et al. (2010). Role of alpha5 nicotinic acetylcholine receptors in pharmacological and behavioral effects of nicotine in mice. *The Journal of Pharmacology and Experimental Therapeutics, 334*, 137–146.

Jackson, K. J., Wang, J. B., Barbier, E., Damaj, M. I., & Chen, X. (2013). The histidine triad nucleotide binding 1 protein is involved in nicotine reward and physical nicotine withdrawal in mice. *Neuroscience Letters, 550*, 129–133.

Keenan, R. M., Hatsukami, D. K., & Anton, D. J. (1989). The effects of short-term smokeless tobacco deprivation on performance. *Psychopharmacology, 98*, 126–130.

Kenney, J. W., Florian, C., Portugal, G. S., Abel, T., & Gould, T. J. (2010). Involvement of hippocampal Jun-N terminal kinase pathway in the enhancement of learning and memory by nicotine. *Neuropsychopharmacology: Official Publication of the American College of Neuropsychopharmacology, 35*, 483–492.

Koenen, K. C., Hitsman, B., Lyons, M. J., Niaura, R., McCaffery, J., Goldberg, J., et al. (2005). A twin registry study of the relationship between posttraumatic stress disorder and nicotine dependence in men. *Archives of General Psychiatry, 62*, 1258–1265.

Kollins, S. H., McClernon, F. J., & Epstein, J. N. (2009). Effects of smoking abstinence on reaction time variability in smokers with and without ADHD: an ex-Gaussian analysis. *Drug and Alcohol Dependence, 100*, 169–172.

Koob, G. F. (2015). The dark side of emotion: the addiction perspective. *European Journal of Pharmacology, 753*, 73–87.

Lawrence, D., Mitrou, F., & Zubrick, S. R. (2009). Smoking and mental illness: results from population surveys in Australia and the United States. *BMC Public Health, 9*.

Lee, A. M., & Messing, R. O. (2011). Protein kinase C epsilon modulates nicotine consumption and dopamine reward signals in the nucleus accumbens. *Proceedings of the National Academy of Sciences USA, 108*, 16080–16085.

Levin, E. D., Petro, A., Rezvani, A. H., Pollard, N., Christopher, N. C., Strauss, M., et al. (2009). Nicotinic alpha7- or beta2-containing receptor knockout: effects on radial-arm maze learning and long-term nicotine consumption in mice. *Behavioural Brain Research, 196*, 207–213.

Lind, P. A., Macgregor, S., Vink, J. M., Pergadia, M. L., Hansell, N. K., de Moor, M. H., et al. (2010). A genomewide association study of nicotine and alcohol dependence in Australian and Dutch populations. *Twin Research and Human Genetics: the Official Journal of the International Society for Twin Studies, 13*, 10–29.

Liu, J. Z., Tozzi, F., Waterworth, D. M., Pillai, S. G., Muglia, P., Middleton, L., et al. (2010). Meta-analysis and imputation refines the association of 15q25 with smoking quantity. *Nature Genetics, 42*, 436–440.

Loughead, J., Ray, R., Wileyto, E. P., Ruparel, K., Sanborn, P., Siegel, S., et al. (2010). Effects of the alpha4beta2 partial agonist varenicline on brain activity and working memory in abstinent smokers. *Biological Psychiatry, 67*, 715–721.

Loukola, A., Wedenoja, J., Keskitalo-Vuokko, K., Broms, U., Korhonen, T., Ripatti, S., et al. (2014). Genome-wide association study on detailed profiles of smoking behavior and nicotine dependence in a twin sample. *Molecular Psychiatry, 19*, 615–624.

Lozada, A. F., Wang, X. L., Gounko, N. V., Massey, K. A., Duan, J. J., Liu, Z. P., et al. (2012a). Glutamatergic synapse formation is promoted by alpha 7-containing nicotinic acetylcholine receptors. *The Journal of Neuroscience: the Official Journal of the Society for Neuroscience, 32*, 7651–7661.

Lozada, A. F., Wang, X. L., Gounko, N. V., Massey, K. A., Duan, J. J., Liu, Z. P., et al. (2012b). Induction of dendritic spines by beta 2-containing nicotinic receptors. *The Journal of Neuroscience: the Official Journal of the Society for Neuroscience, 32*, 8391–8400.

Markou, A., Kosten, T. R., & Koob, G. F. (1998). Neurobiological similarities in depression and drug dependence: a self-medication hypothesis. *Neuropsychopharmacology: Official Publication of the American College of Neuropsychopharmacology, 18*, 135–174.

Marks, M. J., Romm, E., Gaffney, D. K., & Collins, A. C. (1986). Nicotine-induced tolerance and receptor changes in four mouse strains. *The Journal of Pharmacology and Experimental Therapeutics, 237*, 809–819.

Marks, M. J., Stitzel, J. A., & Collins, A. C. (1986). Dose-response analysis of nicotine tolerance and receptor changes in two inbred mouse strains. *The Journal of Pharmacology and Experimental Therapeutics, 239*, 358–364.

Marks, M. J. (2013). Genetic matters: thirty years of progress using mouse models in nicotinic research. *Biochemical Pharmacology, 86*, 1105–1113.

McGranahan, T. M., Patzlaff, N. E., Grady, S. R., Heinemann, S. F., & Booker, T. K. (2011). alpha4beta2 nicotinic acetylcholine receptors on dopaminergic neurons mediate nicotine reward and anxiety relief. *The Journal of Neuroscience: the Official Journal of the Society for Neuroscience, 31*, 10891–10902.

Mexal, S., Jenkins, P. M., Lautner, M. A., Iacob, E., Crouch, E. L., & Stitzel, J. A. (2007). alpha7 nicotinic receptor gene promoter polymorphisms in inbred mice affect expression in a cell type-specific fashion. *Journal of Biological Chemistry, 282*, 13220–13227.

Mineur, Y. S., Brunzell, D. H., Grady, S. R., Lindstrom, J. M., McIntosh, J. M., Marks, M. J., et al. (2009). Localized low-level re-expression of high-affinity mesolimbic nicotinic acetylcholine receptors restores nicotine-induced locomotion but not place conditioning. *Genes, Brain and Behavior, 8*, 257–266.

Morel, C., Fattore, L., Pons, S., Hay, Y. A., Marti, F., Lambolez, B., et al. (2014). Nicotine consumption is regulated by a human polymorphism in dopamine neurons. *Molecular Psychiatry, 19*, 930–936.

Morley, K. I., Lynskey, M. T., Madden, P. A., Treloar, S. A., Heath, A. C., & Martin, N. G. (2007). Exploring the inter-relationship of smoking age-at-onset, cigarette consumption and smoking persistence: genes or environment? *Psychological Medicine, 37*, 1357–1367.

Myers, C. S., Taylor, R. C., Moolchan, E. T., & Heishman, S. J. (2008). Dose-related enhancement of mood and cognition in smokers administered nicotine nasal spray. *Neuropsychopharmacology: Official Publication of the American College of Neuropsychopharmacology, 33*, 588–598.

Navarrete, F., Rodriguez-Arias, M., Martin-Garcia, E., Navarro, D., Garcia-Gutierrez, M. S., Aguilar, M. A., et al. (2013). Role of CB2 cannabinoid receptors in the rewarding, reinforcing, and physical effects of nicotine. *Neuropsychopharmacology: Official Publication of the American College of Neuropsychopharmacology, 38*, 2515–2524.

Orejarena, M. J., Herrera-Solis, A., Pons, S., Maskos, U., Maldonado, R., & Robledo, P. (2012). Selective re-expression of beta 2 nicotinic acetylcholine receptor subunits in the ventral tegmental area of the mouse restores intravenous nicotine self-administration. *Neuropharmacology, 63,* 235–241.

Parikh, V., Ji, J. Z., Decker, M. W., & Sarter, M. (2010). Prefrontal beta 2 subunit-containing and alpha 7 nicotinic acetylcholine receptors differentially control glutamatergic and cholinergic signaling. *The Journal of Neuroscience: the Official Journal of the Society for Neuroscience, 30,* 3518–3530.

Paterson, N. E., & Markou, A. (2007). Animal models and treatments for addiction and depression co-morbidity. *Neurotoxicity Research, 11,* 1–32.

Patterson, F., Jepson, C., Loughead, J., Perkins, K., Strasser, A. A., Siegel, S., et al. (2010). Working memory deficits predict short-term smoking resumption following brief abstinence. *Drug and Alcohol Dependence, 106,* 61–64.

Paylor, R., Nguyen, M., Crawley, J. N., Patrick, J., Beaudet, A., & Orr-Urtreger, A. (1998). Alpha7 nicotinic receptor subunits are not necessary for hippocampal-dependent learning or sensorimotor gating: a behavioral characterization of Acra7-deficient mice. *Learning & Memory, 5,* 302–316.

Picciotto, M. R., Zoli, M., Lena, C., Bessis, A., Lallemand, Y., Le Novere, N., et al. (1995). Abnormal avoidance learning in mice lacking functional high-affinity nicotine receptor in the brain. *Nature, 374,* 65–67.

Plaza-Zabala, A., Flores, A., Maldonado, R., & Berrendero, F. (2012). Hypocretin/Orexin signaling in the hypothalamic paraventricular nucleus is essential for the expression of nicotine withdrawal. *Biological Psychiatry, 71,* 214–223.

Pons, S., Fattore, L., Cossu, G., Tolu, S., Porcu, E., McIntosh, J. M., et al. (2008). Crucial role of alpha 4 and alpha 6 nicotinic acetylcholine receptor subunits from ventral tegmental area in systemic nicotine self-administration. *The Journal of Neuroscience: the Official Journal of the Society for Neuroscience, 28,* 12318–12327.

Portugal, G. S., Kenney, J. W., & Gould, T. J. (2008). Beta2 subunit containing acetylcholine receptors mediate nicotine withdrawal deficits in the acquisition of contextual fear conditioning. *Neurobiology of Learning and Memory, 89,* 106–113.

Ralph, R. J., Paulus, M. P., Fumagalli, F., Caron, M. G., & Geyer, M. A. (2001). Prepulse inhibition deficits and perseverative motor patterns in dopamine transporter knock-out mice: differential effects of D1 and D2 receptor antagonists. *The Journal of Neuroscience: the Official Journal of the Society for Neuroscience, 21,* 305–313.

Raybuck, J. D., & Gould, T. J. (2009). Nicotine withdrawal-induced deficits in trace fear conditioning in C57BL/6 mice–a role for high-affinity beta2 subunit-containing nicotinic acetylcholine receptors. *The European Journal of Neuroscience, 29,* 377–387.

Ren, K., Thinschmidt, J., Liu, J., Ai, L., Papke, R. L., King, M. A., et al. (2007). alpha7 Nicotinic receptor gene delivery into mouse hippocampal neurons leads to functional receptor expression, improved spatial memory-related performance, and tau hyperphosphorylation. *Neuroscience, 145,* 314–322.

Reperant, C., Pons, S., Dufour, E., Rollema, H., Gardier, A. M., & Maskos, U. (2010). Effect of the alpha 4 beta 2*nicotinic acetylcholine receptor partial agonist varenicline on dopamine release in beta 2 knock-out mice with selective re-expression of the beta 2 subunit in the ventral tegmental area. *Neuropharmacology, 58,* 346–350.

Rice, J. P., Hartz, S. M., Agrawal, A., Almasy, L., Bennett, S., Breslau, N., et al. (2012). CHRNB3 is more strongly associated with Fagerstrom test for cigarette dependence-based nicotine dependence than cigarettes per day: phenotype definition changes genome-wide association studies results. *Addiction, 107,* 2019–2028.

Roberts, M. E., Fuemmeler, B. F., McClernon, F. J., & Beckham, J. C. (2008). Association between trauma exposure and smoking in a population-based sample of young adults. *Journal of Adolescent Health, 42,* 266–274.

Romanos, M., Freitag, C., Jacob, C., Craig, D. W., Dempfle, A., Nguyen, T. T., et al. (2008). Genome-wide linkage analysis of ADHD using high-density SNP arrays: novel loci at 5q13.1 and 14q12. *Molecular Psychiatry, 13*, 522–530.

Rose, J. E., Behm, F. M., Drgon, T., Johnson, C., & Uhl, G. R. (2010). Personalized smoking cessation: interactions between nicotine dose, dependence and quit-success genotype score. *Molecular Medicine, 16*, 247–253.

Rudnick, N., Koehler, C., Picciotto, M., & Siegel, S. (2009). Role of beta 2-containing nicotinic acetylcholine receptors in auditory event-related potentials. *Psychopharmacology, 202*, 745–751.

Sacco, K. A., Termine, A., Seyal, A., Dudas, M. M., Vessicchio, J. C., Krishnan-Sarin, S., et al. (2005). Effects of cigarette smoking on spatial working memory and attentional deficits in schizophrenia: involvement of nicotinic receptor mechanisms. *Archives of General Psychiatry, 62*, 649–659.

Saccone, N. L., Saccone, S. F., Hinrichs, A. L., Stitzel, J. A., Duan, W., Pergadia, M. L., et al. (2009). Multiple distinct risk loci for nicotine dependence identified by dense coverage of the complete family of nicotinic receptor subunit (CHRN) genes. *American Journal of Medical Genetics. Part B, Neuropsychiatric Genetics: the Official Publication of the International Society of Psychiatric Genetics, 150B*, 453–466.

Salas, R., & De Biasi, M. (2008). Opposing actions of chronic stress and chronic nicotine on striatal function in mice. *Neuroscience Letters, 440*, 32–34.

Salas, R., Pieri, F., Fung, B., Dani, J. A., & De Biasi, M. (2003). Altered anxiety-related responses in mutant mice lacking the beta4 subunit of the nicotinic receptor. *The Journal of Neuroscience: the Official Journal of the Society for Neuroscience, 23*, 6255–6263.

Salas, R., Main, A., Gangitano, D., & De Biasi, M. (2007). Decreased withdrawal symptoms but normal tolerance to nicotine in mice null for the alpha7 nicotinic acetylcholine receptor subunit. *Neuropharmacology, 53*, 863–869.

Salas, R., Sturm, R., Boulter, J., & De Biasi, M. (2009). Nicotinic receptors in the Habenulo-interpeduncular system are necessary for nicotine withdrawal in mice. *The Journal of Neuroscience: the Official Journal of the Society for Neuroscience, 29*, 3014–3018.

Semenova, S., Contet, C., Roberts, A. J., & Markou, A. (2012). Mice lacking the beta 4 subunit of the nicotinic acetylcholine receptor show memory deficits, altered anxiety- and depression-like behavior, and diminished nicotine-induced analgesia. *Nicotine & Tobacco Research, 14*, 1346–1355.

Snyder, F. R., & Henningfield, J. E. (1989). Effects of nicotine administration following 12 h of tobacco deprivation: assessment on computerized performance tasks. *Psychopharmacology, 97*, 17–22.

Sora, I., Hall, F. S., Andrews, A. M., Itokawa, M., Li, X. F., Wei, H. B., et al. (2001). Molecular mechanisms of cocaine reward: combined dopamine and serotonin transporter knockouts eliminate cocaine place preference. *Proceedings of the National Academy of Sciences USA, 98*, 5300–5305.

Stevens, K. E., Freedman, R., Collins, A. C., Hall, M., Leonard, S., Marks, M. J., et al. (1996). Genetic correlation of inhibitory gating of hippocampal auditory evoked response and alpha-bungarotoxin-binding nicotinic cholinergic receptors in inbred mouse strains. *Neuropsychopharmacology: Official Publication of the American College of Neuropsychopharmacology, 15*, 152–162.

Stevens, K. E., Kem, W. R., Mahnir, V. M., & Freedman, R. (1998). Selective alpha7-nicotinic agonists normalize inhibition of auditory response in DBA mice. *Psychopharmacology, 136*, 320–327.

Stoker, A. K., Olivier, B., & Markou, A. (2012a). Involvement of metabotropic glutamate receptor 5 in brain reward deficits associated with cocaine and nicotine withdrawal and somatic signs of nicotine withdrawal. *Psychopharmacology, 221*, 317–327.

Stoker, A. K., Olivier, B., & Markou, A. (2012b). Role of alpha 7-and beta 4-Containing nicotinic acetylcholine receptors in the affective and somatic aspects of nicotine withdrawal: studies in knockout mice. *Behavior Genetics, 42*, 423–436.

Stoker, A. K., Marks, M. J., & Markou, A. (2015). Null mutation of the beta2 nicotinic ace-tylcholine receptor subunit attenuates nicotine withdrawal-induced anhedonia in mice. *European Journal of Pharmacology, 753,* 146–150.

Sweet, L. H., Mulligan, R. C., Finnerty, C. E., Jerskey, B. A., David, S. P., Cohen, R. A., et al. (2010). Effects of nicotine withdrawal on verbal working memory and associated brain response. *Psychiatry Research, 183,* 69–74.

Tapper, A. R., McKinney, S. L., Marks, M. J., & Lester, H. A. (2007). Nicotine responses in hypersensitive and knockout alpha 4 mice account for tolerance to both hypothermia and locomotor suppression in wild-type mice. *Physiological Genomics, 31,* 422–428.

Thorgeirsson, T. E., Geller, F., Sulem, P., Rafnar, T., Wiste, A., Magnusson, K. P., et al. (2008). A variant associated with nicotine dependence, lung cancer and peripheral arterial disease. *Nature, 452,* 638–642.

Thorgeirsson, T. E., Gudbjartsson, D. F., Surakka, I., Vink, J. M., Amin, N., Geller, F., et al. (2010). Sequence variants at CHRNB3-CHRNA6 and CYP2A6 affect smoking behavior. *Nature Genetics, 42,* 448–453.

Tian, M. K., Bailey, C. D. C., De Biasi, M., Picciotto, M. R., & Lambe, E. K. (2011). Plastic-ity of prefrontal attention circuitry: upregulated muscarinic excitability in response to decreased nicotinic signaling following deletion of alpha 5 or beta 2 subunits. *The Journal of Neuroscience: the Official Journal of the Society for Neuroscience, 31,* 16458–16463.

Tolu, S., Eddine, R., Marti, F., David, V., Graupner, M., Pons, S., et al. (2013). Co-activation of VTA DA and GABA neurons mediates nicotine reinforcement. *Molecular Psychiatry, 18,* 382–393.

Trigo, J. M., Zimmer, A., & Maldonado, R. (2009). Nicotine anxiogenic and rewarding effects are decreased in mice lacking beta-endorphin. *Neuropharmacology, 56,* 1147–1153.

Uchiumi, O., Kasahara, Y., Fukui, A., Hall, F. S., Uhl, G. R., & Sora, I. (2013). Serotonergic involvement in the amelioration of behavioral abnormalities in dopamine transporter knockout mice by nicotine. *Neuropharmacology, 64,* 348–356.

Uhl, G. R., Hall, F. S., & Sora, I. (2002). Cocaine, reward, movement and monoamine trans-porters. *Molecular Psychiatry, 7,* 21–26.

Uhl, G. R., Liu, Q. R., Drgon, T., Johnson, C., Walther, D., & Rose, J. E. (2007). Molecular genetics of nicotine dependence and abstinence: whole genome association using 520,000 SNPs. *BMC Genetics, 8,* 10.

Uhl, G. R., Drgon, T., Johnson, C., Fatusin, O. O., Liu, Q. R., Contoreggi, C., et al. (2008). "Higher order" addiction molecular genetics: convergent data from genome-wide asso-ciation in humans and mice. *Biochemical Pharmacology, 75,* 98–111.

Uhl, G. R., Drgon, T., Johnson, C., Li, C. Y., Contoreggi, C., Hess, J., et al. (2008). Molecu-lar genetics of addiction and related heritable phenotypes: genome-wide association approaches identify "connectivity constellation" and drug target genes with pleiotropic effects. *Annals of the New York Academy of Sciences, 1141,* 318–381.

Uhl, G. R., Liu, Q. R., Drgon, T., Johnson, C., Walther, D., Rose, J. E., et al. (2008). Molecu-lar genetics of successful smoking cessation: convergent genome-wide association study results. *Archives of General Psychiatry, 65,* 683–693.

Uhl, G. R., Drgon, T., Johnson, C., Ramoni, M. F., Behm, F. M., & Rose, J. E. (2010). Genome-wide association for smoking cessation success in a trial of precessation nicotine replace-ment. *Molecular Medicine, 16,* 513–526.

Uhl, G. R., Walther, D., Behm, F. M., & Rose, J. E. (2011). Menthol preference among smokers: association with TRPA1 variants. *Nicotine & Tobacco Research: Official Journal of the Society for Research on Nicotine and Tobacco, 13,* 1311–1315.

Uhl, G. R., Drgonova, J., & Hall, F. S. (2014). Curious cases: altered dose-response relation-ships in addiction genetics. *Pharmacology & Therapeutics, 141,* 335–346.

Varani, A. P., Moutinho, L. M., Bettler, B., & Balerio, G. N. (2012). Acute behavioural responses to nicotine and nicotine withdrawal syndrome are modified in GABA(B1) knockout mice. *Neuropharmacology, 63,* 863–872.

Varani, A. P., Pedron, V. T., Bettler, B., & Balerio, G. N. (2014). Involvement of GABAB receptors in biochemical alterations induced by anxiety-related responses to nicotine in mice: genetic and pharmacological approaches. *Neuropharmacology, 81*, 31–41.

Walters, C. L., Brown, S., Changeux, J. P., Martin, B., & Damaj, M. I. (2006). The beta2 but not alpha7 subunit of the nicotinic acetylcholine receptor is required for nicotine-conditioned place preference in mice. *Psychopharmacology, 184*, 339–344.

Waxmonsky, J. A., Thomas, M. R., Miklowitz, D. J., Allen, M. H., Wisniewski, S. R., Zhang, H. W., et al. (2005). Prevalence and correlates of tobacco use in bipolar disorder: data from the first 2000 participants in the Systematic Treatment Enhancement Program. *General Hospital Psychiatry, 27*, 321–328.

Wehner, J. M., Keller, J. J., Keller, A. B., Picciotto, M. R., Paylor, R., Booker, T. K., et al. (2004). Role of neuronal nicotinic receptors in the effects of nicotine and ethanol on contextual fear conditioning. *Neuroscience, 129*, 11–24.

Weiss, S., Nosten-Bertrand, M., McIntosh, J. M., Giros, B., & Martres, M. P. (2007a). Nicotine improves cognitive deficits of dopamine transporter knockout mice without long-term tolerance. *Neuropsychopharmacology: Official Publication of the American College of Neuropsychopharmacology, 32*, 2465–2478.

Weiss, S., Tzavara, E. T., Davis, R. J., Nomikos, G. G., Michael McIntosh, J., Giros, B., et al. (2007b). Functional alterations of nicotinic neurotransmission in dopamine transporter knock-out mice. *Neuropharmacology, 52*, 1496–1508.

Wilking, J. A., Hesterberg, K. G., Crouch, E. L., Homanics, G. E., & Stitzel, J. A. (2010). Chrna4 A529 knock-in mice exhibit altered nicotine sensitivity. *Pharmacogenetics and Genomics, 20*, 121–130.

Yamashita, M., Fukushima, S., Shen, H. W., Hall, F. S., Uhl, G. R., Numachi, Y., et al. (2006). Norepinephrine transporter blockade can normalize the prepulse inhibition deficits found in dopamine transporter knockout mice. *Neuropsychopharmacology: Official Publication of the American College of Neuropsychopharmacology, 31*, 2132–2139.

Young, J. W., Finlayson, K., Spratt, C., Marston, H. M., Crawford, N., Kelly, J. S., et al. (2004). Nicotine improves sustained attention in mice: evidence for involvement of the alpha7 nicotinic acetylcholine receptor. *Neuropsychopharmacology: Official Publication of the American College of Neuropsychopharmacology, 29*, 891–900.

Young, J. W., Kerr, L. E., Kelly, J. S., Marston, H. M., Spratt, C., Finlayson, K., et al. (2007). The odour span task: a novel paradigm for assessing working memory in mice. *Neuropharmacology, 52*, 634–645.

Young, J. W., Meves, J. M., Tarantino, I. S., Caldwell, S., & Geyer, M. A. (2011). Delayed procedural learning in alpha 7-nicotinic acetylcholine receptor knockout mice. *Genes, Brain and Behavior, 10*, 720–733.

Transmitters and Receptors in Nicotine Withdrawal Syndrome

D.H. Malin, A.N. Anderson, P. Goyarzu

University of Houston-Clear Lake, Houston, TX, United States

Nicotinic cholinergic receptors are located on cells that release a wide variety of transmitters, so that nicotine interacts with multiple neurochemical pathways directly and still others via trans-synaptic connections. Thus, it is not surprising that chronic overstimulation of nicotinic acetylcholine receptors (nAChRs) followed by abrupt reduction of this stimulation results in dysregulation of multiple transmitter and receptor systems. A number of these, in turn, appear to contribute in some way to varied aspects of nicotine withdrawal syndrome.

INFLUENCE OF DIFFERING LABORATORY MODELS OF NICOTINE WITHDRAWAL

The neurochemical mechanisms underlying nicotine withdrawal have repeatedly been shown to vary with the choice of laboratory model (Malin & Goyarzu, 2009). These models can be classified in several ways. First, there is the means of inducing physical dependence on nicotine. This is commonly done by continuous infusion, often via osmotic minipump of nicotine or one of its salts, often nicotine bitartrate (Malin et al., 1992). It can also be performed through a series of chronic injections (Costall et al., 1990a; Isola, Vogelsberg, Wemlinger, Neff, & Hadjiconstantinou, 1999), through adding nicotine to the subjects' diet or drinking water (Halladay et al., 1999), through long-term nicotine self-administration (O'Dell et al., 2007; Paterson & Markou, 2004), and, less commonly, through cutaneous nicotine patches (Cippitelli et al., 2011) or exposure to tobacco smoke (Andersson, Fuxe, Eneroth, Jansson, & Harfstrand, 1989). Second, models

Negative Affective States and Cognitive Impairments in Nicotine Dependence
http://dx.doi.org/10.1016/B978-0-12-802574-1.00008-9

differ in the means of initiating withdrawal. This can be done through "spontaneous withdrawal," which is simply cessation of nicotine administration, with consequent gradual development of withdrawal signs. A withdrawal syndrome may also be rapidly precipitated by injection of a nAChR antagonist. This is most commonly done with mecamylamine, a noncompetitive antagonist that is relatively nonspecific for receptor subtypes (Malin et al., 1994). Certain aspects of nicotine withdrawal syndrome may also be precipitated by antagonists selective for nAChR subtypes or by antagonists of other transmitter systems that are affected by chronic nicotine. This approach may be useful for teasing apart some of the various neurochemical contributors to nicotine withdrawal syndrome.

Third, models may be characterized by the variables used to measure the intensity of the withdrawal syndrome. The withdrawal syndrome observed during smoking cessation has a number of behavioral consequences, such as irritability, depressed mood, anxiety, difficulty concentrating, increased hunger and weight gain, and sleep disturbances (Hughes & Hatsukami, 1986). Therefore, it is not surprising that different rodent models employ a diversity of measures, each generally corresponding to at least one of the features seen in smoking cessation. There are important differences in some underlying neurochemical mechanisms leading to these various measures. The so-called *somatic signs* of nicotine withdrawal are frequently observed as indicators of withdrawal intensity. These include writhes, gasps, shakes, tremors, vacuous chewing, teeth chattering, and ptosis, as well as some less frequent behaviors such as yawning, hind foot scratching, and genital licking (Malin et al., 1992). *Somatic signs* may be misleadingly named. A true somatic sign would be a bodily change, such as altered blood pressure or an enlarged heart. Instead, the somatic signs are actually behaviors initiated by the central nervous system. It is true that some of these behaviors might be a response to internal physiological changes. However, as with the very similar withdrawal signs seen in opiate withdrawal, they likely also reflect increased behavioral and emotional sensitivity to such internal as well as external stimuli. Therefore, these phenomena will here be referred to as "somatically expressed withdrawal behaviors." They thus model the irritability dimension of smoking cessation.

Depression induced by smoking cessation is often modeled by increases in the electrical threshold for intracranial self-stimulation (ICSS), suggesting anhedonia (Epping-Jordan, Watkins, Koob, & Markou, 1998). Another indication of anhedonia is reduced breakpoint in an operant progressive-ratio task (LeSage, Burroughs, & Pentel, 2006). Also, the early cessation of struggling in the forced swim test is sometimes used as an indicator of withdrawal-induced depression (Mannucci, Tedesco, Bellomo, Caputi, & Calapai, 2006), as is reduced locomotor activity (Malin et al., 1992). Withdrawal-induced anxiety may be indicated by avoidance of exposed arms of the elevated plus-maze or by enhanced acoustic startle response (Helton, Modlin, Tizzano, & Rasmussen, 1993). Hyperalgesia (Damaj, Kao, & Martin, 2003) can be detected by standard measures of pain sensitivity, such as the hot plate test. Cognitive impairment is indicated by tests of sustained attention (Shoaib & Bizarro, 2005) and disrupted contextual fear conditioning as an indication of hippocampal dysfunction (Davis & Gould, 2007). Increased hunger and weight gain, particularly in females, is another measurable consequence of nicotine withdrawal (Grunberg, Bowen, & Winders, 1986; Levin, Morgan, Galvez, & Ellison, 1987).

An important issue is whether these various withdrawal effects are aversive enough to be emotionally motivating. This is confirmed by the conditioned place aversion (CPA) test (Suzuki, Ise, Tsuda, Maeda, & Misawa, 1996). Also relevant to this question is an increase in nicotine self-administration induced by nicotine deprivation in dependent rats (O'Dell & Koob, 2007).

CHOLINERGIC MECHANISMS

Since nicotine targets acetylcholine (ACh) receptors, cholinergic mechanisms must be involved. There have been few studies of ACh release during nicotine withdrawal. Withdrawal from continuous nicotine infusion, as in morphine withdrawal, resulted in significantly increased ACh release in the nucleus accumbens (NAcc), concurrent with somatically expressed withdrawal behaviors (Rada, Jensen, & Hoebel, 2001). At the same time, dopamine (DA) release is diminished, so that the transmitter balance in the NAcc was radically altered.

The nAChRs are ligand-gated cation channels for sodium or calcium ions composed of five protein subunits. The alpha subunits contain the actual transmitter binding sites. They are usually combined with beta subunits. There are a variety of alpha and beta protein subtypes and their combinations. The $\alpha 4 \beta 2$ combination is the most abundant in the central nervous system. This receptor type may also assemble with other subunits, such as $\alpha 6$, which may modulate its function. The $\alpha 3 \beta 4$ subtype is also well represented in the brain, as is the $\alpha 7$ receptor type. The latter is composed entirely of five copies of the same $\alpha 7$ protein.

Several specific nicotinic cholinergic receptor subtypes appear to be selectively involved in aspects of nicotine withdrawal syndrome. Such results might guide more specifically targeted nicotine replacement therapies. Nicotine reinforcement and self-administration are primarily mediated by $\alpha 4 \beta 2$ receptors (Picciotto et al., 1998). It is likely that these receptors may have a role in nicotine withdrawal syndrome. The competitive nicotinic receptor antagonist DHβE is relatively selective for $\alpha 4 \beta 2$ receptors. Centrally administered DHβE precipitated nicotine withdrawal, as indicated by somatically expressed behavioral signs (Epping-Jordan et al., 1998; Malin, Lake,

Shenoi et al., 1998). The β4 subunit (as in α3β4) appears to play a prominent role in somatically expressed withdrawal behaviors. In genetically modified mice, somatically expressed withdrawal behaviors were prevented by β4 knockout (Grabus et al., 2005; Salas, Pieri, & De Biasi, 2004; Stoker, Olivier,&Markou,2012),butnotbyα7knockout(Jackson,Martin,Changeux, & Damaj, 2008; Stoker et al., 2012) or β2 knockout (Besson et al., 2006; Jackson et al., 2008; Salas et al., 2004). Also, centrally administered hexamethonium (HMT), a noncompetitive nicotinic receptor antagonist with relative specificity for α3β4 receptors, precipitated somatically expressed nicotine withdrawal signs with enormous potency (Malin et al., 1997), particularly as compared with DHβE, with its relative selectivity for α4β2 receptors (Malin, Lake, Upchurch, et al., 1998). Likewise, the selective α3β4 antagonist α-conotoxin AuIB (AuIB) precipitated these signs (Jackson, Sanjakdar, Muldoon, McIntosh, & Damaj, 2013). The α3β4 selective antagonist HMT, but not the β2 antagonist DHβE, precipitated heightened nociceptive response on the tail flick test (Damaj et al., 2003).

Indicators of nicotine withdrawal-induced anhedonia present a different picture of nAChR involvement. The abundant α4β2 subtype appears to play a prominent role. The β2-selective antagonist DHβE precipitated increased ICSS thresholds (Bruijnzeel & Markou, 2004; Damaj et al., 2003). Conversely, the α4β2/α4α6β2 partial agonists cytisine and varenicline reversed the withdrawal-induced increase in ICSS thresholds.

β2-containing nAChRs also appear to help mediate the effects of nicotine withdrawal on anxiety. DHβE, but not methyllycaconitine (MLA) or HMT, precipitated increased anxiety in nicotine-dependent mice (Damaj et al., 2003). Conversely, withdrawal-induced anxiety was alleviated by the β2 partial agonist ABT-089 and also by the α7 partial agonist ABT-107, but not by the α3β4 antagonist AuIB (Jackson et al., 2013). β2 knockout, but not α7 or α5 knockout, prevented withdrawal-heightened anxiety scores on the plus-maze. A somewhat similar pattern is seen in CPA for nicotine withdrawal. DHβE, but not MLA or HMT, precipitated CPA in nicotine-dependent rats (Jackson, Kota, Martin, & Damaj, 2009). Consistent with this, β2, but not α7 or α5, knockout prevented CPA in nicotine withdrawal (Jackson et al., 2008).

Data suggest that α7 receptors might affect several aspects of nicotine withdrawal syndrome. Knockout of α7, but not β4, prevented mecamylamine-precipitated ICSS threshold elevation. However, both α7 and β4 knockouts delayed, but failed to ultimately prevent, this putative anhedonic effect of spontaneous nicotine withdrawal (Stoker et al., 2012).

The α7 antagonist MLA precipitated a mild withdrawal syndrome in nicotine-dependent rodents with increased somatically expressed behaviors and a degree of suppressed locomotor activity (Alajaji, Bowers, Knackstedt, & Damaj, 2013; Nomikos, Hildebrand, Panagis, & Svensson, 1999). However, interpretation of these results is somewhat complicated by the ability of MLA to cross-react with α3, α6, and β3 subunits. Also, Markou and

Paterson (2001) reported that systemically administered MLA failed to precipitate either somatically expressed withdrawal behaviors or altered ICSS thresholds. MLA did precipitate heightened nociceptive response on the hot-plate test. Also, α7, but not β2 or α5, knockout prevented withdrawal-induced hyperalgesia on the hot-plate test (Damaj et al., 2003).

The entire pattern of results suggests the possibility that α4β2 receptors, with their close connection to reinforcement mechanisms, might be responsible for withdrawal-induced changes in anhedonia and anxiety, while α3β4 receptors might be involved in the heightened irritability leading to somatically expressed nicotine withdrawal signs and hyperalgesia.

DOPAMINE

Rats in withdrawal from continuous nicotine infusion had reduced activity levels and DA content in the striatum and NAcc as well as reduced D2 DA receptors in the NAcc (Fung, Schmid, Anderson, & Lau, 1996). There have been numerous reports of lowered DA output in the NAcc during nicotine withdrawal in rodent models, with a time course roughly parallel with those of various behavioral withdrawal signs (Carboni, Bortone, Giua, & Di Chiara, 2000; Hildebrand, Nomikos, Hertel, Schilstrom, & Svensson, 1998; Lindblom et al., 2005; Rada et al., 2001; Rahman, Zhang, Engleman, & Corrigall, 2004). Decreased release in withdrawal is likely due to adaptations at the origin of the mesolimbic DA pathway in the ventral tegmental area (VTA); both somatically expressed withdrawal signs and inhibited DA output were triggered by mecamylamine injected directly into the VTA, but not into the NAcc (Hildebrand, Panagis, Svensson, & Nomikos, 1999).

Nicotine activation of the mesolimbic DA pathway mediates the reinforcing action of nicotine (Balfour, 2004; Corrigall & Coen, 1991). Adaptations in this pathway may also contribute to aspects of the nicotine abstinence syndrome, particularly its depression/anhedonia-like dimension. Mesolimbic DA activity is essential to intracranial self-stimulation (Zarevics & Setler, 1979). Thus, impaired DA function may mediate the increased ICSS reward thresholds in nicotine withdrawal (Epping-Jordan et al., 1998). This is consistent with the observation that bupropion reversal of withdrawal-induced elevation of ICSS thresholds is closely associated with restoration of mesolimbic DA release (Paterson, Balfour, & Markou, 2007). Another rodent model of depression is early cessation of escape efforts in the forced swim test. Nicotine withdrawal resulted in this sort of effect, which was prevented by L-DOPA and the DA agonist benserazide (Ohmura, Jutkiewicz, & Domino, 2011). Finally, DA may be involved in the connection between nicotine withdrawal and accelerated nicotine reinforcement and addiction. While withdrawal causes reduced

DA activity, this coincides with hypersensitivity to acute DA release in response to nicotine administration (Dani & De Biasi, 2013).

Reduced DA activity is not limited to the NAcc in nicotine withdrawal. Cortical DA and DA metabolite levels are decreased in mecamylamine-precipitated withdrawal (Varani, Moutinho, Calvo, & Balerio, 2011). In spontaneous withdrawal, mouse striatal DA reuptake and DA transporter RNA are raised, while DA overflow is decreased (Hadjiconstantinou, Duchemin, Zhang, & Neff, 2011). Thus, one possible mechanism of reduced DA overflow is heightened transmitter reuptake by transporters (Duchemin, Zhang, Neff, & Hadjiconstantinou, 2009; Hadjiconstantinou et al., 2011).

Conversely, stimulation of DA activity by various means has been reported to attenuate somatically expressed withdrawal signs. The dopamine precursor L-DOPA reduced withdrawal signs, the D1/5 receptor agonist SKF81297 decreased teeth chattering and vacuous chewing but not shaking, and the D2/3 agonist pramipexole relieved all three signs (Ohmura, Jutkiewicz, & Domino, 2011). Furthermore, blockade of the monoamine oxidase B isoform, an intervention that selectively increases brain DA levels, also reduced somatically expressed signs (Malin et al., 2013).

There may be an anatomical dissociation of the role of DA in different withdrawal signs. In contrast to the VTA/NAcc pathway, nicotinic or dopaminergic antagonists injected directly into the amygdala of nicotine-dependent rats fail to increase ICSS thresholds (Jonkman & Markou, 2006). However, mecamylamine-precipitated nicotine withdrawal decreased DA output in the central nucleus of the amygdala, along with somatically expressed withdrawal behaviors (Panagis, Hildebrand, Svensson, & Nomikos, 2000). The central nucleus of the amygdala is implicated in response to aversive or stressful situations (Bohus et al., 1996). Therefore, dopaminergic hypofunction in the central nucleus of the amygdala may possibly be connected to the irritability or anxiety dimensions of nicotine withdrawal syndrome. Acoustic startle activation in withdrawal was reversed by the DA agonist apomorphine, the D1 receptor agonist SKF82958, and the D2 receptor agonist quinpirole (Radke & Gewirtz, 2012). However, despite DA hypofunction, DA signaling may be essential to the aversiveness of withdrawal. The DA antagonist alpha-flupenthixol in rats and D2 receptor knockout in mice interfered with CPA in precipitated withdrawal in nicotine-dependent rodents (Grieder et al., 2010).

SEROTONIN AND NOREPINEPHRINE

Nicotine administration upregulated serotonin (5HT) release in the brain (Ribeiro, Bettiker, Bogdanov, & Wurtman, 1993) and 5HT output from the dorsal raphe nucleus to the NAcc (Chang et al., 2011). Conversely, spontaneous nicotine withdrawal downregulated brain 5HT turnover (Yasuda, Suemaru, Araki, & Gomita, 2002), and mecamylamine-precipitated withdrawal decreased striatal 5HT (Varani et al., 2011). Systemic injection of the immediate 5HT precursor 5HTP attenuated somatically expressed nicotine withdrawal signs (Ohmura, Jutkiewicz, Yoshioka, & Domino, 2011), and oral administration reversed withdrawal-induced immobility in the forced swim test (Mannucci et al., 2006). Also, certain measures of nicotine withdrawal syndrome such as CPA (Suzuki, Ise, Mori, & Misawa, 1997) or anxiety in the light avoidance test (Costall et al., 1990a, 1990b) were reduced by pharmacological stimulation of 5HT3 receptors. Thus, serotonergic hypoactivity in certain pathways may contribute to nicotine abstinence syndrome, while renewed 5HT activity might moderate the syndrome.

5HT1A receptors may also play a role in modulating nicotine withdrawal syndrome. These receptors may inhibit the activation of 5HT neurons, often by acting as autoreceptors (Guilloux et al., 2006). Nicotine withdrawal-induced increases in startle response were reduced by a selective 5HT1A antagonist (Rasmussen et al., 2000). A 5HT1A antagonist combined with the 5HT reuptake inhibitor fluoxetine reversed withdrawal-induced increases in ICSS thresholds (Harrison, Liem, & Markou, 2001). A recent study underscores the complexity of the 5HT1A interactions with nicotine. Acute nicotine administration and nicotine withdrawal induced different and largely opposite anatomical patterns of activation and 5HT1A-dependent inhibition of 5HT neurons within the dorsal and median raphe nuclei (Sperling & Commons, 2011).

Stimulation of 5HT2 receptors may contribute to certain somatically induced behavioral signs. Nicotine withdrawal intensified induction of wet-dog shakes and head twitches induced by a selective 5HT2 agonist (Suemaru, Araki, Kitamura, Yasuda, & Gomita, 2001; Yasuda et al., 2002). However, a selective 5HT2A antagonist exacerbated anhedonic nicotine withdrawal effects (Semenova & Markou, 2010).

There has been surprisingly little study of norepinephrine (NE) in nicotine withdrawal, considering the long-known ability of nicotine to potently release NE from the sympathetic nervous system. Nicotine also releases NE from hippocampal slices via α7 nicotinic receptors. This effect was intensified in slices obtained from rats in nicotine withdrawal (Barik & Wonnacott, 2006). Withdrawal from chronic exposure to cigarette smoke increased NE levels and NE utilization in several hypothalamic regions (Andersson et al., 1989). Inhibition of the enzyme monoamine oxidase A by clorgiline increases levels of NE and intensified somatically expressed withdrawal behaviors (Malin et al., 2013). Desipramine (DMI) is a preferential NE reuptake inhibitor and antidepressant. Chronic, but not acute, DMI administration reduced nicotine withdrawal effects on ICSS and somatically expressed behaviors (Paterson, Semenova, &

Markou, 2008). The α2 adrenoceptor, sometimes occurring as an autoreceptor, limits stimulation of NE synapses. Idazoxan, which blocks this receptor and upregulates NE transmission, reduced the effects of nicotine abstinence on ICSS thresholds as well as some somatically expressed withdrawal behaviors (Semenova & Markou, 2010). Bruijnzeel et al. (2010) reported an interesting dissociation between different adrenergic receptors in mediating anhedonic and somatically expressed withdrawal signs. The α1 receptor antagonist prazosin reduced the ICSS effects but not the somatically expressed withdrawal behaviors. Conversely, the α2 receptor agonist clonidine and the β adrenergic receptor antagonist propranolol reduced the somatically expressed signs, but not the anhedonic effects of withdrawal. Thus, modulation of NE synaptic transmission apparently influences nicotine withdrawal syndrome, but in a complex manner.

GLUTAMATE

Plasticity of excitatory amino acid mechanisms is involved in acquiring dependence on a number of drugs (Siggins et al., 2003). The expression of various subunits of the ionotropic glutamate N-methyl-D-aspartate (NMDA) and α-amino-3-hydroxy-5-methyl-4-isoxazolepropionic acid (AMPA)/kainate receptors was altered during chronic nicotine self-administration and during withdrawal, likely in compensation for changes in glutamate release (Kenny, Chartoff, Roberto, Carlezon, & Markou, 2009; Wang, Chen, Steketee, & Sharp, 2007). Increased activity at the metabotropic mGlu2/3 receptors, which are involved in presynaptic inhibition of glutamate release, intensified nicotine withdrawal-induced elevations of ICSS thresholds. Antagonists to these receptors alleviated reward deficits induced by nicotine withdrawal (Kenny, Gasparini, & Markou, 2003; Liechti & Markou, 2007). Blockade of the ionotropic AMPA/kainate receptor by 6-nitro-7-sulfamoylbenzo(f)quinoxaline-2, 3-dione (NBQX) precipitated ICSS elevations selectively in nicotine-dependent but not nondependent rats (Kenny et al., 2003). Conversely, stimulation of several AMPA/kainate receptors and their positive modulators, metabotropic mGlu5 receptors, prevented or attenuated nicotine withdrawal behavioral signs (Kenny et al., 2003; Liechti & Markou, 2007). Knockout of mGlu5 receptors elevated ICSS thresholds and somatically expressed signs during spontaneous nicotine withdrawal (Stoker et al., 2012).

Glutamate uptake mechanisms may also impact nicotine physical dependence. Chronic nicotine exposure downregulates mechanisms of glutamate transport, increasing extracellular glutamate (Knackstedt et al., 2009). The antibiotic drug ceftriaxone restores levels of the glutamate transporter GLT-1 and the cysteine/glutamate exchanger. Repeated pretreatment with ceftriaxone during the last 4 days of nicotine infusion prevented mecamylamine-precipitated withdrawal in mice, measured by somatically expressed signs, hyperalgesia, and the plus-maze test for anxiety (Alajaji et al., 2013).

GAMMA AMINOBUTYRIC ACID (GABA)

The GABA B agonist baclofen has been reported to reverse somatically expressed signs of nicotine withdrawal in mice. In addition, baclofen reversed the reduction in striatal DA and 5HT induced by nicotine withdrawal (Varani et al., 2011) as well as a mecamylamine-precipitated increase in $\alpha4\beta2$ binding in a number of brain regions (Varani, Antonelli, & Balerio, 2013). However, the somatically expressed nicotine withdrawal behaviors were prevented in GABA B knockout mice (Varani, Moutinho, Bettler, & Balerio, 2012).

The role, if any, of GABA B receptors in the anhedonic aspect of nicotine withdrawal is far from clear. Several GABA agonists did not differentially affect ICSS thresholds in nicotine-dependent as opposed to nondependent rats (Paterson et al., 2005). In contrast, chronic baclofen attenuated the anhedonic effect of nicotine withdrawal through inhibiting dopamine reuptake in the NAcc (Paterson et al., 2007). However, another study found that both GABA B agonists and antagonists exacerbated the anhedonic effect of nicotine withdrawal (Vlachou et al., 2011). The authors raised the possibility that this puzzling finding might be due to differential effects of the test compounds on presynaptic GABA B autoreceptors and postsynaptic receptors.

ENDOGENOUS OPIATE MECHANISMS

Enkephalins and beta-endorphin are released in response to nicotine administration (Gilbert, Meliska, Williams, & Jensen, 1992; Suh et al., 1995). Thus, chronic nicotine exposure could plausibly cause chronic overstimulation of opiate receptors. Abrupt termination or inhibition of nicotine might then sharply reduce overstimulation of opiate receptors, possibly inducing an opiate abstinence-like state. This hypothesis is now supported by an accumulation of evidence, at least in connection with somatically expressed withdrawal behaviors and withdrawal-induced hyperalgesia.

Most nicotine withdrawal signs in the rat (gasps/writhes, shakes/tremors, teeth chatter/vacuous chewing, ptosis, scratches, and spontaneous ejaculation) are all routinely observed in mild to moderate opiate abstinence syndrome (Malin et al., 1990). Somatically expressed withdrawal behaviors are potently reversed by morphine, even at subanalgesic doses (Malin et al., 1994). Morphine also potently reversed hyperalgesia caused by nicotine withdrawal (Schmidt, Tambeli, Gear, & Levine, 2001), and an active beta-endorphin metabolite reduced the aversiveness of precipitated nicotine withdrawal (Göktalay, Cavun, Levendusky, Hamilton, & Millington, 2006).

The competitive opiate receptor antagonist naloxone consistently precipitates a somatically expressed abstinence syndrome in both rats and mice that have been chronically exposed to nicotine (Adams & Cicero, 1998; Biala, Budzynska, & Kruk, 2005; Carboni et al., 2000; Malin, Lake, Carter, Cunningham, & Wilson, 1993; Watkins, Stinus, Koob, & Markou, 2000). Naloxone-precipitated nicotine withdrawal is highly aversive, as indicated by CPA (Ise, Narita, Nagase, & Suzuki, 2000; Watkins et al., 2000), although it does not raise ICSS thresholds (Watkins et al., 2000). Selective mu and delta opiate receptor antagonists also precipitated CPA in nicotine-dependent rats (Ise et al., 2000). Kappa opiate receptors often act in opposition to other opiate receptors. Chronic nicotine increases striatal levels of the endogenous kappa agonist peptide dynorphin, persisting into the period of withdrawal (Isola, Zhang, Tejwani, Neff, & Hadjiconstantinou, 2008). Two different kappa receptor antagonists attenuated somatically expressed withdrawal behaviors, hyperalgesia, CPA, and anxiety measures in nicotine-abstinent mice (Jackson, Carroll, Negus, & Damaj, 2010). In nicotine-dependent rats, kappa opiate activation intensified somatically expressed nicotine withdrawal behaviors, withdrawal-induced anxiety (plus maze), and CPA, and decreased DA release in the NAcc. Conversely, kappa opiate receptor antagonists reduced the aversiveness of mecamylamine-precipitated nicotine withdrawal as indicated by CPA (Ise, Narita, Nagase, & Suzuki, 2002), as well as somatically expressed withdrawal behaviors (Tejeda, Natividad, Orfila, Torres, & O'Dell, 2012).

Nicotine injection promptly alleviates somatically expressed nicotine withdrawal behaviors (Malin et al., 1992). Yet it fails to do so after injection of naloxone to block opiate receptors (Malin, Lake, Short, et al., 1996). This suggests that nicotine relief of these withdrawal behaviors is mediated through release of endogenous opioid peptides.

Somatically expressed nicotine abstinence syndrome was attenuated in knockout mice lacking the gene for mu opiate receptors (Berrendero, Kieffer, & Maldonado, 2002) as well as the gene for the enkephalin precursor preproenkephalin (Berrendero et al., 2005), but not the gene for delta opiate receptors (Berrendero et al., 2012). However, delta receptor coupling and function in the NAcc and the caudate–putamen are disrupted during withdrawal (McCarthy, Zhang, Neff, & Hadjiconstantinou, 2011). Isola et al. (2002) reported alterations in brain regional endogenous opioid peptide levels during nicotine withdrawal in the mouse. Thus, accumulated evidence suggests that opiate mechanisms contribute at least to somatically expressed withdrawal behaviors and hyperalgesia, and thus to irritability and hypersensitivity in nicotine withdrawal.

NONOPIOID PEPTIDES

Cerebrospinal fluid levels of the nonopioid peptide, neuropeptide FF (NPFF), are increased by chronic opiate receptor stimulation. NPFF has potent antiopiate actions in the brain that may contribute to opiate dependence (Malin et al., 1990). Injection of a systemically active NPFF analog precipitated a withdrawal syndrome, not only in morphine-dependent rats (Malin, Lake, Arcangeli, et al., 1993) but also in nicotine-dependent rats (Malin, Lake, Payne, et al., 1996).

Hypothalamic neuropeptide Y (NPY) is involved in appetite regulation. Nicotine withdrawal resulted in increased feeding induced by NPY administration in the paraventricular hypothalamic nucleus (Bishop, Parker, & Coscina, 2002). Nicotine withdrawal also resulted in increased NPY immunoreactivity in several hypothalamic nuclei. Co-administration of an NPY antagonist with nicotine prevented subsequent withdrawal-induced hyperphagia and weight gain. Acute NPY antagonist administration during nicotine withdrawal also reduced withdrawal-induced overeating (Nakhate, Dandekar, Kokare, & Subhedar, 2009). In contrast, NPY itself significantly reduced the somatically expressed withdrawal signs in both precipitated and spontaneous nicotine withdrawal, though not the ICSS threshold elevation in precipitated withdrawal (Rylkova et al., 2008). Following a week of nicotine abstinence, novelty-seeking rats exhibited depletion of hippocampal and amygdala NPY messenger RNA (mRNA) and increased levels of the Y2 NPY receptor mRNA, as well as increased anxiety measured in the social interaction test. An antagonist to the Y2 receptor reversed all these consequences of nicotine withdrawal (Aydin, Oztan, & Isgor, 2011). Also, genetic knockout of alpha calcitonin gene-related peptide, which modulates nAChR function, significantly reduced somatically expressed withdrawal behaviors (Salmon, Evrard, Damaj, & Changeux, 2004). The role of corticotropin-releasing factor (CRF) is explored in "Chapter 10, Critical Role for Brain Stress Systems in the Negative Affective State Associated With Nicotine Withdrawal" of this book.

SIGNAL TRANSDUCTION MECHANISMS

Increases in cyclic adenosine monophosphate (cAMP) and in nitric oxide synthesis are important mechanisms in opiate withdrawal syndrome. Consistent with a hypothesized role of endogenous opioid peptides in nicotine withdrawal syndrome, cAMP is upregulated in the amygdala, possibly contributing to increased anxiety (Tzavara, Monory, Hanoune, & Nomikos, 2002). Likewise, chronic nicotine exposure increases nitric oxide metabolites in a number of brain regions (Pogun et al., 2000). Several nitric oxide synthase inhibitors have prevented mecamylamine-precipitated nicotine withdrawal syndrome or reversed spontaneous withdrawal syndrome, as indicated by somatically expressed behaviors (Adams & Cicero, 1998; Jain, Mukherjee, & Mohan, 2008; Malin, Lake, Shenoi, et al., 1998).

Finally, calcium channels may participate in nicotine withdrawal syndrome. An antagonist against L-type voltage-regulated calcium channels attenuated mecamylamine-precipitated somatically expressed withdrawal behaviors (Biala & Weglinska, 2005; Jackson et al., 2009) and mecamylamine-precipitated CPA (Budzynska, Polak, & Biala, 2012). In addition, a calcium channel blocker attenuated measures of anxiety, depression, cognitive impairment, and hyperalgesia seen during late phases of nicotine withdrawal (Biala, Polak, Michalak, Kruk-Slomka, & Budzynska, 2014).

CONCLUDING THOUGHTS

Prolonged stimulation of various nAChRs followed by decreased nAChR stimulation provokes adaptations of many, and perhaps most, of the major transmitter and receptor systems in the brain. This helps explain the diversity of nicotine withdrawal phenomena, while providing an abundance of potential molecular targets for modulating the distress and discomforts of smoking cessation.

References

Adams, M. L., & Cicero, T. J. (1998). Nitric oxide mediates mecamylamine- and naloxone-precipitated nicotine withdrawal. *European Journal of Pharmacology, 345*(2), R1–R2.

Alajaji, M., Bowers, M. S., Knackstedt, L., & Damaj, M. I. (2013). Effects of the beta-lactam antibiotic ceftriaxone on nicotine withdrawal and nicotine-induced reinstatement of preference in mice. *Psychopharmacology, 228*(3), 419–426. http://dx.doi.org/10.1007/s00213-013-3047-3.

Andersson, K., Fuxe, K., Eneroth, P., Jansson, A., & Harfstrand, A. (1989). Effects of withdrawal from chronic exposure to cigarette smoke on hypothalamic and preoptic catecholamine nerve terminal systems and on the secretion of pituitary hormones in the male rat. *Naunyn-Schmiedeberg's Archives of Pharmacology, 339*(4), 387–396.

Aydin, C., Oztan, O., & Isgor, C. (2011). Vulnerability to nicotine abstinence-related social anxiety-like behavior: molecular correlates in neuropeptide Y, Y2 receptor and corticotropin releasing factor. *Neuroscience Letters, 490*(3), 220–225. http://dx.doi.org/10.1016/j.neulet.2010.12.056.

Balfour, D. J. (2004). The neurobiology of tobacco dependence: a preclinical perspective on the role of the dopamine projections to the nucleus accumbens [corrected]. *Nicotine & Tobacco Research, 6*(6), 899–912.

Barik, J., & Wonnacott, S. (2006). Indirect modulation by alpha7 nicotinic acetylcholine receptors of noradrenaline release in rat hippocampal slices: interaction with glutamate and GABA systems and effect of nicotine withdrawal. *Molecular Pharmacology, 69*(2), 618–628. http://dx.doi.org/10.1124/mol.105.018184.

Berrendero, F., Kieffer, B. L., & Maldonado, R. (2002). Attenuation of nicotine-induced antinociception, rewarding effects, and dependence in mu-opioid receptor knock-out mice. *The Journal of Neuroscience, 22*(24), 10935–10940.

Berrendero, F., Mendizabal, V., Robledo, P., Galeote, L., Bilkei-Gorzo, A., Zimmer, A., & Maldonado, R. (2005). Nicotine-induced antinociception, rewarding effects, and physical dependence are decreased in mice lacking the preproenkephalin gene. *The Journal of Neuroscience, 25*(5), 1103–1112. http://dx.doi.org/10.1523/JNEUROSCI.3008-04.2005.

Berrendero, F., Plaza-Zabala, A., Galeote, L., Flores, A., Bura, S. A., Kieffer, B. L., & Maldonado, R. (2012). Influence of delta-opioid receptors in the behavioral effects of nicotine. *Neuropsychopharmacology, 37*(10), 2332–2344. http://dx.doi.org/10.1038/npp.2012.88.

Besson, M., David, V., Suarez, S., Cormier, A., Cazala, P., Changeux, J. P., & Granon, S. (2006). Genetic dissociation of two behaviors associated with nicotine addiction: beta-2 containing nicotinic receptors are involved in nicotine reinforcement but not in withdrawal syndrome. *Psychopharmacology, 187*(2), 189–199. http://dx.doi.org/10.1007/s00213-006-0418-z.

Biala, G., Budzynska, B., & Kruk, M. (2005). Naloxone precipitates nicotine abstinence syndrome and attenuates nicotine-induced antinociception in mice. *Pharmacological Reports: PR, 57*(6), 755–760.

Biala, G., Polak, P., Michalak, A., Kruk-Slomka, M., & Budzynska, B. (2014). Influence of calcium channel antagonists on nonsomatic signs of nicotine and D-amphetamine withdrawal in mice. *Pharmacological Reports, 66*(2), 212–222. http://dx.doi.org/10.1016/j.pharep.2014.02.003.

Biala, G., & Weglinska, B. (2005). Blockade of the expression of mecamylamine-precipitated nicotine withdrawal by calcium channel antagonists. *Pharmacological Research, 51*(5), 483–488. http://dx.doi.org/10.1016/j.phrs.2004.11.009.

Bishop, C., Parker, G. C., & Coscina, D. V. (2002). Nicotine and its withdrawal alter feeding induced by paraventricular hypothalamic injections of neuropeptide Y in Sprague-Dawley rats. *Psychopharmacology, 162*(3), 265–272. http://dx.doi.org/10.1007/s00213-002-1101-7.

Bohus, B., Koolhaas, J. M., Luiten, P. G., Korte, S. M., Roozendaal, B., & Wiersma, A. (1996). The neurobiology of the central nucleus of the amygdala in relation to neuroendocrine and autonomic outflow. *Progress in Brain Research, 107*, 447–460.

Bruijnzeel, A. W., Bishnoi, M., van Tuijl, I. A., Keijzers, K. F., Yavarovich, K. R., Pasek, T. M., … Yamada, H. (2010). Effects of prazosin, clonidine, and propranolol on the elevations in brain reward thresholds and somatic signs associated with nicotine withdrawal in rats. *Psychopharmacology, 212*(4), 485–499. http://dx.doi.org/10.1007/s00213-010-1970-.

Bruijnzeel, A. W., & Markou, A. (2004). Adaptations in cholinergic transmission in the ventral tegmental area associated with the affective signs of nicotine withdrawal in rats. *Neuropharmacology, 47*(4), 572–579. http://dx.doi.org/10.1016/j.neuropharm.2004.05.005.

Budzynska, B., Polak, P., & Biala, G. (2012). Effects of calcium channel antagonists on the motivational effects of nicotine and morphine in conditioned place aversion paradigm. *Behavioural Brain Research, 228*(1), 144–150. http://dx.doi.org/10.1016/j.bbr.2011.12.003.

Carboni, E., Bortone, L., Giua, C., & Di Chiara, G. (2000). Dissociation of physical abstinence signs from changes in extracellular dopamine in the nucleus accumbens and in the prefrontal cortex of nicotine dependent rats. *Drug and Alcohol Dependence, 58*(1–2), 93–102.

Chang, B., Daniele, C. A., Gallagher, K., Madonia, M., Mitchum, R. D., Barrett, L., … McGehee, D. S. (2011). Nicotinic excitation of serotonergic projections from dorsal raphe to the nucleus accumbens. *Journal of Neurophysiology, 106*(2), 801–808. http://dx.doi.org/10.1152/jn.00575.2010.

Cippitelli, A., Astarita, G., Duranti, A., Caprioli, G., Ubaldi, M., Stopponi, S., & Ciccocioppo, R. (2011). Endocannabinoid regulation of acute and protracted nicotine withdrawal: effect of FAAH inhibition. *PLoS One, 6*(11), http://dx.doi.org/10.1371/journal.pone.0028142.

Corrigall, W. A., & Coen, K. M. (1991). Selective dopamine antagonists reduce nicotine self-administration. *Psychopharmacology, 104*(2), 171–176.

Costall, B., Jones, B. J., Kelly, M. E., Naylor, R. J., Onaivi, E. S., & Tyers, M. B. (1990a). Ondansetron inhibits a behavioural consequence of withdrawing from drugs of abuse. *Pharmacology, Biochemistry, and Behavior, 36*(2), 339–344.

Costall, B., Jones, B. J., Kelly, M. E., Naylor, R. J., Onaivi, E. S., & Tyers, M. B. (1990b). Sites of action of ondansetron to inhibit withdrawal from drugs of abuse. *Pharmacology, Biochemistry, and Behavior, 36*(1), 97–104.

Damaj, M. I., Kao, W., & Martin, B. R. (2003). Characterization of spontaneous and precipitated nicotine withdrawal in the mouse. *The Journal of Pharmacology and Experimental Therapeutics, 307*(2), 526–534. http://dx.doi.org/10.1124/jpet.103.054908.

Dani, J. A., & De Biasi, M. (2013). Mesolimbic dopamine and habenulo-interpeduncular pathways in nicotine withdrawal. *Cold Spring Harbor Perspectives in Medicine, 3*(6). http://dx.doi.org/10.1101/cshperspect.a012138.

Davis, J. A., & Gould, T. J. (2007). Atomoxetine reverses nicotine withdrawal-associated deficits in contextual fear conditioning. *Neuropsychopharmacology, 32*(9), 2011–2019. http://dx.doi.org/10.1038/sj.npp.1301315.

Duchemin, A. M., Zhang, H., Neff, N. H., & Hadjiconstantinou, M. (2009). Increased expression of VMAT2 in dopaminergic neurons during nicotine withdrawal. *Neuroscience Letters, 467*(2), 182–186. http://dx.doi.org/10.1016/j.neulet.2009.10.038.

Epping-Jordan, M. P., Watkins, S. S., Koob, G. F., & Markou, A. (1998). Dramatic decreases in brain reward function during nicotine withdrawal. *Nature, 393*(6680), 76–79. http://dx.doi.org/10.1038/30001.

Fung, Y. K., Schmid, M. J., Anderson, T. M., & Lau, Y. S. (1996). Effects of nicotine withdrawal on central dopaminergic systems. *Pharmacology, Biochemistry, and Behavior, 53*(3), 635–640.

Gilbert, D. G., Meliska, C. J., Williams, C. L., & Jensen, R. A. (1992). Subjective correlates of cigarette-smoking-induced elevations of peripheral beta-endorphin and cortisol. *Psychopharmacology, 106*(2), 275–281.

Göktalay, G., Cavun, S., Levendusky, M. C., Hamilton, J. R., & Millington, W. R. (2006). Glycyl-glutamine inhibits nicotine conditioned place preference and withdrawal. *European Journal of Pharmacology, 530*(1–2), 95–102. http://dx.doi.org/10.1016/j.ejphar.2005.11.034.

Grabus, S. D., Martin, B. R., Batman, A. M., Tyndale, R. F., Sellers, E., & Damaj, M. I. (2005). Nicotine physical dependence and tolerance in the mouse following chronic oral administration. *Psychopharmacology, 178*(2–3), 183–192. http://dx.doi.org/10.1007/s00213-004-2007-3.

Grieder, T. E., Sellings, L. H., Vargas-Perez, H., Ting, A. K. R., Siu, E. C., Tyndale, R. F., & van der Kooy, D. (2010). Dopaminergic signaling mediates the motivational response underlying the opponent process to chronic but not acute nicotine. *Neuropsychopharmacology, 35*(4), 943–954. http://dx.doi.org/10.1038/npp.2009.198.

Grunberg, N. E., Bowen, D. J., & Winders, S. E. (1986). Effects of nicotine on body weight and food consumption in female rats. *Psychopharmacology, 90*(1), 101–105.

Guilloux, J. P., David, D. J., Guiard, B. P., Chenu, F., Reperant, C., Toth, M., … Gardier, A. M. (2006). Blockade of 5-HT1A receptors by (+/−)-pindolol potentiates cortical 5-HT outflow, but not antidepressant-like activity of paroxetine: microdialysis and behavioral approaches in 5-HT1A receptor knockout mice. *Neuropsychopharmacology, 31*(10), 2162–2172. http://dx.doi.org/10.1038/sj.npp.1301019.

Hadjiconstantinou, M., Duchemin, A. M., Zhang, H., & Neff, N. H. (2011). Enhanced dopamine transporter function in striatum during nicotine withdrawal. *Synapse, 65*(2), 91–98. http://dx.doi.org/10.1002/syn.20820.

Halladay, A. K., Schwartz, M., Wagner, G. C., Iba, M. M., Sekowski, A., & Fisher, H. (1999). Efficacy of providing nicotine in a liquid diet to rats. *Proceedings of the Society for Experimental Biology and Medicine, 221*(3), 215–223.

Harrison, A. A., Liem, Y. T., & Markou, A. (2001). Fluoxetine combined with a serotonin-1A receptor antagonist reversed reward deficits observed during nicotine and amphetamine withdrawal in rats. *Neuropsychopharmacology, 25*(1), 55–71. http://dx.doi.org/10.1016/S0893-133X(00)00237-2.

Helton, D. R., Modlin, D. L., Tizzano, J. P., & Rasmussen, K. (1993). Nicotine withdrawal: a behavioral assessment using schedule controlled responding, locomotor activity, and sensorimotor reactivity. *Psychopharmacology, 113*(2), 205–210.

Hildebrand, B. E., Nomikos, G. G., Hertel, P., Schilstrom, B., & Svensson, T. H. (1998). Reduced dopamine output in the nucleus accumbens but not in the medial prefrontal cortex in rats displaying a mecamylamine-precipitated nicotine withdrawal syndrome. *Brain Research, 779*(1–2), 214–225.

Hildebrand, B. E., Panagis, G., Svensson, T. H., & Nomikos, G. G. (1999). Behavioral and biochemical manifestations of mecamylamine-precipitated nicotine withdrawal in the rat: role of nicotinic receptors in the ventral tegmental area. *Neuropsychopharmacology, 21*(4), 560–574. http://dx.doi.org/10.1016/S0893-133X(99)00055-X.

Hughes, J. R., & Hatsukami, D. (1986). Signs and symptoms of tobacco withdrawal. *Archives of General Psychiatry, 43*(3), 289–294.

Ise, Y., Narita, M., Nagase, H., & Suzuki, T. (2000). Modulation of opioidergic system on mecamylamine-precipitated nicotine-withdrawal aversion in rats. *Psychopharmacology, 151*(1), 49–54.

Ise, Y., Narita, M., Nagase, H., & Suzuki, T. (2002). Modulation of kappa-opioidergic systems on mecamylamine-precipitated nicotine-withdrawal aversion in rats. *Neuroscience Letters, 323*(2), 164–166.

Isola, R., Vogelsberg, V., Wemlinger, T. A., Neff, N. H., & Hadjiconstantinou, M. (1999). Nicotine abstinence in the mouse. *Brain Research, 850*(1–2), 189–196.

Isola, R., Zhang, H., Duchemin, A. M., Tejwani, G. A., Neff, N. H., & Hadjiconstantinou, M. (2002). Met-enkephalin and preproenkephalin mRNA changes in the striatum of the nicotine abstinence mouse. *Neuroscience Letters, 325*(1), 67–71.

Isola, R., Zhang, H., Tejwani, G. A., Neff, N. H., & Hadjiconstantinou, M. (2008). Dynorphin and prodynorphin mRNA changes in the striatum during nicotine withdrawal. *Synapse, 62*(6), 448–455. http://dx.doi.org/10.1002/syn.20515.

Jackson, K. J., Carroll, F. I., Negus, S. S., & Damaj, M. I. (2010). Effect of the selective kappa-opioid receptor antagonist JDTic on nicotine antinociception, reward, and withdrawal in the mouse. *Psychopharmacology, 210*(2), 285–294. http://dx.doi.org/10.1007/s00213-010-1803-1.

Jackson, K. J., Kota, D. H., Martin, B. R., & Damaj, M. I. (2009). The role of various nicotinic receptor subunits and factors influencing nicotine conditioned place aversion. *Neuropharmacology, 56*(6–7), 970–974. http://dx.doi.org/10.1016/j.neuropharm.2009.01.023.

Jackson, K. J., Martin, B. R., Changeux, J. P., & Damaj, M. I. (2008). Differential role of nicotinic acetylcholine receptor subunits in physical and affective nicotine withdrawal signs. *The Journal of Pharmacology and Experimental Therapeutics, 325*(1), 302–312. http://dx.doi.org/10.1124/jpet.107.132977.

Jackson, K. J., Sanjakdar, S. S., Muldoon, P. P., McIntosh, J. M., & Damaj, M. I. (2013). The alpha3beta4* nicotinic acetylcholine receptor subtype mediates nicotine reward and physical nicotine withdrawal signs independently of the alpha5 subunit in the mouse. *Neuropharmacology, 70*, 228–235. http://dx.doi.org/10.1016/j.neuropharm.2013.01.017.

Jain, R., Mukherjee, K., & Mohan, D. (2008). Effects of nitric oxide synthase inhibitors in attenuating nicotine withdrawal in rats. *Pharmacology, Biochemistry, and Behavior, 88*(4), 473–480. http://dx.doi.org/10.1016/j.pbb.2007.09.021.

Jonkman, S., & Markou, A. (2006). Blockade of nicotinic acetylcholine or dopamine D1-like receptors in the central nucleus of the amygdala or the bed nucleus of the stria terminalis does not precipitate nicotine withdrawal in nicotine-dependent rats. *Neuroscience Letters, 400*(1–2), 140–145. http://dx.doi.org/10.1016/j.neulet.2006.02.030.

Kenny, P. J., Chartoff, E., Roberto, M., Carlezon, W. A., Jr., & Markou, A. (2009). NMDA receptors regulate nicotine-enhanced brain reward function and intravenous nicotine self-administration: role of the ventral tegmental area and central nucleus of the amygdala. *Neuropsychopharmacology, 34*(2), 266–281. http://dx.doi.org/10.1038/npp.2008.58.

Kenny, P. J., Gasparini, F., & Markou, A. (2003). Group II metabotropic and alpha-amino-3-hydroxy-5-methyl-4-isoxazole propionate (AMPA)/kainate glutamate receptors regulate the deficit in brain reward function associated with nicotine withdrawal in rats. *The Journal of Pharmacology and Experimental Therapeutics, 306*(3), 1068–1076. http://dx.doi.org/10.1124/jpet.103.052027.

Knackstedt, L. A., LaRowe, S., Mardikian, P., Malcolm, R., Upadhyaya, H., Hedden, S., ... Kalivas, P. W. (2009). The role of cystine-glutamate exchange in nicotine dependence in rats and humans. *Biological Psychiatry, 65*(10), 841–845. http://dx.doi.org/10.1016/j.biopsych.2008.10.040.

LeSage, M. G., Burroughs, D., & Pentel, P. R. (2006). Effects of nicotine withdrawal on performance under a progressive-ratio schedule of sucrose pellet delivery in rats. *Pharmacology, Biochemistry, and Behavior, 83*(4), 585–591. http://dx.doi.org/10.1016/j.pbb.2006.03.021.

Levin, E. D., Morgan, M. M., Galvez, C., & Ellison, G. D. (1987). Chronic nicotine and withdrawal effects on body weight and food and water consumption in female rats. *Physiology & Behavior, 39*(4), 441–444.

Liechti, M. E., & Markou, A. (2007). Interactive effects of the mGlu5 receptor antagonist MPEP and the mGlu2/3 receptor antagonist LY341495 on nicotine self-administration and reward deficits associated with nicotine withdrawal in rats. *European Journal of Pharmacology, 554*(2–3), 164–174. http://dx.doi.org/10.1016/j.ejphar.2006.10.011.

Lindblom, N., de Villiers, S. H., Semenova, S., Kalayanov, G., Gordon, S., Schilstrom, B., ... Svensson, T. H. (2005). Active immunisation against nicotine blocks the reward facilitating effects of nicotine and partially prevents nicotine withdrawal in the rat as measured by dopamine output in the nucleus accumbens, brain reward thresholds and somatic signs. *Naunyn-Schmiedeberg's Archives of Pharmacology, 372*(3), 182–194. http://dx.doi.org/10.1007/s00210-005-0019-0.

Malin, D. H., & Goyarzu, P. (2009). Rodent models of nicotine withdrawal syndrome. *Handbook of Experimental Pharmacology, 192,* 401–434. http://dx.doi.org/10.1007/978-3-540-69248-5_14.

Malin, D. H., Lake, J. R., Arcangeli, K. R., Deshotel, K. D., Hausam, D. D., Witherspoon, W. E., ... Burgess, K. (1993). Subcutaneous injection of an analog of neuropeptide FF precipitates morphine abstinence syndrome. *Life Sciences, 53*(17), PL261–PL266.

Malin, D. H., Lake, J. R., Carter, V. A., Cunningham, J. S., Hebert, K. M., Conrad, D. L., & Wilson, O. B. (1994). The nicotinic antagonist mecamylamine precipitates nicotine abstinence syndrome in the rat. *Psychopharmacology, 115*(1–2), 180–184.

Malin, D. H., Lake, J. R., Carter, V. A., Cunningham, J. S., & Wilson, O. B. (1993). Naloxone precipitates nicotine abstinence syndrome in the rat. *Psychopharmacology, 112*(2–3), 339–342.

Malin, D. H., Lake, J. R., Hammond, M. V., Fowler, D. E., Rogillio, R. B., Brown, S. L., ... Yang, H. Y. (1990). FMRF-NH2-like mammalian octapeptide: possible role in opiate dependence and abstinence. *Peptides, 11*(5), 969–972.

Malin, D. H., Lake, J. R., Newlin-Maultsby, P., Roberts, L. K., Lanier, J. G., Carter, V. A., ... Wilson, O. B. (1992). Rodent model of nicotine abstinence syndrome. *Pharmacology, Biochemistry, and Behavior, 43*(3), 779–784.

Malin, D. H., Lake, J. R., Payne, M. C., Short, P. E., Carter, V. A., Cunningham, J. S., & Wilson, O. B. (1996). Nicotine alleviation of nicotine abstinence syndrome is naloxone-reversible. *Pharmacology, Biochemistry, and Behavior, 53*(1), 81–85.

Malin, D. H., Lake, J. R., Schopen, C. K., Kirk, J. W., Sailer, E. E., Lawless, B. A., ... Rajan, N. (1997). Nicotine abstinence syndrome precipitated by central but not peripheral hexamethonium. *Pharmacology, Biochemistry, and Behavior, 58*(3), 695–699.

Malin, D. H., Lake, J. R., Shenoi, M., Upchurch, T. P., Johnson, S. C., Schweinle, W. E., & Cadle, C. D. (1998). The nitric oxide synthesis inhibitor nitro-L-arginine (L-NNA) attenuates nicotine abstinence syndrome in the rat. *Psychopharmacology, 140*(3), 371–377.

Malin, D. H., Lake, J. R., Short, P. E., Blossman, J. B., Lawless, B. A., Schopen, C. K., … Wilson, O. B. (1996). Nicotine abstinence syndrome precipitated by an analog of neuropeptide FF. *Pharmacology, Biochemistry, and Behavior, 54*(3), 581–585.

Malin, D. H., Lake, J. R., Upchurch, T. P., Shenoi, M., Rajan, N., & Schweinle, W. E. (1998). Nicotine abstinence syndrome precipitated by the competitive nicotinic antagonist dihydro-beta-erythroidine. *Pharmacology, Biochemistry, and Behavior, 60*(3), 609–613.

Malin, D. H., Moon, W. D., Goyarzu, P., Barclay, E., Magallanes, N., Vela, A. J., … Mills, W. R. (2013). Inhibition of monoamine oxidase isoforms modulates nicotine withdrawal syndrome in the rat. *Life Sciences, 93*(12–14), 448–453. http://dx.doi.org/10.1016/j.lfs.2013.08.006.

Mannucci, C., Tedesco, M., Bellomo, M., Caputi, A. P., & Calapai, G. (2006). Long-term effects of nicotine on the forced swimming test in mice: an experimental model for the study of depression caused by smoke. *Neurochemistry International, 49*(5), 481–486. http://dx.doi.org/10.1016/j.neuint.2006.03.010.

Markou, A., & Paterson, N. E. (2001). The nicotinic antagonist methyllycaconitine has differential effects on nicotine self-administration and nicotine withdrawal in the rat. *Nicotine & Tobacco Research, 3*(4), 361–373. http://dx.doi.org/10.1080/14622200110073380.

McCarthy, M. J., Zhang, H., Neff, N. H., & Hadjiconstantinou, M. (2011). Desensitization of delta-opioid receptors in nucleus accumbens during nicotine withdrawal. *Psychopharmacology, 213*(4), 735–744. http://dx.doi.org/10.1007/s00213-010-2028-z.

Nakhate, K. T., Dandekar, M. P., Kokare, D. M., & Subhedar, N. K. (2009). Involvement of neuropeptide Y Y(1) receptors in the acute, chronic and withdrawal effects of nicotine on feeding and body weight in rats. *European Journal of Pharmacology, 609*(1–3), 78–87. http://dx.doi.org/10.1016/j.ejphar.2009.03.008.

Nomikos, G. G., Hildebrand, B. E., Panagis, G., & Svensson, T. H. (1999). Nicotine withdrawal in the rat: role of alpha7 nicotinic receptors in the ventral tegmental area. *Neuroreport, 10*(4), 697–702.

O'Dell, L. E., Chen, S. A., Smith, R. T., Specio, S. E., Balster, R. L., Paterson, N. E., … Koob, G. F. (2007). Extended access to nicotine self-administration leads to dependence: circadian measures, withdrawal measures, and extinction behavior in rats. *The Journal of Pharmacology and Experimental Therapeutics, 320*(1), 180–193. http://dx.doi.org/10.1124/jpet.106.105270.

O'Dell, L. E., & Koob, G. F. (2007). 'Nicotine deprivation effect' in rats with intermittent 23-hour access to intravenous nicotine self-administration. *Pharmacology, Biochemistry, and Behavior, 86*(2), 346–353. http://dx.doi.org/10.1016/j.pbb.2007.01.004.

Ohmura, Y., Jutkiewicz, E. M., & Domino, E. F. (2011). L-DOPA attenuates nicotine withdrawal-induced behaviors in rats. *Pharmacology, Biochemistry, and Behavior, 98*(4), 552–558. http://dx.doi.org/10.1016/j.pbb.2011.02.007.

Ohmura, Y., Jutkiewicz, E. M., Yoshioka, M., & Domino, E. F. (2011). 5-Hydroxytryptophan attenuates somatic signs of nicotine withdrawal. *Journal of Pharmacological Sciences, 117*(2), 121–124.

Panagis, G., Hildebrand, B. E., Svensson, T. H., & Nomikos, G. G. (2000). Selective c-fos induction and decreased dopamine release in the central nucleus of amygdala in rats displaying a mecamylamine-precipitated nicotine withdrawal syndrome. *Synapse, 35*(1), 15–25. http://dx.doi.org/10.1002/(SICI)1098-2396(200001)35:1<15::AID-SYN3>3.0.CO;2-C.

Paterson, N. E., Balfour, D. J., & Markou, A. (2007). Chronic bupropion attenuated the anhedonic component of nicotine withdrawal in rats via inhibition of dopamine reuptake in the nucleus accumbens shell. *The European Journal of Neuroscience, 25*(10), 3099–3108. http://dx.doi.org/10.1111/j.1460-9568.2007.05546.x.

Paterson, N. E., Bruijnzeel, A. W., Kenny, P. J., Wright, C. D., Froestl, W., & Markou, A. (2005). Prolonged nicotine exposure does not alter GABA(B) receptor-mediated regulation of brain reward function. *Neuropharmacology, 49*(7), 953–962. http://dx.doi.org/10.1016/j.neuropharm.2005.04.031.

Paterson, N. E., & Markou, A. (2004). Prolonged nicotine dependence associated with extended access to nicotine self-administration in rats. *Psychopharmacology, 173*(1–2), 64–72. http://dx.doi.org/10.1007/s00213-003-1692-7.

Paterson, N. E., Semenova, S., & Markou, A. (2008). The effects of chronic versus acute desipramine on nicotine withdrawal and nicotine self-administration in the rat. *Psychopharmacology, 198*(3), 351–362. http://dx.doi.org/10.1007/s00213-008-1144-5.

Picciotto, M. R., Zoli, M., Rimondini, R., Lena, C., Marubio, L. M., Pich, E. M., … Changeux, J. P. (1998). Acetylcholine receptors containing the beta2 subunit are involved in the reinforcing properties of nicotine. *Nature, 391*(6663), 173–177. http://dx.doi.org/10.1038/34413.

Pogun, S., Demirgoren, S., Taskiran, D., Kanit, L., Yilmaz, O., Koylu, E. O., … London, E. D. (2000). Nicotine modulates nitric oxide in rat brain. *European Neuropsychopharmacology, 10*(6), 463–472.

Rada, P., Jensen, K., & Hoebel, B. G. (2001). Effects of nicotine and mecamylamine-induced withdrawal on extracellular dopamine and acetylcholine in the rat nucleus accumbens. *Psychopharmacology, 157*(1), 105–110.

Radke, A. K., & Gewirtz, J. C. (2012). Increased dopamine receptor activity in the nucleus accumbens shell ameliorates anxiety during drug withdrawal. *Neuropsychopharmacology, 37*(11), 2405–2415. http://dx.doi.org/10.1038/npp.2012.97.

Rahman, S., Zhang, J., Engleman, E. A., & Corrigall, W. A. (2004). Neuroadaptive changes in the mesoaccumbens dopamine system after chronic nicotine self-administration: a microdialysis study. *Neuroscience, 129*(2), 415–424. http://dx.doi.org/10.1016/j.neuroscience.2004.08.010.

Rasmussen, K., Calligaro, D. O., Czachura, J. F., Dreshfield-Ahmad, L. J., Evans, D. C., Hemrick-Luecke, S. K., … Xu, Y. C. (2000). The novel 5-Hydroxytryptamine(1A) antagonist LY426965: effects on nicotine withdrawal and interactions with fluoxetine. *The Journal of Pharmacology and Experimental Therapeutics, 294*(2), 688–700.

Ribeiro, E. B., Bettiker, R. L., Bogdanov, M., & Wurtman, R. J. (1993). Effects of systemic nicotine on serotonin release in rat brain. *Brain Research, 621*(2), 311–318.

Rylkova, D., Boissoneault, J., Isaac, S., Prado, M., Shah, H. P., & Bruijnzeel, A. W. (2008). Effects of NPY and the specific Y1 receptor agonist [D-His(26)]-NPY on the deficit in brain reward function and somatic signs associated with nicotine withdrawal in rats. *Neuropeptides, 42*(3), 215–227. http://dx.doi.org/10.1016/j.npep.2008.03.004.

Salas, R., Pieri, F., & De Biasi, M. (2004). Decreased signs of nicotine withdrawal in mice null for the beta4 nicotinic acetylcholine receptor subunit. *The Journal of Neuroscience, 24*(45), 10035–10039. http://dx.doi.org/10.1523/JNEUROSCI.1939-04.2004.

Salmon, A. M., Evrard, A., Damaj, I., & Changeux, J. P. (2004). Reduction of withdrawal signs after chronic nicotine exposure of alpha-calcitonin gene-related peptide knock-out mice. *Neuroscience Letters, 360*(1–2), 73–76. http://dx.doi.org/10.1016/j.neulet.2004.02.031.

Schmidt, B. L., Tambeli, C. H., Gear, R. W., & Levine, J. D. (2001). Nicotine withdrawal hyperalgesia and opioid-mediated analgesia depend on nicotine receptors in nucleus accumbens. *Neuroscience, 106*(1), 129–136.

Semenova, S., & Markou, A. (2010). The alpha2 adrenergic receptor antagonist idazoxan, but not the serotonin-2A receptor antagonist M100907, partially attenuated reward deficits associated with nicotine, but not amphetamine, withdrawal in rats. *European Neuropsychopharmacology, 20*(10), 731–746. http://dx.doi.org/10.1016/j.euroneuro.2010.05.003.

Shoaib, M., & Bizarro, L. (2005). Deficits in a sustained attention task following nicotine withdrawal in rats. *Psychopharmacology, 178*(2–3), 211–222. http://dx.doi.org/10.1007/s00213-004-2004-6.

Siggins, G. R., Martin, G., Roberto, M., Nie, Z., Madamba, S., & De Lecea, L. (2003). Glutamatergic transmission in opiate and alcohol dependence. *Annals of the New York Academy of Sciences, 1003*, 196–211.

Sperling, R., & Commons, K. G. (2011). Shifting topographic activation and 5-HT1A receptor-mediated inhibition of dorsal raphe serotonin neurons produced by nicotine exposure and withdrawal. *The European Journal of Neuroscience, 33*(10), 1866–1875. http://dx.doi.org/10.1111/j.1460-9568.2011.07677.x.

Stoker, A. K., Olivier, B., & Markou, A. (2012). Role of alpha7- and beta4-containing nicotinic acetylcholine receptors in the affective and somatic aspects of nicotine withdrawal: studies in knockout mice. *Behavior Genetics, 42*(3), 423–436. http://dx.doi.org/10.1007/s10519-011-9511-0.

Suemaru, K., Araki, H., Kitamura, Y., Yasuda, K., & Gomita, Y. (2001). Cessation of chronic nicotine administration enhances wet-dog shake responses to 5-HT2 receptor stimulation in rats. *Psychopharmacology, 159*(1), 38–41. http://dx.doi.org/10.1007/s002130100866.

Suh, H. W., Hudson, P. M., McMillian, M. K., Das, K. P., Wilson, B. C., Wu, G. C., & Hong, J. S. (1995). Long-term stimulation of nicotinic receptors is required to increase proenkephalin A mRNA levels and the delayed secretion of [Met5]-enkephalin in bovine adrenal medullary chromaffin cells. *The Journal of Pharmacology and Experimental Therapeutics, 275*(3), 1663–1670.

Suzuki, T., Ise, Y., Mori, T., & Misawa, M. (1997). Attenuation of mecamylamine-precipitated nicotine-withdrawal aversion by the 5-HT3 receptor antagonist ondansetron. *Life Sciences, 61*(16), PL249–254.

Suzuki, T., Ise, Y., Tsuda, M., Maeda, J., & Misawa, M. (1996). Mecamylamine-precipitated nicotine-withdrawal aversion in rats. *European Journal of Pharmacology, 314*(3), 281–284.

Tejeda, H. A., Natividad, L. A., Orfila, J. E., Torres, O. V., & O'Dell, L. E. (2012). Dysregulation of kappa-opioid receptor systems by chronic nicotine modulate the nicotine withdrawal syndrome in an age-dependent manner. *Psychopharmacology, 224*(2), 289–301. http://dx.doi.org/10.1007/s00213-012-2752-7.

Tzavara, E. T., Monory, K., Hanoune, J., & Nomikos, G. G. (2002). Nicotine withdrawal syndrome: behavioural distress and selective up-regulation of the cyclic AMP pathway in the amygdala. *The European Journal of Neuroscience, 16*(1), 149–153.

Varani, A. P., Antonelli, M. C., & Balerio, G. N. (2013). Mecamylamine-precipitated nicotine withdrawal syndrome and its prevention with baclofen: an autoradiographic study of alpha4beta2 nicotinic acetylcholine receptors in mice. *Progress in Neuro-Psychopharmacology & Biological Psychiatry, 44*, 217–225. http://dx.doi.org/10.1016/j.pnpbp.2013.02.016.

Varani, A. P., Moutinho, L. M., Bettler, B., & Balerio, G. N. (2012). Acute behavioural responses to nicotine and nicotine withdrawal syndrome are modified in GABA(B1) knockout mice. *Neuropharmacology, 63*(5), 863–872. http://dx.doi.org/10.1016/j.neuropharm.2012.06.006.

Varani, A. P., Moutinho, L. M., Calvo, M., & Balerio, G. N. (2011). Ability of baclofen to prevent somatic manifestations and neurochemical changes during nicotine withdrawal. *Drug and Alcohol Dependence, 119*(1–2), e5–12. http://dx.doi.org/10.1016/j.drugalcdep.2011.05.017.

Vlachou, S., Paterson, N. E., Guery, S., Kaupmann, K., Froestl, W., Banerjee, D., … Markou, A. (2011). Both GABA(B) receptor activation and blockade exacerbated anhedonic aspects of nicotine withdrawal in rats. *European Journal of Pharmacology, 655*(1–3), 52–58. http://dx.doi.org/10.1016/j.ejphar.2011.01.009.

Wang, F., Chen, H., Steketee, J. D., & Sharp, B. M. (2007). Upregulation of ionotropic glutamate receptor subunits within specific mesocorticolimbic regions during chronic nicotine self-administration. *Neuropsychopharmacology, 32*(1), 103–109. http://dx.doi.org/10.1038/sj.npp.1301033.

Watkins, S. S., Stinus, L., Koob, G. F., & Markou, A. (2000). Reward and somatic changes during precipitated nicotine withdrawal in rats: centrally and peripherally mediated effects. *The Journal of Pharmacology and Experimental Therapeutics, 292*(3), 1053–1064.

Yasuda, K., Suemaru, K., Araki, H., & Gomita, Y. (2002). Effect of nicotine cessation on the central serotonergic systems in mice: involvement of 5-HT(2) receptors. *Naunyn-Schmiedeberg's Archives of Pharmacology, 366*(3), 276–281. http://dx.doi.org/10.1007/s00210-002-0592-4.

Zarevics, P., & Setler, P. E. (1979). Simultaneous rate-independent and rate-dependent assessment of intracranial self-stimulation: evidence for the direct involvement of dopamine in brain reinforcement mechanisms. *Brain Research, 169*(3), 499–512.

The Cannabinoid System in Nicotine Dependence and Withdrawal

M.E. McIlwain[1,2], A. Minassian[2], W. Perry[2]

[1]University of Auckland, Auckland, New Zealand; [2]University of California San Diego, La Jolla, CA, United States

Receptors	
CB1	Cannabinoid receptor type 1
CB2	Cannabinoid receptor type 2
nAChR	Nicotinic acetylcholine receptor
PPAR-α	Peroxisome proliferator-activated receptor
Endocannabinoids	
AEA	N-arachidonoylethanolamine, anandamide
2-AG	2-Arachidonylglycerol
OEA	Oleoylethanolamine; monosaturated analog of anandamide
PEA	Palmitoylethanolamide; enhances anandamide activity through "entourage effect," not strictly an endocannabinoid as no CB1/CB2 receptor affinity
Exogenous Ligands	
THC	Δ^9-tetrahydrocannabinol, CB1 agonist
CBD	Cannabidiol, CB1/CB2 inverse agonist/antagonist
Rimonabant/SR141716a	CB1 receptor inverse agonist/antagonist
AM251	CB1 receptor inverse agonist/antagonist

Negative Affective States and Cognitive Impairments in Nicotine Dependence
http://dx.doi.org/10.1016/B978-0-12-802574-1.00009-0

Exogenous Ligands	
WIN55,212-2	Nonselective CB1/CB2 agonist
JWH133	CB2 agonist
AM1241	CB2 agonist
AM630	CB2 antagonist
SR144528	CB2 antagonist
Mecamylamine	Nicotinic receptor antagonist

Enzymes	
FAAH	Fatty acid amide hydrolase (degrades AEA)
MAGL	Monoacylglycerol lipase (degrades 2-AG)

Enzyme Inhibitors	
URB597	FAAH inhibitor; increases AEA levels
JZL184	MAGL inhibitor; increases 2-AG levels

Endocannabinoid Uptake Inhibitors	
AM404	Anandamide uptake inhibitor
VDM11	Anandamide uptake inhibitor

INTRODUCTION TO THE CANNABINOID SYSTEM

The cannabinoid system is comprised of CB1 and CB2 receptors, endogenous cannabinoids, and the pathways responsible for their biosynthesis, uptake, and metabolism. The active constituent of cannabis, Δ^9-tetrahydrocannabinol (THC) was first characterized in 1964, two and a half decades before the existence of its site of action, the CB1 receptor, was known (Devane, Dysarz, Johnson, Melvin, & Howlett, 1988; Gaoni & Mechoulam, 1964). Originally, it was believed that the CB1 receptor was the brain cannabinoid receptor because it is one of the most abundant G protein–coupled receptors (GPCRs) in the central nervous system (CNS); however, CB1 receptors are present in numerous peripheral organs (Herkenham et al., 1990; Howlett et al., 2002). The CB2 receptor, also a GPCR, was identified shortly after CB1 (Munro, Thomas, & Abu-Shaar, 1993). CB2 was thought of as the peripheral cannabinoid receptor present mainly in cells of the immune system until it was identified throughout the CNS, albeit at lower levels than CB1 (Onaivi et al., 2006).

One of the major functions of the cannabinoid system is the inhibition of neurotransmitter release that accounts for the ability of cannabinoids to modify the synaptic efficacy of neuronal circuits involved in reward and other processes (Freund, Katona, & Piomelli, 2003). CB1 receptors are located pre-synaptically and when activated cause a decrease in cyclic adenosine monophosphate (cAMP) accumulation and inhibition of cAMP-dependent protein kinase (PKA). Stimulation of mitogen-activated protein kinase activity by CB1 receptor activation affects synaptic plasticity, cell migration, and potentially neuronal growth (Howlett et al., 2002). Inhibition of glutamatergic or GABAergic neurotransmission in the mesocorticolimbic system is particularly relevant in drug addiction processes (Katona et al., 2001; Melis et al., 2004; Robbe, Alonso, Duchamp, Bockaert, & Manzoni, 2001).

2-arachidonoylglycerol (2-AG) and anandamide (also known as arachidonoyl ethanolamide; AEA) are the two main endogenous cannabinoid agonists; other potential endocannabinoid molecules have been identified, but they have not been well characterized, and some may be artifacts (Devane et al., 1992; Mechoulam & Parker, 2013). 2-AG is a full agonist at CB1 receptors, while anandamide is a CB1 partial agonist and, in the presence of 2-AG, is thought to act as a competitive antagonist (Howlett & Mukhopadhyay, 2000). Most of the physiological actions of endocannabinoids are mediated by 2-AG, including regulation of dopamine neuron function in the ventral tegmental area (VTA) (Sugiura, Kobayashi, Oka, & Waku, 2002; Ueda, Tsuboi, Uyama, & Ohnishi, 2011).

Endocannabinoids do not possess the typical properties of neurotransmitters. They are synthesized from membranous, lipidic precursors when and where they are required and are released by diffusing across membranes unlike other neurotransmitters, such as dopamine and serotonin, which are stored in vesicles (Di Marzo, Melck, Bisogno, & De Petrocellis, 1998; Piomelli, Giuffrida, Calignano, & de Fonseca, 2000). Endocannabinoids are released by postsynaptic neurons and act as fast retrograde messengers inhibiting neurotransmitter release by the presynaptic neuron (Howlett et al., 2002). The mechanisms by which this is accomplished are depolarization-induced suppression of "inhibition" (DSI) and depolarization-induced suppression of "excitation" (DSE). Both DSI and DSE are forms of short-term synaptic plasticity of GABAergic and glutamatergic neurotransmission, respectively. Following postsynaptic depolarization, a rise in calcium levels occurs in the postsynaptic neuron that triggers the release of endocannabinoids. The consequent activation of presynaptic CB1 receptors inhibits the release of GABA in the case of DSI or glutamate in the case of DSE (Kreitzer & Regehr, 2001; Ohno-Shosaku, Maejima, & Kano, 2001; Wilson & Nicoll, 2001).

Anandamide and 2-AG levels are tightly regulated by the enzymes responsible for their synthesis and degradation. Fatty acid amide hydrolase

(FAAH) is the primary enzyme involved in breaking down anandamide, while monoacylglycerol lipase (MAGL) degrades 2-AG (Cravatt et al., 1996; Dinh et al., 2002). The cessation of endocannabinoid signaling is mediated by a two-step elimination process in which the neurotransmitter is first internalized by neurons and astrocytes and then hydrolyzed (Beltramo et al., 1997; Cravatt et al., 2001; Fu et al., 2011). Endocannabinoids are rapidly removed from the synapse by a membrane transport system, unlike THC, which is metabolized over a period of several hours and either excreted or stored as one of its metabolites (Fu et al., 2011). Once inside the cell, anandamide is hydrolyzed by FAAH, while 2-AG is metabolized by both FAAH and monoacyl hydrolases, mainly MAGL (Blankman, Simon, & Cravatt, 2007; Hillard, Edgemond, & Campbell, 1995; Tsou et al., 1998). The action of endocannabinoids can be indirectly enhanced by blocking these enzymes, and compounds such as FAAH inhibitors have been investigated as potential treatments for anxiety and depression (Gaetani et al., 2009).

THE CANNABINOID SYSTEM AND THE REWARD PATHWAY

All addictive drugs, including THC, as well as several normal adaptive behaviors (eg, eating, drinking, and sex), activate the mesolimbic dopamine pathway. Dopamine neurons project from the VTA to the nucleus accumbens (NAcc) where dopamine release results in positive reinforcing feelings of joy and accomplishment in the case of "natural highs" or more intense euphoria as a consequence of "artificial highs" (Gardner, 2011; Koob, 2009a). The psychological effects of THC are biphasic and depend on dose and the individual's personality. In healthy subjects, THC can cause relaxation and euphoria or anxiety and dysphoria (D'Souza et al., 2004; Wade, Robson, House, Makela, & Aram, 2003). Transient dopamine events in the NAcc also occur in response to conditioned stimuli or cues that predict drug availability; this is thought to mediate secondary reinforcing effects (Owesson-White et al., 2009; Phillips, Stuber, Heien, Wightman, & Carelli, 2003). On the other hand, drug withdrawal and the accompanying negative affective state is associated with a decrease in mesolimbic dopamine function that may result in compulsive drug seeking behaviors (Koob, 2009b; Weiss et al., 2001).

It was originally thought and argued in the experimental literature that cannabinoids, such as THC, did not increase dopamine in the mesolimbic system like other drugs of abuse (Castaneda, Moss, Oddie, & Whishaw, 1991; Gardner & Lowinson, 1991; Oleson & Cheer, 2012a; Wickelgren, 1997). However, this misconception has now been disproved by several studies that show that cannabinoids do increase dopamine concentrations in the NAcc in a CB1 receptor-dependent manner (Chen, Marmur, Pulles, Paredes, & Gardner, 1993; Chen et al., 1990; Chen, Paredes, Lowinson, & Gardner, 1991; Gessa, Melis, Muntoni, & Diana, 1998; Malone & Taylor, 1999; Ng Cheong Ton et al., 1988; Tanda, Pontieri, & Di Chiara, 1997). Single unit recording techniques have demonstrated that the increase in accumbal dopamine levels occurs via an increase in the mean firing rate of dopamine neurons within the VTA (French, 1997; French, Dillon, & Wu, 1997; Gessa et al., 1998; Wu & French, 2000). Administration of the CB1 receptor agonist WIN55,212-2 confirmed that CB1 receptor activation increases the frequency of dopamine neural firing, and this effect was abolished by CB1 receptor antagonism (Gessa et al., 1998).

The cannabinoid system has an important role in modulating meso-limbic dopamine levels during reward- and reinforcement-related behaviors in response to drugs of abuse including nicotine (Wang & Lupica, 2014). In recent years the disruption of cannabinoid signaling has emerged as a potential pharmacotherapeutic target in the treatment of addiction. Sanofi-Aventis were the first to develop and market a CB1 receptorinverseagonist/antagonist,rimonabant(a.k.a.SR141716A)(Rinaldi-Carmona et al., 1994). The drug was originally developed to treat obesity since CB1 receptor agonists enhance appetite, a well-known effect of THC consumption (Gaoni & Mechoulam, 1964). In placebo-controlled clinical trials, rimonabant did indeed produce significant weight loss (Christensen, Kristensen, Bartels, Bliddal, & Astrup, 2007) and showed promise for other indications including nicotine addiction by improving smoking cessation rates (Cahill & Ussher, 2007; Le Foll, Forget, Aubin, & Goldberg, 2008). However, rimonabant produced significant psychiatric side effects; patients were two and a half times more likely to discontinue treatment due to depressive mood disorders and three times more likely due to anxiety symptoms (Christensen et al., 2007). The Food and Drug Administration ruled against the approval of rimonabant due to these side effects and increased risk of suicidality; consequentially, rimonabant was withdrawn from the market in 2008 (Le Foll, Gorelick, & Goldberg, 2009).

THE CANNABINOID SYSTEM AND NICOTINE DEPENDENCE

Multiple neurotransmitters are affected by nicotine consumption, including acetylcholine (Wilkie, Hutson, Stephens, Whiting, & Wonnacott, 1993), noradrenaline (Clarke & Reuben, 1996), dopamine (Pontieri, Tanda, Orzi, & Di Chiara, 1996), GABA (Yang, Criswell, & Breese, 1996), serotonin (Kenny, File, & Neal, 2000), glutamate (McGehee, Heath, Gelber, Devay, & Role, 1995), and opioids (Berrendero, Robledo, Trigo, Martin-Garcia, & Maldonado, 2010). Nicotine activates nicotinic acetylcholine receptors (nAChRs) present in several brain regions; the $\alpha4\beta2$ subtype has the highest affinity for nicotine (Balfour, 2015). Activation of $\alpha4\beta2$ nAChRs in the VTA stimulates dopamine release in the NAcc and is central to the rewarding effects of nicotine consumption (Pidoplichko, DeBiasi, Williams, & Dani, 1997). The overlapping distribution of cannabinoid receptors and nAChRs in the brain is thought to facilitate interactions between the two systems. For instance, cannabinoid receptors and nAChRs in the midbrain mediate the reinforcing effects of nicotine, while those in the hippocampus and amygdala enable nicotine-associated memory (Le Foll & Goldberg, 2005; Picciotto, Caldarone, King, & Zachariou, 2000; Schlicker & Kathmann, 2001).

CB1 RECEPTORS

CB1 and nicotinic receptors are expressed on glutamatergic and GABAergic neurons in multiple brain regions. On glutamatergic neurons, presynaptic CB1 and $\alpha7$ nAChRs modulate glutamate release. Activation of $\alpha7$ nAChR enhances excitatory glutamate release (Mansvelder, Keath, & McGehee, 2002), and CB1 activation decreases glutamate release (Melis et al., 2004). Similarly, GABAergic neurons express both CB1 receptors and nAChRs including $\alpha6\beta2$ and $\alpha7$ but predominantly $\alpha4\beta2$ nAChRs. Stimulation of nAChRs on GABAergic neurons enhances, whereas CB1 receptor activation diminishes, GABAergic neurotransmission (Mansvelder et al., 2002; Szabo, Siemes, & Wallmichrath, 2002).

Experimental data reveal that the CB1 receptor has a bidirectional role in regulating the reward/reinforcement of nicotine-seeking behavior and on the reinstatement of nicotine-seeking behavior following periods of abstinence (see Table 9.1). Overall, activation of CB1 receptors increases the rewarding effects of nicotine as measured by increased nicotine-induced conditioned place preference (CPP) (Valjent, Mitchell, Besson, Caboche, & Maldonado, 2002), increased nicotine self-administration, discriminative stimulus effects of low-dose nicotine, and reinstatement following abstinence (Gamaleddin, Wertheim, et al., 2012). Genetic deletion or pharmacological blockade of CB1 receptors produces the opposite effect and decreases the rewarding and reinforcing properties of nicotine. CB1 knockout mice fail to develop nicotine-induced CPP, as do mice treated with CB1 receptor antagonists (Castane et al., 2002; Merritt, Martin, Walters, Lichtman, & Damaj, 2008). CB1 antagonists in studies of rats decrease nicotine-induced CPP (Forget, Hamon, & Thiebot, 2005; Le Foll & Goldberg, 2004). CB1 antagonists also decrease nicotine self-administration in rats (Cohen, Perrault, Voltz, Steinberg, & Soubrie, 2002; Shoaib, 2008; Simonnet, Cador, & Caille, 2013); however, one study did not detect this effect in CB1 knockout mice (Cossu et al., 2001).

TABLE 9.1 Preclinical Studies of CB1 Receptor Activation and Antagonism

	CB1 Receptor Activation	CB1 Receptor Antagonism
Reward and reinforcement	↑ Nicotine self-administration (Gamaleddin, Wertheim, et al., 2012)	↓ Nicotine self-administration decreased in rats (Cohen et al., 2002; Shoaib, 2008; Simonnet et al., 2013)
		↓ Breakpoint/motivation to self-administer nicotine in the progressive ratio schedule of reinforcement (Forget et al., 2009)
	↑ CPP in rats (Hashemizadeh, Sardari, & Rezayof, 2014) and mice (Valjent et al., 2002)♦	↓ Nicotine-induced elevations in extracellular dopamine release in the NAcc (Cohen et al., 2002)
	↑ Anxiolytic effects following co-administration of subthreshold doses THC and nicotine (Valjent et al., 2002)♦	⊗ Blocks the development of nicotine-induced CPP in rats (Forget et al., 2005; Hashemizadeh et al., 2014; Le Foll & Goldberg, 2004) and Mice (Merritt et al., 2008)♦
Relapse/reinstatement	↑ Cue-induced reinstatement of nicotine-seeking behavior (Gamaleddin, Wertheim, et al., 2012)	⊗ Blocks the reinstatement of extinguished nicotine-seeking behavior (Cohen et al., 2005; De Vries et al., 2005; Diergaarde et al., 2008; Forget et al., 2009)

All studies were conducted in rats unless otherwise specified. ♦ = study conducted in mice.

This discrepancy may reflect interspecies variation. Several studies have shown the ability of CB1 antagonists to decrease reinstatement of nicotine-seeking behavior (Cohen, Perrault, Griebel, & Soubrie, 2005; DeVries, de Vries, Janssen, & Schoffelmeer, 2005; Diergaarde, de Vries, Raaso, Schoffelmeer, & DeVries, 2008; Forget, Coen, & Le Foll, 2009). Clinical data were in agreement with these results when rimonabant was introduced to the market to aid weight loss and smoking cessation before it was withdrawn due to psychiatric side effects (Cahill & Ussher, 2007; Christensen et al., 2007; US Food and Drug Administration & Endocrinologic and Metabolic Drugs Advisory Committee, 2008).

Cannabidiol (CBD) is the non-psychoactive component of cannabis and acts as an antagonist at CB1 and CB2 receptors, and it inhibits the uptake and degradation of anandamide (Leweke et al., 2012; Pertwee, 2008; Thomas et al., 2007). CBD has been shown to have anxiolytic (Crippa et al., 2011) and antipsychotic properties (Leweke et al., 2012).

With the additional advantage of a superior safety profile to that of rimonabant, one small trial has tested CBD in humans as a smoking cessation treatment (Bergamaschi, Queiroz, Zuardi, & Crippa, 2011; Morgan, Das, Joye, Curran, & Kamboj, 2013). Morgan, Das, Joye, Curan, and Kamboj (2013) noted that cannabidiol treatment over a 1-week period reduced the number of cigarettes smoked by 40% compared to placebo. These results may also be accounted for by CBD's ability to act as an antagonist at α7 nAChRs (Mahgoub et al., 2013); however, larger scale studies with longer follow-up are required to confirm the results of this trial.

Intravenous self-administration (IVSA) of nicotine was blocked by central infusions of the CB1 antagonist AM251; however, nicotine IVSA was unaltered by intra-NAcc delivery of AM251 (Simonnet et al., 2013). These results suggest that CB1 receptors in the VTA specifically control nicotine-taking behaviors, ie, self-administration. However, it should be noted that electrophysiological recording of dopaminergic neurons in the VTA of anesthetized rats did not detect a change in activity following treatment with rimonabant (Melis et al., 2008). Further studies are required to elucidate the role of VTA CB1 receptors in the reinforcing effects of nicotine. Additionally, blockade of CB1 receptors in other brain regions such as the shell of the NAcc, basolateral amygdala, prelimbic cortex, and the bed nucleus of the stria terminalis has been shown to decrease nicotine-seeking behavior (Kodas, Cohen, Louis, & Griebel, 2007; Reisiger et al., 2014).

CB2 RECEPTORS

Recent studies using genetic and pharmacological models suggest that CB2 receptors may modulate the addictive properties of drugs of abuse. For instance, CB2 receptor activation has been shown to decrease cocaine self-administration in wild-type and CB1 knockout mice but not in CB2 knockout mice (Zhang et al., 2014). Likewise, mice overexpressing CB2 receptors showed decreased cocaine self-administration (Aracil-Fernandez et al., 2012). Administration of the CB2 agonist JWH133 inhibited cocaine self-administration and decreased extracellular dopamine in the NAcc, and these effects were blocked by the CB2 antagonist AM630 (Xi et al., 2011).

The role of CB2 receptors in nicotine addiction specifically is less clear. The α-3 and α-4-nAChR subtypes are localized in the same neurons as CB2 receptors in the VTA and the shell of the NAcc (Navarrete et al., 2013). Despite overlapping receptor distributions with cholinergic receptors, CB2 receptors appear to have a less prominent role in the rewarding and reinforcing effects of nicotine than CB1 receptors (Table 9.2). To

TABLE 9.2　Preclinical Studies of CB2 Receptor Activation and Antagonism

	CB2 Receptor Activation	CB2 Receptor Antagonism
Reward and reinforcement	= No effect of AM1241 on nicotine self-administration in rats (Gamaleddin, Zvonok, et al., 2012) O-1966 with subthreshold nicotine doses induced CPP in mice (Ignatowska-Jankowska et al., 2013)	= No effect of AM630 on nicotine self-administration in rats (Gamaleddin, Zvonok, et al., 2012) ↓ Nicotine self-administration with AM630 in mice (Navarrete et al., 2013) ⊗ AM630-treated and CB2 knockout mice did not show nicotine-induced CPP (Navarrete et al., 2013) ⊗ SR144528 blocked nicotine-induced CPP in mice (Ignatowska-Jankowska et al., 2013)
Relapse	= No effect of AM1241 on cue- or nicotine-induced reinstatement (Gamaleddin, Zvonok, et al., 2012)	= No effect of AM630 on cue- or nicotine-induced reinstatement of nicotine seeking in rats (Gamaleddin, Zvonok, et al., 2012)

date, three studies have investigated the role of CB2 on the rewarding properties of nicotine. Using fixed and progressive ratio schedules of reinforcement, Gamaleddin, Zvonok, Makriyannis, Goldberg, and Le Foll, 2012 evaluated the effects of AM1241 (CB2 agonist) and AM630 in rats. Neither drug affected nicotine self-administration or nicotine- or cue-induced reinstatement of nicotine-seeking in either of the reinforcement schedules.

Although the findings in rats suggest that the CB2 receptor is relatively less important in nicotine addiction, studies in mice suggest otherwise and highlight the issue of interspecies variability.

CB2 knockout mice and wild-type mice treated with AM630 did not develop nicotine-induced CPP and showed reduced nicotine self-administration (Navarrete et al., 2013). Ignatowska-Jankowska, Muldoon, Lichtman, and Damaj (2013) reported similar findings in CB2 knockout mice and wild-type mice treated with the CB2 antagonist SR144528. In contrast, the CB2 receptor agonist O-1966 in combination with subthreshold doses of nicotine did induce CPP.

ENDOCANNABINOIDS AND NICOTINE DEPENDENCE

FAAH Inhibitors

Given that CB1 receptor activation enhances the rewarding and reinforcing properties of nicotine, it stands to reason that increasing anandamide levels in the brain may have similar effects (Valjent et al., 2002).

TABLE 9.3   Preclinical Studies of FAAH Inhibition and Anandamide Reuptake Inhibitors on Nicotine Dependence

	FAAH Inhibition (Increases Anandamide Levels)	Anandamide Uptake Inhibitors
Reward/reinforcement	↑ CPP in FAAH knockout mice (Merritt et al., 2008) ↑ CPP in mice pretreated with URB597 (Merritt et al., 2008) ↓ CPP in rats (Scherma et al., 2008) ↓ nicotine self-administration in rats (Scherma et al., 2008)	↓ CPP in rats (Gamaleddin et al., 2013; Scherma et al., 2012) ↓ Nicotine self-administration in rats (Scherma et al., 2012) = No effect of AM404 on nicotine self-administration in rats (Gamaleddin et al., 2013)
Relapse/reinstatement	↓ in rats (Forget et al., 2009; Scherma et al., 2008)	↓ in rats (Gamaleddin et al., 2011, 2013)

Merritt et al. (2008) observed increased nicotine-induced CPP in both FAAH knockout mice and mice pretreated with the FAAH inhibitor URB597 (Table 9.3). Studies conducted in rats produced the opposite results; FAAH inhibition prevented the development of nicotine-induced CPP, decreased nicotine self-administration, and inhibited cue- or nicotine-induced reinstatement of nicotine-seeking behavior (Forget et al., 2009; Scherma et al., 2008). While the differences in these findings could be ascribed to the use of mice versus rats, URB597-induced increases in anandamide are not significantly different between the species; these results are more likely due to the role of PPAR-α ligands discussed subsequently (Fegley et al., 2005).

Anandamide Uptake Inhibitors

Administration of the anandamide uptake inhibitor, VDM11, yielded results similar to those of FAAH inhibitors. VDM11 decreased cue- and nicotine-induced reinstatement of nicotine-seeking behavior in rats but failed to affect responding for nicotine fixed- and progressive-ratio reinforcement schedules (Gamaleddin, Guranda, Goldberg, & Le Foll, 2011). Another anandamide uptake inhibitor, AM404, blocked the development of nicotine-induced CPP and reinstatement (Gamaleddin et al., 2013; Scherma et al., 2012). Effects on nicotine self-administration varied in the two studies using AM404: no effect on nicotine-taking (Gamaleddin et al., 2013) and decreased nicotine-taking (Scherma et al., 2012) were reported. These findings are in line with reduced encoding of reward-predictive cues in the NAcc of rats treated with VDM11 (Oleson & Cheer, 2012b).

PPARs

Oleoylethanolamine (OEA) and palmitoylethanolamide (PEA) are members of the extended endocannabinoid family and ligands at non-cannabinoid peroxisome proliferator-activated receptors (PPAR-α). These receptors are expressed throughout tissues in the body and in many brain regions and have neuroprotective, anti-inflammatory, and lipid-regulating actions (Moreno, Farioli-Vecchioli, & Ceru, 2004; O'Sullivan, 2007; Pistis & Melis, 2010). Electrophysiology studies revealed that OEA and PEA suppress nicotine-induced excitation of dopamine cells (Melis et al., 2008). In rats and squirrel monkeys, exogenous PPAR-α agonists were found to reduce nicotine self-administration specifically as opposed to cocaine or food self-administration (Mascia et al., 2011; Panlilio et al., 2012). This effect was reversed by MK886, a PPAR antagonist. Nicotine- and cue-induced reinstatement of nicotine-seeking behavior was blocked by exogenous PPAR-α agonists (Mascia et al., 2011; Panlilio et al., 2012). Additionally, the divergent findings of FAAH inhibitors in mice and rats may be explained by the involvement of PPAR-α receptors. While URB597 increases anandamide to similar levels in mice and rats, OEA and PEA increase anandamide by twofold in mice compared to four to fivefold in rats (Fegley et al., 2005).

THE CANNABINOID SYSTEM AND NICOTINE WITHDRAWAL

During waking hours, smokers maintain a constant level of saturation of $\alpha 4\beta 2$ nAChRs; as a consequence, these receptors become desensitized and upregulated. Withdrawal symptoms occur when $\alpha 4\beta 2$ nAChRs become sensitive once more following cessation of chronic nicotine intake, causing hyperexcitability of the cholinergic system (Balfour, 1994; Dani & Heinemann, 1996). The aversive symptoms of nicotine withdrawal and craving can be countered by recommencing smoking; in this way, smoking behaviors are negatively reinforced (Dani & Heinemann, 1996).

The ability of the cannabinoid system to modulate nicotine reward and dependence has been well documented, but far less is known about the role of this system in nicotine withdrawal (Gamaleddin et al., 2015). The majority of preclinical studies investigating the effects of nicotine have been performed in nicotine naïve versus dependent animals (Hall et al., 2015). Like other drugs of abuse, nicotine withdrawal is associated with a decrease in dopamine levels in the NAcc (Di Chiara, 2000; Tapper et al., 2004). Given the ability of cannabinoid system to modulate dopamine neuron firing in the VTA, it has been suggested that modulation of this system may be a therapeutic target for nicotine withdrawal in addition to dependence.

CB1 RECEPTORS AND NICOTINE WITHDRAWAL

Since CB1 antagonists such as rimonabant decrease the rewarding effects of nicotine, it has been suggested that CB1 agonists may alleviate nicotine withdrawal symptoms. Few studies have examined the interaction of the two systems in the context of nicotine abstinence following dependence (Table 9.4). In an early study, co-administration of nicotine and THC in rats was shown to potentiate the acute depressant effects of THC in the conditioned avoidance paradigm, and decreased heart rate, body temperature, locomotion, and motor coordination (Pryor, Larsen, Husain, & Braude, 1978). A subsequent study replicated some of these findings, reporting that nicotine strongly facilitated hypothermia, antinociception, and hypolocomotion following acute THC administration. When the co-treated mice were challenged with rimonabant, the result was an increased withdrawal syndrome (Valjent et al., 2002).

Studies of CB1 knockout mice have reported either no effect on nicotine withdrawal symptoms (Castane et al., 2002; Merritt et al., 2008) or decreased nicotine withdrawal-associated anxiety (Bura, Burokas, Martin-Garcia, & Maldonado, 2010). Castane et al. (2002) did not observe a difference in the severity of mecamylamine (nonspecific nAChR antagonist)-induced nicotine withdrawal between CB1 knockout mice and wild types; however, the CB1 knockout mice also did not exhibit the rewarding effects of nicotine. Similarly, no differences were observed between CB1 knockout mice and wild types following spontaneous nicotine withdrawal (Merritt et al., 2008). Bura et al. (2010) observed that CB1 knockout mice displayed less nicotine withdrawal-associated anxiety than wild types; however, this finding may reflect a ceiling effect since the CB1 knockouts displayed a lower level of exploration at baseline.

THC administration to nicotine-dependent mice decreased the somatic expressions and dysphoric manifestations of nicotine withdrawal (Balerio, Aso, Berrendero, Murtra, & Maldonado, 2004). Acute THC pretreatment decreased the somatic effects precipitated by mecamylamine and naloxone, suggesting an interaction between the cannabinoid and nicotine systems. Cannabinoid agonists have been shown to modulate cholinergic neurotransmission in areas of the brain involved in the behavioral responses to nicotine. Elevated acetylcholine (ACh) release in response to cannabinoid agonists has been reported in the hippocampus, cortex, and striatum (Acquas, Pisanu, Marrocu, & Di Chiara, 2000; Tripathi, Vocci, Brase, & Dewey, 1987), in addition to decreased ACh turnover in these regions (Revuelta, Moroni, Cheney, & Costa, 1978; Tripathi et al., 1987). To clarify the role of CB1 receptors in this finding, Balerio et al. (2004) administered rimonabant to mice co-treated with THC and nicotine. At low doses (1–3 mg/kg), rimonabant displayed intrinsic activity of its own, obscuring

TABLE 9.4   Studies Examining Cannabinoid System Modulation of Nicotine Withdrawal

CB1 Receptor Activation	Decreased CB1 Receptor Activity
↓ Signs of somatic withdrawal following THC administration in nicotine-dependent mice (Balerio et al., 2004)	*Genetic deletion:* = No difference between CB1 KO mice and wild-type in severity of withdrawal symptoms (Castane et al., 2002; Merritt et al., 2008) ↓ Withdrawal in CB1 KO mice (Bura et al., 2010) *Pharmacological antagonism:* ↑ Withdrawal following treatment with rimonabant in mice co-treated with nicotine and THC (Valjent et al., 2002) ↑ Withdrawal following treatment with rimonabant at a high dose (10 mg/kg) in nicotine-dependent mice (Balerio et al., 2004) = No difference in withdrawal symptoms following treatment with rimonabant at low/moderate dose (1–3 mg/kg) in nicotine-dependent mice (Balerio et al., 2004) ↓ Withdrawal in wild-type mice following treatment with rimonabant (3 mg/kg) (Merritt et al., 2008)
CB2 receptor activation	**CB2 receptor genetic deletion/antagonism**
N.A.	= No difference in CB2 (+/+) and (−/−) nicotine-dependent mice in withdrawal responses (Ignatowska-Jankowska et al., 2013) ⊗ CB2 knockout mice did not develop nicotine withdrawal (Navarrete et al., 2013) ⊗ AM630 blocks nicotine withdrawal syndrome (Navarrete et al., 2013)
MAGL inhibition (increases 2-AG levels)	**FAAH inhibition (increases anandamide levels)**
↓ Somatic and aversive withdrawal signs following administration of JZL184 to nicotine-dependent mice; this protective effect was blocked by rimonabant (Muldoon et al., 2015)	↑ Withdrawal in mice following genetic deletion or with URB597 at high doses (10 mg/kg) only (Merritt et al., 2008) = No change in somatic signs of nicotine withdrawal following treatment with URB597 (Cippitelli et al., 2011) ↓ Nicotine withdrawal associated anxiety following treatment with URB597 (Cippitelli et al., 2011)

the results; however, at a high dose (10 mg/kg), rimonabant was able to precipitate withdrawal syndrome in nicotine-dependent mice. In contrast, Merritt et al. (2008) observed that acute administration of rimonabant ameliorated somatic signs of nicotine withdrawal, but this was observed using a relatively lower dose of 3 mg/kg, which may account for these conflicting results.

CB2 RECEPTORS AND NICOTINE WITHDRAWAL

As in nicotine dependence, CB2 receptors do not appear to play a major role in nicotine withdrawal; however, few studies have been performed on this topic. Nicotine-dependent CB2 wild-type and CB2 knockout mice exhibited almost identical precipitated withdrawal responses (Ignatowska-Jankowska et al., 2013). On the other hand, somatic signs of nicotine withdrawal (rearings, groomings, scratches, teeth chattering, and body tremors) were absent in CB2 knockout mice, and the administration of AM630 (CB2 antagonist) blocked the nicotine withdrawal syndrome (Navarrete et al., 2013). The discrepancy in these findings may be due to differences in nAChR expression between these studies. The CB2 knockout mice studied by Navarrete et al. had significantly reduced gene expression of $\alpha3$ and $\alpha4$ nAChRs in the VTA, but this was not observed in the study by Ignatowska-Janowska et al.

ENDOCANNABINOIDS AND NICOTINE WITHDRAWAL

CB1 agonists appear to alleviate nicotine withdrawal symptoms (Balerio et al., 2004); however, their use is associated with side effects (Darmani, 2001; Lichtman & Martin, 1991; Martin, Mechoulam, & Razdan, 1999). Several studies suggest that increasing endocannabinoid levels with FAAH and MAGL inhibitors may provide the beneficial effects of exogenous CB1 agonists, such as THC, with fewer side effects (Ahn, McKinney, & Cravatt, 2008; Cravatt et al., 1996; Justinova et al., 2008; Long, Li, et al., 2009; Long, Nomura, & Cravatt, 2009; Solinas et al., 2007). Yet the utility of FAAH inhibitors as a potential treatment for nicotine withdrawal remains unclear based on the preclinical data (see Table 9.4). FAAH inhibition appears to differentially modulate affective nicotine withdrawal symptoms in mice and rats (Cippitelli et al., 2011; Merritt et al., 2008). FAAH knockout mice exhibited more pronounced nicotine withdrawal somatic symptoms and nicotine withdrawal–induced place aversion than wild types. In the same study, high doses (10 mg/kg) of the FAAH inhibitor URB597 worsened withdrawal symptoms, though this effect was not seen at lower doses (Merritt et al., 2008). In rats, URB597 treatment had no effect on somatic withdrawal symptoms but decreased withdrawal-related anxiety, suggesting important interspecies variation (Cippitelli et al., 2011).

2-AG is regarded as the main endocannabinoid responsible for retrograde signaling in the CNS (Pan et al., 2009). As a full agonist at both CB1 and CB2 receptors, 2-AG is approximately 200-fold more abundant than anandamide in the brain (Gonsiorek et al., 2000; Savinainen, Jarvinen, Laine, & Laitinen, 2001). 2-AG is the main endocannabinoid that regulates the firing activity of

VTA dopamine neurons in particular. As of 2016, only one study has evaluated the role of 2-AG in nicotine dependence (Muldoon et al., 2015). Muldoon et al. conducted a series of experiments investigating MAGL mRNA expression and using the MAGL knockout mice and an MAGL inhibitor. The results from these multiple lines of evidence supported the hypothesis that decreased MAGL levels (and thereby increased 2-AG levels) in the brain attenuated withdrawal responses. Following chronic nicotine exposure, mecamylamine-induced somatic withdrawal signs showed a significant positive correlation with basal MAGL mRNA expression. Administration of the MAGL inhibitor JZL184 dose-dependently decreased somatic and aversive withdrawal signs. Furthermore, this protective effect of JZL184 was blocked by rimonabant, suggesting a CB1-mediated mechanism. A diminished nicotine withdrawal syndrome was also observed in MAGL knockout mice.

CONCLUSIONS

CB1 receptor activation appears to be a prerequisite for the rewarding effects of nicotine exposure, and the blockade of CB1 receptors is clearly associated with decreased nicotine-taking and nicotine-seeking behavior. Conversely, CB1 receptor agonists improve symptoms of nicotine withdrawal. The effect of blocking CB1 receptor activity in nicotine withdrawal has produced conflicting results with increased withdrawal symptoms observed with high doses of rimonabant and no effect or even decreased withdrawal symptoms with low doses of rimonabant and in CB1 knockout mice. CB2 receptors do not play a major role in the rewarding or reinforcing effects of nicotine, and limited evidence suggests that CB2 receptors may be involved in nicotine withdrawal. The usefulness of FAAH inhibitors remains uncertain, though initial studies propose that CBD, PPAR-α agonists, and MAGL inhibitors may be novel therapeutic strategies for smoking cessation and nicotine withdrawal.

Modulation of the cannabinoid system in nicotine dependence and withdrawal is particularly important in the context of psychiatric illness for three main reasons. First, stimulation of CB1 receptors increases dopaminergic, serotonergic, and noradrenergic neurotransmission—systems affected in psychiatric patients (for review, see Esteban & Garcia-Sevilla, 2012). Second, patients with schizophrenia, bipolar disorder, major depression, and anxiety disorder exhibit greatly increased rates of cannabis and nicotine dependence, which may reflect self-medication of uncomfortable symptoms that are at least temporarily alleviated by these substances (Lev-Ran, Imtiaz, Rehm, & Le Foll, 2013). As such, this vulnerable patient group stands to benefit most from smoking cessation interventions. Third, the emerging evidence reveals that the endocannabinoid system is deeply involved in the underlying neurobiological processes of these psychiatric conditions (Leweke & Koethe, 2008).

The pharmacotherapeutic challenge going forward is to untangle the intricate interactions of these systems in patients with mental illness and develop treatments that ameliorate nicotine addiction and potentially improve—or at least not exacerbate—psychiatric symptoms.

References

Acquas, E., Pisanu, A., Marrocu, P., & Di Chiara, G. (2000). Cannabinoid CB(1) receptor agonists increase rat cortical and hippocampal acetylcholine release in vivo. *European Journal of Pharmacology, 401*(2), 179–185. pii:S0014-2999(00)00403-9.

Ahn, K., McKinney, M. K., & Cravatt, B. F. (2008). Enzymatic pathways that regulate endocannabinoid signaling in the nervous system. *Chemical Reviews, 108*(5), 1687–1707. http://dx.doi.org/10.1021/cr0782067.

Aracil-Fernandez, A., Trigo, J. M., Garcia-Gutierrez, M. S., Ortega-Alvaro, A., Ternianov, A., Navarro, D., … Manzanares, J. (2012). Decreased cocaine motor sensitization and self-administration in mice overexpressing cannabinoid CB(2) receptors. *Neuropsychopharmacology: Official Publication of the American College of Neuropsychopharmacology, 37*(7), 1749–1763. http://dx.doi.org/10.1038/npp.2012.22.

Balerio, G. N., Aso, E., Berrendero, F., Murtra, P., & Maldonado, R. (2004). Delta9-tetrahydrocannabinol decreases somatic and motivational manifestations of nicotine withdrawal in mice. *The European Journal of Neuroscience, 20*(10), 2737–2748. pii:EJN3714.

Balfour, D. J. (1994). Neural mechanisms underlying nicotine dependence. *Addiction (Abingdon, England), 89*(11), 1419–1423.

Balfour, D. J. (2015). The role of mesoaccumbens dopamine in nicotine dependence. *Current Topics in Behavioral Neurosciences, 24*, 55–98. http://dx.doi.org/10.1007/978-3-319-13482-6-3.

Beltramo, M., Stella, N., Calignano, A., Lin, S. Y., Makriyannis, A., & Piomelli, D. (1997). Functional role of high-affinity anandamide transport, as revealed by selective inhibition. *Science (New York, N.Y.), 277*(5329), 1094–1097.

Bergamaschi, M. M., Queiroz, R. H., Zuardi, A. W., & Crippa, J. A. (2011). Safety and side effects of cannabidiol, a cannabis sativa constituent. *Current Drug Safety, 6*(4), 237–249. pii:BSP/CDS/6/4/0237.

Berrendero, F., Robledo, P., Trigo, J. M., Martin-Garcia, E., & Maldonado, R. (2010). Neurobiological mechanisms involved in nicotine dependence and reward: participation of the endogenous opioid system. *Neuroscience and Biobehavioral Reviews, 35*(2), 220–231. http://dx.doi.org/10.1016/j.neubiorev.2010.02.006.

Blankman, J. L., Simon, G. M., & Cravatt, B. F. (2007). A comprehensive profile of brain enzymes that hydrolyze the endocannabinoid 2-arachidonoylglycerol. *Chemistry & Biology, 14*(12), 1347–1356. pii:S1074-5521(07)00399-7.

Bura, S. A., Burokas, A., Martin-Garcia, E., & Maldonado, R. (2010). Effects of chronic nicotine on food intake and anxiety-like behaviour in CB(1) knockout mice. *European Neuropsychopharmacology: The Journal of the European College of Neuropsychopharmacology, 20*(6), 369–378. http://dx.doi.org/10.1016/j.euroneuro.2010.02.003.

Cahill, K., & Ussher, M. (2007). Cannabinoid type 1 receptor antagonists (rimonabant) for smoking cessation. *The Cochrane Database of Systematic Reviews, 4*(4), CD005353. http://dx.doi.org/10.1002/14651858.CD005353.pub3.

Castane, A., Valjent, E., Ledent, C., Parmentier, M., Maldonado, R., & Valverde, O. (2002). Lack of CB1 cannabinoid receptors modifies nicotine behavioural responses, but not nicotine abstinence. *Neuropharmacology, 43*(5), 857–867. pii:S0028390802001181.

Castaneda, E., Moss, D. E., Oddie, S. D., & Whishaw, I. Q. (1991). THC does not affect striatal dopamine release: microdialysis in freely moving rats. *Pharmacology, Biochemistry, and Behavior, 40*(3), 587–591. pii:0091-3057(91)90367-B.

Chen, J., Marmur, R., Pulles, A., Paredes, W., & Gardner, E. L. (1993). Ventral tegmental microinjection of delta 9-tetrahydrocannabinol enhances ventral tegmental somato-dendritic dopamine levels but not forebrain dopamine levels: evidence for local neural action by marijuana's psychoactive ingredient. *Brain Research, 621*(1), 65–70. pii:0006-8993(93)90298-2.

Chen, J. P., Paredes, W., Li, J., Smith, D., Lowinson, J., & Gardner, E. L. (1990). Delta 9-tet-rahydrocannabinol produces naloxone-blockable enhancement of presynaptic basal dopamine efflux in nucleus accumbens of conscious, freely-moving rats as measured by intracerebral microdialysis. *Psychopharmacology, 102*(2), 156–162.

Chen, J. P., Paredes, W., Lowinson, J. H., & Gardner, E. L. (1991). Strain-specific facilitation of dopamine efflux by delta 9-tetrahydrocannabinol in the nucleus accumbens of rat: an in vivo microdialysis study. *Neuroscience Letters, 129*(1), 136–180.

Christensen, R., Kristensen, P. K., Bartels, E. M., Bliddal, H., & Astrup, A. (2007). Efficacy and safety of the weight-loss drug rimonabant: a meta-analysis of randomised trials. *Lancet (London, England), 370*(9600), 1706–1713. pii:S0140-6736(07)61721-8.

Cippitelli, A., Astarita, G., Duranti, A., Caprioli, G., Ubaldi, M., Stopponi, S., … Ciccocioppo, R. (2011). Endocannabinoid regulation of acute and protracted nicotine withdrawal: effect of FAAH inhibition. *PLoS One, 6*(11), e28142. http://dx.doi.org/10.1371/journal. pone.0028142.

Clarke, P. B., & Reuben, M. (1996). Release of [3H]-noradrenaline from rat hippocampal syn-aptosomes by nicotine: mediation by different nicotinic receptor subtypes from striatal [3H]-dopamine release. *British Journal of Pharmacology, 117*(4), 595–606.

Cohen, C., Perrault, G., Griebel, G., & Soubrie, P. (2005). Nicotine-associated cues maintain nicotine-seeking behavior in rats several weeks after nicotine withdrawal: reversal by the cannabinoid (CB1) receptor antagonist, rimonabant (SR141716). *Neuropsychopharmacology: Official Publication of the American College of Neuropsychopharmacology, 30*(1), 145–155. http://dx.doi.org/10.1038/sj.npp.1300541.

Cohen, C., Perrault, G., Voltz, C., Steinberg, R., & Soubrie, P. (2002). SR141716, a central can-nabinoid (CB(1)) receptor antagonist, blocks the motivational and dopamine-releasing effects of nicotine in rats. *Behavioural Pharmacology, 13*(5–6), 451–463.

Cossu, G., Ledent, C., Fattore, L., Imperato, A., Bohme, G. A., Parmentier, M., & Fratta, W. (2001). Cannabinoid CB1 receptor knockout mice fail to self-administer morphine but not other drugs of abuse. *Behavioural Brain Research, 118*(1), 61–65. pii:S0166-4328(00)00311-9.

Cravatt, B. F., Demarest, K., Patricelli, M. P., Bracey, M. H., Giang, D. K., Martin, B. R., & Lichtman, A. H. (2001). Supersensitivity to anandamide and enhanced endogenous can-nabinoid signaling in mice lacking fatty acid amide hydrolase. *Proceedings of the National Academy of Sciences of the United States of America, 98*(16), 9371–9376. http://dx.doi. org/10.1073/pnas.161191698.

Cravatt, B., Giang, D., Mayfield, S., Boger, D., Lerner, R., & Gilula, N. (1996). Molecular char-acterization of an enzyme that degrades neuromodulatory fatty-acid amides. *Nature, 384*(6604), 83–87. http://dx.doi.org/10.1038/384083a0.

Crippa, J. A., Derenusson, G. N., Ferrari, T. B., Wichert-Ana, L., Duran, F. L., Martin-Santos, R., … Hallak, J. E. (2011). Neural basis of anxiolytic effects of cannabidiol (CBD) in gener-alized social anxiety disorder: a preliminary report. *Journal of Psychopharmacology (Oxford, England), 25*(1), 121–130. http://dx.doi.org/10.1177/0269881110379283.

Dani, J. A., & Heinemann, S. (1996). Molecular and cellular aspects of nicotine abuse. *Neuron, 16*(5), 905–908. pii:S0896-6273(00)80112-9.

Darmani, N. A. (2001). Delta-9-tetrahydrocannabinol differentially suppresses cisplatin-induced emesis and indices of motor function via cannabinoid CB(1) receptors in the least shrew. *Pharmacology, Biochemistry, and Behavior, 69*(1–2), 239–249. pii:S0091-3057(01)00531-7.

De Vries, T. J., de Vries, W., Janssen, M. C., & Schoffelmeer, A. N. (2005). Suppression of conditioned nicotine and sucrose seeking by the cannabinoid-1 receptor antagonist SR141716A. *Behavioural Brain Research, 161*(1), 164–168. pii:S0166-4328(05)00067-7.

Devane, W. A., Dysarz, F. A., 3rd, Johnson, M. R., Melvin, L. S., & Howlett, A. C. (1988). Determination and characterization of a cannabinoid receptor in rat brain. *Molecular Pharmacology, 34*(5), 605–613.

Devane, W. A., Hanus, L., Breuer, A., Pertwee, R. G., Stevenson, L. A., Griffin, G., … Mechoulam, R. (1992). Isolation and structure of a brain constituent that binds to the cannabinoid receptor. *Science (New York, N.Y.), 258*(5090), 1946–1949.

Di Chiara, G. (2000). Role of dopamine in the behavioural actions of nicotine related to addiction. *European Journal of Pharmacology, 393*(1–3), 295–314. pii:S0014-2999(00)00122-9.

Di Marzo, V., Melck, D., Bisogno, T., & De Petrocellis, L. (1998). Endocannabinoids: endogenous cannabinoid receptor ligands with neuromodulatory action. *Trends in Neurosciences, 21*(12), 521–528.

Diergaarde, L., de Vries, W., Raaso, H., Schoffelmeer, A. N., & De Vries, T. J. (2008). Contextual renewal of nicotine seeking in rats and its suppression by the cannabinoid-1 receptor antagonist rimonabant (SR141716A). *Neuropharmacology, 55*(5), 712–716. http://dx.doi.org/10.1016/j.neuropharm.2008.06.003.

Dinh, T. P., Carpenter, D., Leslie, F. M., Freund, T. F., Katona, I., Sensi, S. L., … Piomelli, D. (2002). Brain monoglyceride lipase participating in endocannabinoid inactivation. *Proceedings of the National Academy of Sciences, 99*(16), 10819–10824. http://dx.doi.org/10.1073/pnas.152334899.

D'Souza, D. C., Perry, E., MacDougall, L., Ammerman, Y., Cooper, T., Wu, Y. T., … Krystal, J. H. (2004). The psychotomimetic effects of intravenous delta-9-tetrahydrocannabinol in healthy individuals: implications for psychosis. *Neuropsychopharmacology: Official Publication of the American College of Neuropsychopharmacology, 29*(8), 1558–1572. http://dx.doi.org/10.1038/sj.npp.1300496.

Esteban, S., & Garcia-Sevilla, J. A. (2012). Effects induced by cannabinoids on monoaminergic systems in the brain and their implications for psychiatric disorders. *Progress in Neuro-Psychopharmacology & Biological Psychiatry, 38*(1), 78–87. http://dx.doi.org/10.1016/j.pnpbp.2011.11.007.

Fegley, D., Gaetani, S., Duranti, A., Tontini, A., Mor, M., Tarzia, G., & Piomelli, D. (2005). Characterization of the fatty acid amide hydrolase inhibitor cyclohexyl carbamic acid 3'-carbamoyl-biphenyl-3-yl ester (URB597): effects on anandamide and oleoylethanolamide deactivation. *The Journal of Pharmacology and Experimental Therapeutics, 313*(1), 352–358. pii:jpet.104.078980.

Forget, B., Coen, K. M., & Le Foll, B. (2009). Inhibition of fatty acid amide hydrolase reduces reinstatement of nicotine seeking but not break point for nicotine self-administration–comparison with CB(1) receptor blockade. *Psychopharmacology, 205*(4), 613–624. http://dx.doi.org/10.1007/s00213-009-1569-5.

Forget, B., Hamon, M., & Thiebot, M. H. (2005). Cannabinoid CB1 receptors are involved in motivational effects of nicotine in rats. *Psychopharmacology, 181*(4), 722–734. http://dx.doi.org/10.1007/s00213-005-0015-6.

French, E. D. (1997). Delta9-tetrahydrocannabinol excites rat VTA dopamine neurons through activation of cannabinoid CB1 but not opioid receptors. *Neuroscience Letters, 226*(3), 159–162. pii:S0304-3940(97)00278-4.

French, E. D., Dillon, K., & Wu, X. (1997). Cannabinoids excite dopamine neurons in the ventral tegmentum and substantia nigra. *Neuroreport, 8*(3), 649–652.

Freund, T. F., Katona, I., & Piomelli, D. (2003). Role of endogenous cannabinoids in synaptic signaling. *Physiological Reviews, 83*(3), 1017–1066. http://dx.doi.org/10.1152/physrev.00004.2003.

Fu, J., Bottegoni, G., Sasso, O., Bertorelli, R., Rocchia, W., Masetti, M., … Piomelli, D. (2011). A catalytically silent FAAH-1 variant drives anandamide transport in neurons. *Nature Neuroscience, 15*(1), 64–69. http://dx.doi.org/10.1038/nn.2986.

Gaetani, S., Dipasquale, P., Romano, A., Righetti, L., Cassano, T., Piomelli, D., & Cuomo, V. (2009). The endocannabinoid system as a target for novel anxiolytic and antidepressant drugs. *International Review of Neurobiology, 85*, 57–72. http://dx.doi.org/10.1016/S0074-7742(09)85005-8.

Gamaleddin, I., Guranda, M., Goldberg, S. R., & Le Foll, B. (2011). The selective anandamide transport inhibitor VDM11 attenuates reinstatement of nicotine seeking behaviour, but does not affect nicotine intake. *British Journal of Pharmacology, 164*(6), 1652–1660. http://dx.doi.org/10.1111/j.1476-5381.2011.01440.x.

Gamaleddin, I., Guranda, M., Scherma, M., Fratta, W., Makriyannis, A., Vadivel, S. K., ... Le Foll, B. (2013). AM404 attenuates reinstatement of nicotine seeking induced by nicotine-associated cues and nicotine priming but does not affect nicotine- and food-taking. *Journal of Psychopharmacology (Oxford, England), 27*(6), 564–571. http://dx.doi.org/10.1177/0269881113477710.

Gamaleddin, I., Trigo, J. M., Gueye, A. B., Zvonok, A., Makriyannis, A., Goldberg, S. R., & Le Foll, B. (2015). Role of the endogenous cannabinoid system in nicotine addiction: novel insights. *Frontiers in Psychiatry, 6*, 41. http://dx.doi.org/10.3389/fpsyt.2015.00041.

Gamaleddin, I., Wertheim, C., Zhu, A. Z., Coen, K. M., Vemuri, K., Makryannis, A., ... Le Foll, B. (2012). Cannabinoid receptor stimulation increases motivation for nicotine and nicotine seeking. *Addiction Biology, 17*(1), 47–61. http://dx.doi.org/10.1111/j.1369-1600.2011.00314.x.

Gamaleddin, I., Zvonok, A., Makriyannis, A., Goldberg, S. R., & Le Foll, B. (2012). Effects of a selective cannabinoid CB2 agonist and antagonist on intravenous nicotine self administration and reinstatement of nicotine seeking. *PLoS One, 7*(1), e29900. http://dx.doi.org/10.1371/journal.pone.0029900.

Gaoni, Y., & Mechoulam, R. (1964). Isolation, structure, and partial synthesis of an active constituent of hashish. *Journal of the American Chemical Society, 86*(8), 1646–1647.

Gardner, E. L. (2011). Addiction and brain reward and antireward pathways. *Advances in Psychosomatic Medicine, 30*, 22–60. http://dx.doi.org/10.1159/000324065.

Gardner, E. L., & Lowinson, J. H. (1991). Marijuana's interaction with brain reward systems: update 1991. *Pharmacology, Biochemistry, and Behavior, 40*(3), 571–580 pii:0091-3057(91)90365-9.

Gessa, G. L., Melis, M., Muntoni, A. L., & Diana, M. (1998). Cannabinoids activate mesolimbic dopamine neurons by an action on cannabinoid CB1 receptors. *European Journal of Pharmacology, 341*(1), 39–44. pii:S0014299997014428.

Gonsiorek, W., Lunn, C., Fan, X., Narula, S., Lundell, D., & Hipkin, R. W. (2000). Endocannabinoid 2-arachidonyl glycerol is a full agonist through human type 2 cannabinoid receptor: antagonism by anandamide. *Molecular Pharmacology, 57*(5), 1045–1050.

Hall, F. S., Der-Avakian, A., Gould, T. J., Markou, A., Shoaib, M., & Young, J. W. (2015). Negative affective states and cognitive impairments in nicotine dependence. *Neuroscience and Biobehavioral Reviews.* http://dx.doi.org/10.1016/j.neubiorev.2015.06.004.

Hashemizadeh, S., Sardari, M., & Rezayof, A. (2014). Basolateral amygdala CB1 cannabinoid receptors mediate nicotine-induced place preference. *Progress in Neuro-Psychopharmacology and Biological Psychiatry, 51*, 65–71.

Herkenham, M., Lynn, A. B., Little, M. D., Johnson, M. R., Melvin, L. S., de Costa, B. R., & Rice, K. C. (1990). Cannabinoid receptor localization in brain. *Proceedings of the National Academy of Sciences of the United States of America, 87*(5), 1932–1936.

Hillard, C. J., Edgemond, W. S., & Campbell, W. B. (1995). Characterization of ligand binding to the cannabinoid receptor of rat brain membranes using a novel method: application to anandamide. *Journal of Neurochemistry, 64*(2), 677–683.

Howlett, A. C., & Mukhopadhyay, S. (2000). Cellular signal transduction by anandamide and 2-arachidonoylglycerol. *Chemistry and Physics of Lipids, 108*(1–2), 53–70. pii:S0009308400001870.

Howlett, A. C., Barth, F., Bonner, T. I., Cabral, G., Casellas, P., Devane, W. A., ... Pertwee, R. G. (2002). International union of pharmacology. XXVII. classification of cannabinoid receptors. *Pharmacological Reviews, 54*(2), 161–202.

Ignatowska-Jankowska, B. M., Muldoon, P. P., Lichtman, A. H., & Damaj, M. I. (2013). The cannabinoid CB2 receptor is necessary for nicotine-conditioned place preference, but not other behavioral effects of nicotine in mice. *Psychopharmacology, 229*(4), 591–601. http://dx.doi.org/10.1007/s00213-013-3117-6.

Justinova, Z., Mangieri, R. A., Bortolato, M., Chefer, S. I., Mukhin, A. G., Clapper, J. R., … Goldberg, S. R. (2008). Fatty acid amide hydrolase inhibition heightens anandamide signaling without producing reinforcing effects in primates. *Biological Psychiatry*, *64*(11), 930–937. http://dx.doi.org/10.1016/j.biopsych.2008.08.008.

Katona, I., Rancz, E. A., Acsady, L., Ledent, C., Mackie, K., Hajos, N., & Freund, T. F. (2001). Distribution of CB1 cannabinoid receptors in the amygdala and their role in the control of GABAergic transmission. *The Journal of Neuroscience: The Official Journal of the Society for Neuroscience*, *21*(23), 9506–9518. pii:21/23/9506.

Kenny, P. J., File, S. E., & Neal, M. J. (2000). Evidence for a complex influence of nicotinic acetylcholine receptors on hippocampal serotonin release. *Journal of Neurochemistry*, *75*(6), 2409–2414.

Kodas, E., Cohen, C., Louis, C., & Griebel, G. (2007). Cortico-limbic circuitry for conditioned nicotine-seeking behavior in rats involves endocannabinoid signaling. *Psychopharmacology*, *194*(2), 161–171. http://dx.doi.org/10.1007/s00213-007-0813-0.

Koob, G. F. (2009a). Dynamics of neuronal circuits in addiction: reward, antireward, and emotional memory. *Pharmacopsychiatry*, *42*(Suppl. 1), S32–S41. http://dx.doi.org/10.1055/s-0029-1216356.

Koob, G. F. (2009b). Neurobiological substrates for the dark side of compulsivity in addiction. *Neuropharmacology*, *56*(Suppl. 1), 18–31. http://dx.doi.org/10.1016/j.neuropharm.2008.07.043.

Kreitzer, A. C., & Regehr, W. G. (2001). Retrograde inhibition of presynaptic calcium influx by endogenous cannabinoids at excitatory synapses onto purkinje cells. *Neuron*, *29*(3), 717–727.

Le Foll, B., & Goldberg, S. R. (2004). Rimonabant, a CB1 antagonist, blocks nicotine-conditioned place preferences. *Neuroreport*, *15*(13), 2139–2143. pii:00001756-200409150-00028.

Le Foll, B., & Goldberg, S. R. (2005). Cannabinoid CB1 receptor antagonists as promising new medications for drug dependence. *The Journal of Pharmacology and Experimental Therapeutics*, *312*(3), 875–883. pii:jpet.104.077974.

Le Foll, B., Forget, B., Aubin, H. J., & Goldberg, S. R. (2008). Blocking cannabinoid CB1 receptors for the treatment of nicotine dependence: insights from pre-clinical and clinical studies. *Addiction Biology*, *13*(2), 239–252. http://dx.doi.org/10.1111/j.1369-1600.2008.00113.x.

Le Foll, B., Gorelick, D. A., & Goldberg, S. R. (2009). The future of endocannabinoid-oriented clinical research after CB1 antagonists. *Psychopharmacology*, *205*(1), 171–174. http://dx.doi.org/10.1007/s00213-009-1506-7.

Lev-Ran, S., Imtiaz, S., Rehm, J., & Le Foll, B. (2013). Exploring the association between lifetime prevalence of mental illness and transition from substance use to substance use disorders: results from the national epidemiologic survey of alcohol and related conditions (NESARC). *The American Journal on Addictions/American Academy of Psychiatrists in Alcoholism and Addictions*, *22*(2), 93–98. http://dx.doi.org/10.1111/j.1521-0391.2013.00304.x.

Leweke, F. M., & Koethe, D. (2008). Cannabis and psychiatric disorders: it is not only addiction. *Addiction Biology*, *13*(2), 264–275. http://dx.doi.org/10.1111/j.1369-1600.2008.00106.x.

Leweke, F. M., Piomelli, D., Pahlisch, F., Muhl, D., Gerth, C. W., Hoyer, C., … Koethe, D. (2012). Cannabidiol enhances anandamide signaling and alleviates psychotic symptoms of schizophrenia. *Translational Psychiatry*, *2*, e94. http://dx.doi.org/10.1038/tp.2012.15.

Lichtman, A. H., & Martin, B. R. (1991). Spinal and supraspinal components of cannabinoid-induced antinociception. *The Journal of Pharmacology and Experimental Therapeutics*, *258*(2), 517–523.

Long, J. Z., Li, W., Booker, L., Burston, J. J., Kinsey, S. G., Schlosburg, J. E., … Cravatt, B. F. (2009). Selective blockade of 2-arachidonoylglycerol hydrolysis produces cannabinoid behavioral effects. *Nature Chemical Biology*, *5*(1), 37–44. http://dx.doi.org/10.1038/nchembio.129.

Long, J. Z., Nomura, D. K., & Cravatt, B. F. (2009). Characterization of monoacylglycerol lipase inhibition reveals differences in central and peripheral endocannabinoid metabolism. *Chemistry & Biology*, *16*(7), 744–753. http://dx.doi.org/10.1016/j.chembiol.2009.05.009.

Mahgoub, M., Keun-Hang, S. Y., Sydorenko, V., Ashoor, A., Kabbani, N., Al Kury, L., … Galadari, S. (2013). Effects of cannabidiol on the function of α 7-nicotinic acetylcholine receptors. *European Journal of Pharmacology*, *720*(1), 310–319.

Malone, D. T., & Taylor, D. A. (1999). Modulation by fluoxetine of striatal dopamine release following delta9-tetrahydrocannabinol: a microdialysis study in conscious rats. *British Journal of Pharmacology*, 128(1), 21–26. http://dx.doi.org/10.1038/sj.bjp.0702753.

Mansvelder, H. D., Keath, J. R., & McGehee, D. S. (2002). Synaptic mechanisms underlie nicotine-induced excitability of brain reward areas. *Neuron*, 33(6), 905–919. pii:S0896627302006256.

Martin, B. R., Mechoulam, R., & Razdan, R. K. (1999). Discovery and characterization of endogenous cannabinoids. *Life Sciences*, 65(6–7), 573–595.

Mascia, P., Pistis, M., Justinova, Z., Panlilio, L. V., Luchicchi, A., Lecca, S., … Goldberg, S. R. (2011). Blockade of nicotine reward and reinstatement by activation of alpha-type peroxisome proliferator-activated receptors. *Biological Psychiatry*, 69(7), 633–641. http://dx.doi.org/10.1016/j.biopsych.2010.07.009.

McGehee, D. S., Heath, M. J., Gelber, S., Devay, P., & Role, L. W. (1995). Nicotine enhancement of fast excitatory synaptic transmission in CNS by presynaptic receptors. *Science (New York, N.Y.)*, 269(5231), 1692–1696.

Mechoulam, R., & Parker, L. A. (2013). The endocannabinoid system and the brain. *Annual Review of Psychology*, 64, 21–47. http://dx.doi.org/10.1146/annurev-psych-113011-143739.

Melis, M., Pistis, M., Perra, S., Muntoni, A. L., Pillolla, G., & Gessa, G. L. (2004). Endocannabinoids mediate presynaptic inhibition of glutamatergic transmission in rat ventral tegmental area dopamine neurons through activation of CB1 receptors. *The Journal of Neuroscience: The Official Journal of the Society for Neuroscience*, 24(1), 53–62. http://dx.doi.org/10.1523/JNEUROSCI.4503-03.2004.

Melis, M., Pillolla, G., Luchicchi, A., Muntoni, A. L., Yasar, S., Goldberg, S. R., & Pistis, M. (2008). Endogenous fatty acid ethanolamides suppress nicotine-induced activation of mesolimbic dopamine neurons through nuclear receptors. *The Journal of Neuroscience: The Official Journal of the Society for Neuroscience*, 28(51), 13985–13994. http://dx.doi.org/10.1523/JNEUROSCI.3221-08.2008.

Merritt, L. L., Martin, B. R., Walters, C., Lichtman, A. H., & Damaj, M. I. (2008). The endogenous cannabinoid system modulates nicotine reward and dependence. *The Journal of Pharmacology and Experimental Therapeutics*, 326(2), 483–492. http://dx.doi.org/10.1124/jpet.108.138321.

Moreno, S., Farioli-Vecchioli, S., & Ceru, M. P. (2004). Immunolocalization of peroxisome proliferator-activated receptors and retinoid X receptors in the adult rat CNS. *Neuroscience*, 123(1), 131–145. pii:S0306452203006377.

Morgan, C. J., Das, R. K., Joye, A., Curran, H. V., & Kamboj, S. K. (2013). Cannabidiol reduces cigarette consumption in tobacco smokers: preliminary findings. *Addictive Behaviors*, 38(9), 2433–2436. http://dx.doi.org/10.1016/j.addbeh.2013.03.011.

Muldoon, P. P., Chen, J., Harenza, J. L., Abdullah, R. A., Sim-Selley, L. J., Cravatt, B. F., … Damaj, M. I. (2015). Inhibition of monoacylglycerol lipase reduces nicotine withdrawal. *British Journal of Pharmacology*, 172(3), 869–882. http://dx.doi.org/10.1111/bph.12948.

Munro, S., Thomas, K. L., & Abu-Shaar, M. (1993). Molecular characterization of a peripheral receptor for cannabinoids. *Nature*, 365(6441), 61–65.

Navarrete, F., Rodriguez-Arias, M., Martin-Garcia, E., Navarro, D., Garcia-Gutierrez, M. S., Aguilar, M. A., … Manzanares, J. (2013). Role of CB2 cannabinoid receptors in the rewarding, reinforcing, and physical effects of nicotine. *Neuropsychopharmacology: Official Publication of the American College of Neuropsychopharmacology*, 38(12), 2515–2524. http://dx.doi.org/10.1038/npp.2013.157.

Ng Cheong Ton, J. M., Gerhardt, G. A., Friedemann, M., Etgen, A. M., Rose, G. M., Sharpless, N. S., & Gardner, E. L. (1988). The effects of delta 9-tetrahydrocannabinol on potassium-evoked release of dopamine in the rat caudate nucleus: an in vivo electrochemical and in vivo microdialysis study. *Brain Research*, 451(1–2), 59–68.

Ohno-Shosaku, T., Maejima, T., & Kano, M. (2001). Endogenous cannabinoids mediate retrograde signals from depolarized postsynaptic neurons to presynaptic terminals. *Neuron*, 29(3), 729–738.

Oleson, E. B., & Cheer, J. F. (2012a). A brain on cannabinoids: the role of dopamine release in reward seeking. *Cold Spring Harbor Perspectives in Medicine, 2*(8). http://dx.doi.org/10.1101/cshperspect.a012229.

Oleson, E. B., & Cheer, J. F. (2012b). Paradoxical effects of the endocannabinoid uptake inhibitor VDM11 on accumbal neural encoding of reward predictive cues. *Synapse (New York, N.Y.), 66*(11), 984–988. http://dx.doi.org/10.1002/syn.21587.

Onaivi, E. S., Ishiguro, H., Gong, J., Patel, S., Perchuk, A., Meozzi, P. A., ... Gardner, E. (2006). Discovery of the presence and functional expression of cannabinoid CB2 receptors in brain. *Annals of the New York Academy of Sciences, 1074*(1), 514–536.

O'Sullivan, S. E. (2007). Cannabinoids go nuclear: evidence for activation of peroxisome proliferator-activated receptors. *British Journal of Pharmacology, 152*(5), 576–582. pii:0707423.

Owesson-White, C. A., Ariansen, J., Stuber, G. D., Cleaveland, N. A., Cheer, J. F., Wightman, R. M., & Carelli, R. M. (2009). Neural encoding of cocaine-seeking behavior is coincident with phasic dopamine release in the accumbens core and shell. *The European Journal of Neuroscience, 30*(6), 1117–1127. http://dx.doi.org/10.1111/j.1460-9568.2009.06916.x.

Pan, B., Wang, W., Long, J. Z., Sun, D., Hillard, C. J., Cravatt, B. F., & Liu, Q. S. (2009). Blockade of 2-arachidonoylglycerol hydrolysis by selective monoacylglycerol lipase inhibitor 4-nitrophenyl 4-(dibenzo[d][1,3]dioxol-5-yl(hydroxy)methyl)piperidine-1-carboxylate (JZL184) enhances retrograde endocannabinoid signaling. *The Journal of Pharmacology and Experimental Therapeutics, 331*(2), 591–597. http://dx.doi.org/10.1124/jpet.109.158162.

Panlilio, L. V., Justinova, Z., Mascia, P., Pistis, M., Luchicchi, A., Lecca, S., ... Goldberg, S. R. (2012). Novel use of a lipid-lowering fibrate medication to prevent nicotine reward and relapse: preclinical findings. *Neuropsychopharmacology: Official Publication of the American College of Neuropsychopharmacology, 37*(8), 1838–1847. http://dx.doi.org/10.1038/npp.2012.31.

Pertwee, R. G. (2008). The diverse CB1 and CB2 receptor pharmacology of three plant cannabinoids: delta9-tetrahydrocannabinol, cannabidiol and delta9-tetrahydrocannabivarin. *British Journal of Pharmacology, 153*(2), 199–215. pii:0707442.

Phillips, P. E., Stuber, G. D., Heien, M. L., Wightman, R. M., & Carelli, R. M. (2003). Subsecond dopamine release promotes cocaine seeking. *Nature, 422*(6932), 614–618. http://dx.doi.org/10.1038/nature01476.

Picciotto, M. R., Caldarone, B. J., King, S. L., & Zachariou, V. (2000). Nicotinic receptors in the brain. links between molecular biology and behavior. *Neuropsychopharmacology: Official Publication of the American College of Neuropsychopharmacology, 22*(5), 451–465. pii:S0893-133X(99)00146-3.

Pidoplichko, V. I., DeBiasi, M., Williams, J. T., & Dani, J. A. (1997). Nicotine activates and desensitizes midbrain dopamine neurons. *Nature, 390*(6658), 401–404. http://dx.doi.org/10.1038/37120.

Piomelli, D., Giuffrida, A., Calignano, A., & de Fonseca, F. R. (2000). The endocannabinoid system as a target for therapeutic drugs. *Trends in Pharmacological Sciences, 21*(6), 218–224.

Pistis, M., & Melis, M. (2010). From surface to nuclear receptors: the endocannabinoid family extends its assets. *Current Medicinal Chemistry, 17*(14), 1450–1467. pii:BSP/CMC/E-Pub/095.

Pontieri, F. E., Tanda, G., Orzi, F., & Di Chiara, G. (1996). Effects of nicotine on the nucleus accumbens and similarity to those of addictive drugs. *Nature, 382*(6588), 255–257. http://dx.doi.org/10.1038/382255a0.

Pryor, G. T., Larsen, F. F., Husain, S., & Braude, M. C. (1978). Interactions of delta9-tetrahydrocannabinol with D-amphetamine, cocaine, and nicotine in rats. *Pharmacology, Biochemistry, and Behavior, 8*(3), 295–318. pii:0091-3057(78)90320-9.

Reisiger, A. R., Kaufling, J., Manzoni, O., Cador, M., Georges, F., & Caille, S. (2014). Nicotine self-administration induces CB1-dependent LTP in the bed nucleus of the stria terminalis. *The Journal of Neuroscience: The Official Journal of the Society for Neuroscience, 34*(12), 4285–4292. http://dx.doi.org/10.1523/JNEUROSCI.3149-13.2014.

Revuelta, A. V., Moroni, F., Cheney, D. L., & Costa, E. (1978). Effect of cannabinoids on the turnover rate of acetylcholine in rat hippocampus, striatum and cortex. *Naunyn-Schmiedeberg's Archives of Pharmacology*, *304*(2), 107–110.

Rinaldi-Carmona, M., Barth, F., Héaulme, M., Shire, D., Calandra, B., Congy, C., ... Caput, D. (1994). SR141716A, a potent and selective antagonist of the brain cannabinoid receptor. *FEBS Letters*, *350*(2), 240–244.

Robbe, D., Alonso, G., Duchamp, F., Bockaert, J., & Manzoni, O. J. (2001). Localization and mechanisms of action of cannabinoid receptors at the glutamatergic synapses of the mouse nucleus accumbens. *The Journal of Neuroscience: The Official Journal of the Society for Neuroscience*, *21*(1), 109–116. pii:21/1/109.

Savinainen, J. R., Jarvinen, T., Laine, K., & Laitinen, J. T. (2001). Despite substantial degradation, 2-arachidonoylglycerol is a potent full efficacy agonist mediating CB(1) receptor-dependent G-protein activation in rat cerebellar membranes. *British Journal of Pharmacology*, *134*(3), 664–672. http://dx.doi.org/10.1038/sj.bjp.0704297.

Scherma, M., Justinova, Z., Zanettini, C., Panlilio, L. V., Mascia, P., Fadda, P., ... Goldberg, S. R. (2012). The anandamide transport inhibitor AM404 reduces the rewarding effects of nicotine and nicotine-induced dopamine elevations in the nucleus accumbens shell in rats. *British Journal of Pharmacology*, *165*(8), 2539–2548. http://dx.doi.org/10.1111/j.1476-5381.2011.01467.x.

Scherma, M., Panlilio, L. V., Fadda, P., Fattore, L., Gamaleddin, I., Le Foll, B., ... Goldberg, S. R. (2008). Inhibition of anandamide hydrolysis by cyclohexyl carbamic acid 3′-carbamoyl-3-yl ester (URB597) reverses abuse-related behavioral and neurochemical effects of nicotine in rats. *The Journal of Pharmacology and Experimental Therapeutics*, *327*(2), 482–490. http://dx.doi.org/10.1124/jpet.108.142224.

Schlicker, E., & Kathmann, M. (2001). Modulation of transmitter release via presynaptic cannabinoid receptors. *Trends in Pharmacological Sciences*, *22*(11), 565–572 pii:S0165-6147(00)01805-8.

Shoaib, M. (2008). The cannabinoid antagonist AM251 attenuates nicotine self-administration and nicotine-seeking behaviour in rats. *Neuropharmacology*, *54*(2), 438–444. pii:S0028-3908(07)00333-4.

Simonnet, A., Cador, M., & Caille, S. (2013). Nicotine reinforcement is reduced by cannabinoid CB1 receptor blockade in the ventral tegmental area. *Addiction Biology*, *18*(6), 930–936. http://dx.doi.org/10.1111/j.1369-1600.2012.00476.x.

Solinas, M., Tanda, G., Justinova, Z., Wertheim, C. E., Yasar, S., Piomelli, D., ... Goldberg, S. R. (2007). The endogenous cannabinoid anandamide produces delta-9-tetrahydrocannabinol-like discriminative and neurochemical effects that are enhanced by inhibition of fatty acid amide hydrolase but not by inhibition of anandamide transport. *The Journal of Pharmacology and Experimental Therapeutics*, *321*(1), 370–380. pii:jpet.106.114124.

Sugiura, T., Kobayashi, Y., Oka, S., & Waku, K. (2002). Biosynthesis and degradation of anandamide and 2-arachidonoylglycerol and their possible physiological significance. *Prostaglandins, Leukotrienes, and Essential Fatty Acids*, *66*(2–3), 173–192. http://dx.doi.org/10.1054/plef.2001.0356.

Szabo, B., Siemes, S., & Wallmichrath, I. (2002). Inhibition of GABAergic neurotransmission in the ventral tegmental area by cannabinoids. *The European Journal of Neuroscience*, *15*(12), 2057–2061. pii:2041.

Tanda, G., Pontieri, F. E., & Di Chiara, G. (1997). Cannabinoid and heroin activation of mesolimbic dopamine transmission by a common mu1 opioid receptor mechanism. *Science (New York, N.Y.)*, *276*(5321), 2048–2050.

Tapper, A. R., McKinney, S. L., Nashmi, R., Schwarz, J., Deshpande, P., Labarca, C., ... Lester, H. A. (2004). Nicotine activation of alpha4* receptors: sufficient for reward, tolerance, and sensitization. *Science (New York, N.Y.)*, *306*(5698), 1029–1032. pii:306/5698/1029.

Thomas, A., Baillie, G. L., Phillips, A. M., Razdan, R. K., Ross, R. A., & Pertwee, R. G. (2007). Cannabidiol displays unexpectedly high potency as an antagonist of CB1 and CB2 receptor agonists in vitro. *British Journal of Pharmacology*, *150*(5), 613–623. pii:0707133.

Tripathi, H. L., Vocci, F. J., Brase, D. A., & Dewey, W. L. (1987). Effects of cannabinoids on levels of acetylcholine and choline and on turnover rate of acetylcholine in various regions of the mouse brain. *Alcohol and Drug Research, 7*(5–6), 525–532.

Tsou, K., Nogueron, M. I., Muthian, S., Sanudo-Pena, M. C., Hillard, C. J., Deutsch, D. G., & Walker, J. M. (1998). Fatty acid amide hydrolase is located preferentially in large neurons in the rat central nervous system as revealed by immunohistochemistry. *Neuroscience Letters, 254*(3), 137–140. pii:S0304394098007009.

Ueda, N., Tsuboi, K., Uyama, T., & Ohnishi, T. (2011). Biosynthesis and degradation of the endocannabinoid 2-arachidonoylglycerol. *BioFactors (Oxford, England), 37*(1), 1–7. http://dx.doi.org/10.1002/biof.131.

US Food and Drug Administration, & Endocrinologic and Metabolic Drugs Advisory Committee. (2008). June 13, 2007. Briefing Information. NDA 21-888. ZIMULTI®(Rimonabant)–Sanofi-Aventis.

Valjent, E., Mitchell, J. M., Besson, M. J., Caboche, J., & Maldonado, R. (2002). Behavioural and biochemical evidence for interactions between delta 9-tetrahydrocannabinol and nicotine. *British Journal of Pharmacology, 135*(2), 564–578. http://dx.doi.org/10.1038/sj.bjp.0704479.

Wade, D. T., Robson, P., House, H., Makela, P., & Aram, J. (2003). A preliminary controlled study to determine whether whole-plant cannabis extracts can improve intractable neurogenic symptoms. *Clinical Rehabilitation, 17*(1), 21–29.

Wang, H., & Lupica, C. R. (2014). Release of endogenous cannabinoids from ventral tegmental area dopamine neurons and the modulation of synaptic processes. *Progress in Neuro-Psychopharmacology & Biological Psychiatry, 52*, 24–27. http://dx.doi.org/10.1016/j.pnpbp.2014.01.019.

Weiss, F., Ciccocioppo, R., Parsons, L. H., Katner, S., Liu, X., Zorrilla, E. P., … Richter, R. R. (2001). Compulsive drug-seeking behavior and relapse. Neuroadaptation, stress, and conditioning factors. *Annals of the New York Academy of Sciences, 937*, 1–26.

Wickelgren, I. (1997). Marijuana: harder than thought? *Science (New York, N.Y.), 276*(5321), 1967–1968.

Wilkie, G. I., Hutson, P. H., Stephens, M. W., Whiting, P., & Wonnacott, S. (1993). Hippocampal nicotinic autoreceptors modulate acetylcholine release. *Biochemical Society Transactions, 21*(2), 429–431.

Wilson, R. I., & Nicoll, R. A. (2001). Endogenous cannabinoids mediate retrograde signalling at hippocampal synapses. *Nature, 410*(6828), 588–592.

Wu, X., & French, E. D. (2000). Effects of chronic delta9-tetrahydrocannabinol on rat midbrain dopamine neurons: an electrophysiological assessment. *Neuropharmacology, 39*(3), 391–398. pii:S0028390899001409.

Xi, Z. X., Peng, X. Q., Li, X., Song, R., Zhang, H. Y., Liu, Q. R., … Gardner, E. L. (2011). Brain cannabinoid CB(2) receptors modulate cocaine's actions in mice. *Nature Neuroscience, 14*(9), 1160–1166. http://dx.doi.org/10.1038/nn.2874.

Yang, X., Criswell, H. E., & Breese, G. R. (1996). Nicotine-induced inhibition in medial septum involves activation of presynaptic nicotinic cholinergic receptors on gamma-aminobutyric acid-containing neurons. *The Journal of Pharmacology and Experimental Therapeutics, 276*(2), 482–489.

Zhang, H. Y., Gao, M., Liu, Q. R., Bi, G. H., Li, X., Yang, H. J., … Xi, Z. X. (2014). Cannabinoid CB2 receptors modulate midbrain dopamine neuronal activity and dopamine-related behavior in mice. *Proceedings of the National Academy of Sciences of the United States of America, 111*(46), E5007–E5015. http://dx.doi.org/10.1073/pnas.1413210111.

10

Critical Role for Brain Stress Systems in the Negative Affective State Associated With Nicotine Withdrawal

X. Qi, D. Bruijnzeel, A.W. Bruijnzeel

University of Florida, Gainesville, FL, United States

INTRODUCTION

Nicotine is one of the most widely abused drugs in the world. Worldwide, there are about one billion men who smoke and 250 million women (WHO, 2011). Smoking increases the risk for a wide range of life-threatening diseases, including cancer, chronic obstructive pulmonary disease, cardiovascular diseases, and brain disorders such as dementia and Alzheimer's disease (Ott et al., 1998; Pirie, Peto, Reeves, Green, & Beral, 2013; Postma, Bush, & van den Berge, 2014; Thun et al., 2013). About half the smokers will die prematurely as a consequence of their addiction. Worldwide, about 5.4 million people die each year from smoking or secondhand smoke exposure, including 520,000 people in the United States and 640,000 people in Europe (ASPECT-Consortium, 2005; Thun et al., 2013; WHO, 2011). Research by the World Health Organization (WHO) indicates that the tobacco pandemic is moving from Western countries to developing nations and that about 80% of the people who die from smoking live in low to middle-income countries (WHO, 2011). Several smoking cessation treatments have been developed, but relapse rates are still very high among people receiving treatment for nicotine addiction. Therefore, a better understanding of the factors that contribute to the development and maintenance of nicotine addiction is warranted.

Negative Affective States and Cognitive Impairments in Nicotine Dependence
http://dx.doi.org/10.1016/B978-0-12-802574-1.00010-7

The positive reinforcing effects of nicotine play a pivotal role in the initiation of smoking (Finkenauer, Pomerleau, Snedecor, & Pomerleau, 2009). The positive reinforcing effects of smoking include mild euphoria, relaxation, and improved attention and working memory (Ague, 1973; Benowitz, 1988; Wesnes & Warburton, 1983). Although there are many psychoactive compounds in tobacco smoke, nicotine is considered the main component of tobacco smoke that leads to the development of tobacco addiction. This is also supported by the rapid increase in the use of *electronic nicotine delivery systems* (ENDS, also referred to as e-cigarettes) in young people who have never smoked conventional cigarettes (Corey, Wang, Johnson, Apelberg, & Husten, 2013; Johnston, O'Malley, Miech, Bachman, & Schulenberg, 2015). The ENDS deliver nicotine but not any of the other tobacco smoke ingredients (Pellegrino et al., 2012). It should be noted, however, that there are some compounds in tobacco smoke that may potentiate the rewarding effects of nicotine. Burning tobacco leads to the formation of acetaldehyde, which is self-administered by rodents, induces conditioned place preference, and potentiates the rewarding effects of nicotine (Belluzzi, Wang, & Leslie, 2005; Brown, Amit, & Rockman, 1979; Myers, Ng, & Singer, 1982; Smith, Amit, & Splawinsky, 1984). This might explain why some ENDS users transition to smoking conventional cigarettes.

Smoking cessation leads to negative affective symptoms such as depressed mood, anxiety, and impaired memory and attention (Hughes, Gust, Skoog, Keenan, & Fenwick, 1991; Hughes & Hatsukami, 1986). The negative affective symptoms associated with smoking cessation may increase the risk for relapse to smoking (Bruijnzeel & Gold, 2005). Nicotine is the main component of tobacco that prevents people from quitting smoking (Bardo, Green, Crooks, & Dwoskin, 1999; Stolerman & Jarvis, 1995). Studies with ENDS and nicotine patches show that nicotine decreases the desire to smoke conventional cigarettes, improves memory during abstinence, and diminishes withdrawal signs (Dawkins, Turner, Hasna, & Soar, 2012; Harrell et al., 2015; Shiffman, Ferguson, Gwaltney, Balabanis, & Shadel, 2006).

DYSPHORIA AND NICOTINE WITHDRAWAL

During the last several decades, a wide range of animal models and test procedures have been used to investigate the negative mood state associated with smoking cessation. In most of these experiments, the animals were made nicotine dependent by using intermittent injection protocols or by using osmotic minipumps that continuously deliver nicotine. Cessation of chronic nicotine administration decreases responding for food pellets under both fixed-ratio and progressive-ratio schedules of reinforcement, which might be indicative of a negative mood state (Corrigall, Herling, & Coen, 1989; LeSage, Burroughs, & Pentel, 2006). Cessation of nicotine administration has also been shown to increase immobility in the forced swim test (Mannucci, Tedesco, Bellomo, Caputi, & Calapai, 2006; Roni & Rahman, 2014). Interestingly, the increase in immobility in the forced swim test has been observed up to 60 days after the cessation of nicotine administration (Mannucci et al., 2006). The forced swim test has been widely used to screen drugs for antidepressant activity, and antidepressant drugs decrease immobility and increase swimming or climbing (Cryan, Valentino, & Lucki, 2005). It should be noted that it has been argued that the forced swim test is not an animal model for depression but merely a screening tool for antidepressant activity of compounds (Nestler & Hyman, 2010). Thus, withdrawal or stress-induced behavioral changes in the forced swim test may not necessarily reflect depressive-like behavior. The conditioned place aversion procedure has also been used to assess the aversive state associated with precipitated nicotine withdrawal. In this test, the negative motivational properties of drug withdrawal (unconditioned stimulus) are paired with a neutral test environment. After pairing, the previously neutral environment acts as a conditioned stimulus and induces avoidance behavior (Tzschentke, 1998). The nicotinic receptor antagonist mecamylamine induces place aversion in rats chronically treated with nicotine but not in saline control rats (Suzuki, Ise, Tsuda, Maeda, & Misawa, 1996). Finally, the intracranial self-stimulation (ICSS) procedure has been widely used to investigate the negative mood state associated with drug withdrawal (Epping-Jordan, Watkins, Koob, & Markou, 1998). In the discrete trial ICSS procedure, the animals are prepared with electrodes in the lateral hypothalamus/medial forebrain bundle, and when placed in the test chamber they can self-stimulate their brain reward system. By systematically changing the intensity of the electrical current and determining the lowest current that supports self-stimulation, the state of the brain reward system can be assessed (Der-Avakian & Markou, 2012). The acute administration of drugs of abuse increases sensitivity to the electrical stimuli and lowers brain reward/ICSS thresholds, which is indicative of a potentiation of brain reward function. In contrast, cessation of chronic drug administration leads to an increase in ICSS thresholds, which is indicative of a negative mood state. The administration of nonselective nicotine receptor antagonists to nicotine-dependent animals or cessation of chronic nicotine administration leads to elevations in brain reward thresholds (Epping-Jordan et al., 1998; Johnson, Hollander, & Kenny, 2008). One of the main advantages of the ICSS procedure is that it provides a quantitative measure of the emotional state of the brain reward system during withdrawal. The ICSS procedure is a well-validated test to assess the negative mood state associated with nicotine withdrawal.

The US Food and Drug Administration (FDA) has approved two non-nicotine treatments for smoking cessation. The first drug to be approved for smoking cessation was bupropion. This drug was originally approved in 1985 for the treatment of depression. The mechanism by which bupropion improves smoking cessation rates is not completely clear yet. However, bupropion and its metabolites may improve smoking cessation rates by noncompetitive blockade of α4β2* and α3β4* nicotinic acetylcholine receptors (nAChRs), inhibiting reuptake of dopamine, norepinephrine, and serotonin, or by inhibiting the firing of noradrenergic neurons (Carroll et al., 2014; Cryan, Gasparini, van Heeke, & Markou, 2003). Varenicline was approved in 1997, the second smoking cessation drug to be approved by the FDA. Varenicline is a partial agonist at α4β2* and α6β2* nAChRs and a full agonist at α7 and α3β4* nAChRs (Grady et al., 2010). Both bupropion and varenicline have been shown to prevent the elevations in ICSS thresholds associated with nicotine withdrawal (Cryan et al., 2003; Igari et al., 2013). Therefore, this animal model has face and predictive validity for identifying treatments that diminish the negative mood state associated with smoking cessation in humans.

Although the roles of age and sex in nicotine withdrawal are rather unexplored, there is some evidence that suggests that these factors affect nicotine withdrawal. A study with adolescent male rats showed that adolescents display fewer somatic signs during withdrawal than adult rats (O'Dell et al., 2006). In addition, mecamylamine elevated ICSS thresholds of adult rats chronically treated with nicotine but did not affect ICSS thresholds of adolescent rats. This suggests that the somatic and affective nicotine withdrawal signs are diminished in adolescent rats compared to adult rats. Several animal studies have also investigated the role of sex in nicotine withdrawal. The studies suggest that female rats display more somatic nicotine withdrawal signs than male rats (Hamilton, Berger, Perry, & Grunberg, 2009; Nesil, Kanit, Ugur, & Pogun, 2015). Furthermore, a study by O'Dell and colleagues showed that precipitated nicotine withdrawal induces greater conditioned place aversion in female compared to male rats (O'Dell & Torres, 2014). Taken together, these findings suggest that the negative mood state associated with nicotine withdrawal is diminished in adolescent rats and more severe in female rats.

CRF AND DYSPHORIA ASSOCIATED WITH NICOTINE WITHDRAWAL

The 41-amino-acid neuropeptide corticotropin-releasing factor (CRF) was first isolated from sheep hypothalami (Vale, Spiess, Rivier, & Rivier, 1981). CRF-positive neurons have been detected in the paraventricular nucleus of the hypothalamus and in other brain areas such as the central nucleus of the amygdala (CeA), bed nucleus of the stria terminalis (BNST), ventral tegmental area, and locus coeruleus (LC) (Grieder et al., 2014; Swanson, Sawchenko, Rivier, & Vale, 1983). Scattered CRF neurons have also been found throughout the neocortex (Swanson et al., 1983). Hypothalamic CRF neurons project to the median eminence and play an important role in the release of ACTH from the anterior pituitary. ACTH is transported via the blood to the adrenal cortex and stimulates the release of corticosterone into the circulation. Corticosterone prepares the body for stressors by mobilizing energy stores and suppressing physiological processes that are not necessary for immediate survival (McEwen, 2000; Sapolsky, 1992). Extrahypothalamic CRF orchestrates behavioral and autonomic responses to stressors (Koob & Heinrichs, 1999; Nijsen, Croiset, Diamant, De Wied, & Wiegant, 2001), and many of these effects are independent of CRF's effects on the hypothalamic–pituitary–adrenal axis (Eaves, Thatcher-Britton, Rivier, Vale, & Koob, 1985; Sutton, Koob, Le Moal, Rivier, & Vale, 1982). Two CRF receptors have been cloned, the CRF_1 and CRF_2 receptors (Chen, Lewis, Perrin, & Vale, 1993; Lovenberg et al., 1995; Perrin, Donaldson, Chen, Lewis, & Vale, 1993). The CRF_1 and CRF_2 receptors are G-protein-coupled receptors and are positively coupled to adenylyl cyclase (Chalmers, Lovenberg, Grigoriadis, Behan, & De Souza, 1996; Lewis et al., 2001). Pharmacological studies suggest that CRF serves as an endogenous ligand for the CRF_1 receptor and that urocortin 2 and 3 are endogenous ligands for the CRF_2 receptor (Lewis et al., 2001). Urocortin 1 binds with a somewhat higher affinity to the CRF_1 than the CRF_2 receptor (Lewis et al., 2001). Stress-induced psychopathology and drug withdrawal-induced behavioral and physiological changes are predominantly mediated via activation of CRF_1 receptors (Bruijnzeel & Gold, 2005; Koob, 1999; Steckler & Holsboer, 1999). Conflicting findings have been reported regarding the role of CRF_2 receptors in stress-induced behavioral changes and drug addiction (Bruijnzeel & Gold, 2005). It is not yet known if the urocortins affect nicotine withdrawal.

In our laboratory, we have extensively investigated the role of CRF in the negative mood state associated with nicotine withdrawal. We started this line of research by investigating if blockade of CRF receptors with the nonspecific CRF_1/CRF_2 receptor antagonist D-Phe $CRF_{(12-41)}$ diminishes the elevations in ICSS thresholds associated with mecamylamine-precipitated and spontaneous nicotine withdrawal (Bruijnzeel, Zislis, Wilson, & Gold, 2007). Spontaneous nicotine withdrawal was induced by removing osmotic minipumps that chronically delivered nicotine after a 14-day period. It was shown that a high dose of D-Phe $CRF_{(12-41)}$ (20 µg) administered directly into the lateral ventricles diminished the mecamylamine-induced elevations in brain reward thresholds in nicotine-dependent rats. None of the doses of D-Phe $CRF_{(12-41)}$ affected the brain reward thresholds of the saline control rats. At the end of the experiment, we investigated if the same dose of D-Phe CRF$_{(12-41)}$ would diminish the negative mood state associated with spontaneous nicotine withdrawal. In this experiment, the CRF antagonist was administered immediately before the 6 h time point (post pump removal). In contrast to the precipitated withdrawal experiment, in the spontaneous nicotine withdrawal experiment, blockade of the CRF receptors did not diminish the negative mood state associated with nicotine withdrawal. This pattern of results suggests that CRF receptor antagonists can prevent the negative mood state associated with drug withdrawal when they are administered prior to the onset of withdrawal but do not reverse the negative mood state when they are administered after the onset of withdrawal. In a follow-up experiment, the role of CRF$_1$ and CRF$_2$ receptors in the negative mood state associated with precipitated nicotine withdrawal was investigated (Bruijnzeel, Prado, & Isaac, 2009). In order to block CRF$_1$ receptors, the highly selective CRF$_1$ receptor antagonist R278995/CRA0450 was used and CRF$_2$ receptors were blocked with the CRF$_2$ receptor antagonist astressin-2B. The CRF$_1$ receptor antagonist prevented the elevations in brain reward thresholds associated with precipitated nicotine withdrawal. In contrast, the CRF$_2$ receptor antagonist astressin-2B did not diminish the elevations in brain reward thresholds associated with precipitated nicotine withdrawal. These studies suggest that CRF$_1$, but not CRF$_2$, receptors play a role in the negative mood state associated with nicotine withdrawal.

We then investigated which brain areas play a role in the negative mood state associated with precipitated nicotine withdrawal (Marcinkiewcz et al., 2009). In our studies, we investigated the role of CRF receptors in the CeA, BNST, and nucleus accumbens (Nacc) shell. Administration of the nonselective CRF$_1$/CRF$_2$ receptor antagonist D-Phe CRF$_{(12-41)}$ into the CeA or the Nacc shell prevented mecamylamine-induced elevations in brain reward thresholds in nicotine-dependent rats. In contrast, administration of D-Phe CRF$_{(12-41)}$ in the lateral BNST did not prevent elevations in ICSS thresholds associated with nicotine withdrawal. This suggests that CRF receptors in the CeA and Nacc shell play a critical role in the negative mood state associated with nicotine withdrawal. In order to investigate if CRF$_1$ receptors in the CeA play a role in nicotine withdrawal, we conducted an additional study with the highly selective CRF$_1$ receptor antagonist R278995/CRA0450 (Bruijnzeel et al., 2012). This study showed that blockade of CRF$_1$ receptors in the CeA diminishes the negative mood state associated with nicotine withdrawal. To further explore the role of CRF in the CeA in the regulation of mood states and withdrawal, the effect of the overexpression of CRF in the CeA on the negative mood state associated with nicotine withdrawal was investigated. CRF was overexpressed in the CeA by using an adeno-associated virus (AAV), with AAV2 terminal repeats and AAV5 capsids (AAV2/5), that selectively and efficiently transduces neurons in the brain (Burger et al., 2004). In this experiment, the control animals received green fluorescent protein (GFP) instead of CRF. The rats were trained on the ICSS paradigm, and when the thresholds were stable, they received the viral vectors that delivered GFP or CRF, and brain reward thresholds were assessed for 28 days. Previous studies suggest that increased release of CRF in the CeA contributes to negative mood states (Bruijnzeel et al., 2012; Marcinkiewcz et al., 2009). However, in the present study, the overexpression of CRF in the CeA did not affect ICSS thresholds. This suggests that the overexpression of CRF does not lead to a negative mood state. We then investigated if the overexpression of CRF in the CeA affects the negative mood state associated with mecamyl-amine-precipitated and spontaneous nicotine withdrawal (Qi et al., 2014). The administration of mecamylamine to nicotine-dependent rats and the removal of the nicotine pumps led to large elevations in brain reward thresholds, and this effect was diminished in the rats that overexpressed CRF. Therefore, this suggests that the overexpression of CRF in the CeA diminishes the negative mood state associated with nicotine withdrawal. At the end of the experiment, we investigated the effect of administration of the AAV–CRF vector on CRF, CRF_1 receptor, and CRF_2 receptor levels. It was shown that administration of the AAV–CRF vector led to an increase in CRF levels, a decrease in CRF_1 receptor levels, and an increase in CRF_2 receptor levels. Considering the critical role of CRF_1 receptors in negative mood states, we speculate that the overexpression of CRF in the CeA diminished negative mood states associated with nicotine withdrawal by downregulating CRF_1 receptors in the CeA. However, it should be noted that there is some evidence that stimulation of CRF_2 receptors has antide-pressant-like effects (Chen et al., 2006; Tanaka & Telegdy, 2008). Therefore, the upregulation of CRF_2 receptors might have contributed to the diminished negative mood state in the nicotine-withdrawing rats as well.

NOREPINEPHRINE AND DYSPHORIA ASSOCIATED WITH NICOTINE WITHDRAWAL

There is extensive evidence for a role of noradrenergic systems in psychiatric disorders, but the role of norepinephrine in the negative mood state associated with nicotine withdrawal is relatively unexplored. Two noradrenergic cell groups have been located in the rodent and human brain (Dahlström & Fuxe, 1964). The noradrenergic neurons in the LC and sub-coeruleus give rise to the dorsal noradrenergic bundle, which projects to cortical areas, the hippocampus, amygdala, and other forebrain areas. The LC provides most of the norepinephrine input to the forebrain areas and plays an important role in attention, arousal, waking, and learning and memory (Aston-Jones, 2005). Noradrenergic cell groups (A1, A2, A5, and A7) located in the lateral tegmentum give rise to the ventral noradrenergic bundle. These projections innervate the hypothalamus, the septum, and subcomponents of the extended amygdala such as the CeA and BNST (Moore & Card, 1984).

In our studies, we investigated the effects of the α1-adrenoceptor antagonist prazosin, the α2-adrenoceptor agonist clonidine, and the nonselective β_1- and β_2-adrenoceptor antagonist propranolol on the negative mood state and somatic signs associated with precipitated nicotine withdrawal (Bruijnzeel et al., 2010). All these compounds inhibit noradrenergic transmission in the brain, either by blocking α1 or β-adrenergic receptors or by stimulating presynaptic α2-adrenergic receptors. The α1-adrenoceptor antagonist prazosin attenuated the elevations in brain reward thresholds associated with precipitated nicotine withdrawal. Prazosin had a U-shaped dose-dependent effect on the negative mood state in nicotine-withdrawing rats. The administration of an intermediate dose (0.125 mg/kg) was more effective in preventing the mecamylamine-precipitated elevations in brain reward thresholds in the nicotine group than lower or higher doses of this compound. The α2-adrenoceptor agonist clonidine or the nonselective β-adrenoceptor antagonist propranolol did not affect the elevations in brain reward thresholds associated with precipitated nicotine withdrawal. These drugs had opposite effects on somatic withdrawal signs. Prazosin, which diminished the negative mood state, did not affect the somatic signs associated with nicotine withdrawal. Clonidine and propranolol did not diminish the negative mood state associated with nicotine withdrawal but decreased the total number of somatic signs associated with nicotine withdrawal. It is interesting to note that some drugs affect somatic withdrawal signs but do not change affective withdrawal signs. This clearly indicates that different neuronal mechanisms mediate affective and somatic withdrawal signs. Clinical studies suggest that the negative mood state associated with drug withdrawal and craving is the main cause of relapse to drug use (Bruijnzeel, 2012; Bruijnzeel & Gold, 2005). In contrast, there is little evidence that somatic withdrawal signs contribute to relapse. Therefore, this suggests that drugs that decrease somatic withdrawal signs may not diminish affective withdrawal signs and are therefore unlikely to affect withdrawal in people who try to quit smoking.

We showed that the α1-adrenoceptor antagonist prazosin diminished the negative mood state associated with nicotine withdrawal (Bruijnzeel et al., 2010), but this compound may also attenuate the positive reinforcing properties of nicotine. It has been reported that prazosin diminishes the self-administration of nicotine and also attenuates nicotine-prime-induced reinstatement of extinguished nicotine seeking (Forget et al., 2010). Prazosin might diminish nicotine intake and nicotine-prime-induced reinstatement by attenuating nicotine-induced dopamine release in the Nacc shell (Forget et al., 2010). This brain region plays a critical role in signaling the rewarding effects of drugs of abuse.

In conclusion, the studies that we discussed here suggest that increased activity in brain stress systems plays a critical role in the negative mood state associated with smoking cessation. Nicotine withdrawal in rats leads to a negative mood state, and this is prevented by pretreatment with the FDA-approved smoking cessation drugs bupropion and varenicline. These drugs have significant side effects, and therefore we investigated the effects of drugs that prevent the activation of brain stress systems during withdrawal. The studies that are presented here show that drugs that block CRF_1 receptors or α1-adrenoceptors prevent the negative mood state associated with nicotine withdrawal. This suggests that drugs that block CRF_1 receptors or α1-adrenoceptors may prevent the negative mood state in people trying to quit smoking and thereby decrease the risk for relapse after a period of abstinence.

References

Ague, C. (1973). Nicotine and smoking: effects upon subjective changes in mood. *Psychopharmacologia, 30*(4), 323–328.

ASPECT-Consortium. (2005). *Tobacco or health in the European Union: Past, present and future.*

Aston-Jones, G. (2005). Brain structures and receptors involved in alertness. *Sleep Medicine, 6*(Suppl. 1), S3–S7.

Bardo, M. T., Green, T. A., Crooks, P. A., & Dwoskin, L. P. (1999). Nornicotine is self-administered intravenously by rats. *Psychopharmacology (Berlin), 146*(3), 290–296.

Belluzzi, J. D., Wang, R., & Leslie, F. M. (2005). Acetaldehyde enhances acquisition of nicotine self-administration in adolescent rats. *Neuropsychopharmacology, 30*(4), 705–712.

Benowitz, N. L. (1988). Drug therapy. Pharmacologic aspects of cigarette smoking and nicotine addition. *The New England Journal of Medicine, 319*(20), 1318–1330.

Brown, Z. W., Amit, Z., & Rockman, G. E. (1979). Intraventricular self-administration of acetaldehyde, but not ethanol, in naive laboratory rats. *Psychopharmacology (Berlin), 64*(3), 271–276.

Bruijnzeel, A. W. (2012). Tobacco addiction and the dysregulation of brain stress systems. *Neuroscience & Biobehavioral Reviews, 36*, 1418–1441.

Bruijnzeel, A. W., Bishnoi, M., van Tuijl, I. A., Keijzers, K. F., Yavarovich, K. R., Pasek, T. M., … Yamada, H. (2010). Effects of prazosin, clonidine, and propranolol on the elevations in brain reward thresholds and somatic signs associated with nicotine withdrawal in rats. *Psychopharmacology (Berlin), 212*(4), 485–499.

Bruijnzeel, A. W., Ford, J., Rogers, J. A., Scheick, S., Ji, Y., Bishnoi, M., & Alexander, J. C. (2012). Blockade of CRF1 receptors in the central nucleus of the amygdala attenuates the dysphoria associated with nicotine withdrawal in rats. *Pharmacology Biochemistry and Behavior, 101*(1), 62–68.

Bruijnzeel, A. W., & Gold, M. S. (2005). The role of corticotropin-releasing factor-like peptides in cannabis, nicotine, and alcohol dependence. *Brain Research. Brain Research Reviews, 49*(3), 505–528.

Bruijnzeel, A. W., Prado, M., & Isaac, S. (2009). Corticotropin-releasing factor-1 receptor activation mediates nicotine withdrawal-induced deficit in brain reward function and stress-induced relapse. *Biological Psychiatry, 66*, 110–117.

Bruijnzeel, A. W., Zislis, G., Wilson, C., & Gold, M. S. (2007). Antagonism of CRF receptors prevents the deficit in brain reward function associated with precipitated nicotine withdrawal in rats. *Neuropsychopharmacology, 32*(4), 955–963.

Burger, C., Gorbatyuk, O. S., Velardo, M. J., Peden, C. S., Williams, P., Zolotukhin, S., ... Muzyczka, N. (2004). Recombinant AAV viral vectors pseudotyped with viral capsids from serotypes 1, 2, and 5 display differential efficiency and cell tropism after delivery to different regions of the central nervous system. *Molecular Therapy, 10*(2), 302–317.

Carroll, F. I., Blough, B. E., Mascarella, S. W., Navarro, H. A., Lukas, R. J., & Damaj, M. I. (2014). Bupropion and bupropion analogs as treatments for CNS disorders. *Advances in Pharmacology, 69*, 177–216. http://dx.doi.org/10.1016/b978-0-12-420118-7.00005-6.

Chalmers, D. T., Lovenberg, T. W., Grigoriadis, D. E., Behan, D. P., & De Souza, E. B. (1996). Corticotrophin-releasing factor receptors: from molecular biology to drug design. *Trends in Pharmacological Sciences, 17*(4), 166–172.

Chen, R., Lewis, K. A., Perrin, M. H., & Vale, W. W. (1993). Expression cloning of a human corticotropin-releasing-factor receptor. *Proceedings of the National Academy of Sciences of the United States of America, 90*(19), 8967–8971.

Chen, A., Zorrilla, E., Smith, S., Rousso, D., Levy, C., Vaughan, J., ... Vale, W. (2006). Urocortin 2-deficient mice exhibit gender-specific alterations in circadian hypothalamus-pituitary-adrenal axis and depressive-like behavior. *The Journal of Neuroscience: the Official Journal of the Society for Neuroscience, 26*(20), 5500–5510. http://dx.doi.org/10.1523/jneurosci.3955-05.2006.

Corey, C., Wang, B., Johnson, S. E., Apelberg, B., & Husten, C. (2013). Notes from the field: electronic cigarette use among middle and high school students – United States, 2011–2012. *MMWR (Morbidity and Mortality Weekly Report), 62*(35), 729–730.

Corrigall, W. A., Herling, S., & Coen, K. M. (1989). Evidence for a behavioral deficit during withdrawal from chronic nicotine treatment. *Pharmacology, Biochemistry, and Behavior, 33*(3), 559–562.

Cryan, J. F., Bruijnzeel, A. W., Skjei, K. L., & Markou, A. (2003). Bupropion enhances brain reward function and reverses the affective and somatic aspects of nicotine withdrawal in the rat. *Psychopharmacology (Berlin), 168*(3), 347–358.

Cryan, J. F., Gasparini, F., van Heeke, G., & Markou, A. (2003). Non-nicotinic neuropharmacological strategies for nicotine dependence: beyond bupropion. *Drug Discovery Today, 8*, 1025–1034.

Cryan, J. F., Valentino, R. J., & Lucki, I. (2005). Assessing substrates underlying the behavioral effects of antidepressants using the modified rat forced swimming test. *Neuroscience and Biobehavioral Reviews, 29*(4–5), 547–569. http://dx.doi.org/10.1016/j.neubiorev.2005.03.008.

Dahlström, A., & Fuxe, K. (1964). Evidence for the existence of monamine-containing neurons in the central nervous system. I. Demonstration of monamines in the cell bodies of brain stem neurons. *Archives of General Psychiatry* (Suppl. 232), 1–55.

Dawkins, L., Turner, J., Hasna, S., & Soar, K. (2012). The electronic-cigarette: effects on desire to smoke, withdrawal symptoms and cognition. *Addictive Behaviors, 37*(8), 970–973. http://dx.doi.org/10.1016/j.addbeh.2012.03.004.

Der-Avakian, A., & Markou, A. (2012). The neurobiology of anhedonia and other reward-related deficits. *Trends in Neurosciences, 35*(1), 68–77. http://dx.doi.org/10.1016/j.tins.2011.11.005.

Eaves, M., Thatcher-Britton, K., Rivier, J., Vale, W., & Koob, G. F. (1985). Effects of corticotropin releasing factor on locomotor activity in hypophysectomized rats. *Peptides, 6*(5), 923–926.

Epping-Jordan, M. P., Watkins, S. S., Koob, G. F., & Markou, A. (1998). Dramatic decreases in brain reward function during nicotine withdrawal. *Nature, 393*(6680), 76–79.

Finkenauer, R., Pomerleau, C. S., Snedecor, S. M., & Pomerleau, O. F. (2009). Race differences in factors relating to smoking initiation. *Addictive Behaviors, 34*, 1056–1059.

Forget, B., Wertheim, C., Mascia, P., Pushparaj, A., Goldberg, S. R., & Le, F. B. (2010). Noradrenergic alpha1 receptors as a novel target for the treatment of nicotine addiction. *Neuropsychopharmacology, 35*(8), 1751–1760.

Grady, S. R., Drenan, R. M., Breining, S. R., Yohannes, D., Wageman, C. R., Fedorov, N. B., ... Marks, M. J. (2010). Structural differences determine the relative selectivity of nicotinic compounds for native alpha 4 beta 2*-, alpha 6 beta 2*-, alpha 3 beta 4*- and alpha 7-nicotine acetylcholine receptors. *Neuropharmacology*, *58*(7), 1054–1066.

Grieder, T. E., Herman, M. A., Contet, C., Tan, L. A., Vargas-Perez, H., Cohen, A., ... George, O. (2014). VTA CRF neurons mediate the aversive effects of nicotine withdrawal and promote intake escalation. *Nature Neuroscience*, *17*(12), 1751–1758. http://dx.doi.org/10.1038/nn.3872.

Hamilton, K. R., Berger, S. S., Perry, M. E., & Grunberg, N. E. (2009). Behavioral effects of nicotine withdrawal in adult male and female rats. *Pharmacology, Biochemistry, and Behavior*, *92*(1), 51–59. http://dx.doi.org/10.1016/j.pbb.2008.10.010.

Harrell, P. T., Marquinez, N. S., Correa, J. B., Meltzer, L. R., Unrod, M., Sutton, S. K., ... Brandon, T. H. (2015). Expectancies for cigarettes, e-cigarettes, and nicotine replacement therapies among e-cigarette users (aka vapers). *Nicotine & Tobacco Research: Official Journal of the Society for Research on Nicotine and Tobacco*, *17*(2), 193–200. http://dx.doi.org/10.1093/ntr/ntu149.

Hughes, J. R., Gust, S. W., Skoog, K., Keenan, R. M., & Fenwick, J. W. (1991). Symptoms of tobacco withdrawal. A replication and extension. *Archives of General Psychiatry*, *48*(1), 52–59.

Hughes, J. R., & Hatsukami, D. (1986). Signs and symptoms of tobacco withdrawal. *Archives of General Psychiatry*, *43*(3), 289–294.

Igari, M., Alexander, J. C., Ji, Y., Qi, X., Papke, R. L., & Bruijnzeel, A. W. (2013). Varenicline and cytisine diminish the dysphoric-like state associated with spontaneous nicotine withdrawal in rats. *Neuropsychopharmacology*, *39*, 455–465.

Johnson, P. M., Hollander, J. A., & Kenny, P. J. (2008). Decreased brain reward function during nicotine withdrawal in C57BL6 mice: evidence from intracranial self-stimulation (ICSS) studies. *Pharmacology Biochemistry and Behavior*, *90*(3), 409–415.

Johnston, L. D., O'Malley, P. M., Miech, R. A., Bachman, J. G., & Schulenberg, J. E. (2015). *Monitoring the future national survey results on drug use: 1975–2014: Overview, key findings on adolescent drug use*. Ann Arbor: Institute for Social Research, The University of Michigan.

Koob, G. F. (1999). Stress, corticotropin-releasing factor, and drug addiction. *Annals of the New York Academy of Sciences*, *897*, 27–45.

Koob, G. F., & Heinrichs, S. C. (1999). A role for corticotropin releasing factor and urocortin in behavioral responses to stressors. *Brain Research*, *848*, 141–152.

LeSage, M. G., Burroughs, D., & Pentel, P. R. (2006). Effects of nicotine withdrawal on performance under a progressive-ratio schedule of sucrose pellet delivery in rats. *Pharmacology, Biochemistry, and Behavior*, *83*(4), 585–591. http://dx.doi.org/10.1016/j.pbb.2006.03.021.

Lewis, K., Li, C., Perrin, M. H., Blount, A., Kunitake, K., Donaldson, C., ... Vale, W. W. (2001). Identification of urocortin III, an additional member of the corticotropin-releasing factor (CRF) family with high affinity for the CRF2 receptor. *Proceedings of the National Academy of Sciences of the United States of America*, *98*(13), 7570–7575.

Lovenberg, T. W., Liaw, C. W., Grigoriadis, D. E., Clevenger, W., Chalmers, D. T., De Souza, E. B., & Oltersdorf, T. (1995). Cloning and characterization of a functionally distinct corticotropin-releasing factor receptor subtype from rat brain. *Proceedings of the National Academy of Sciences of the United States of America*, *92*(3), 836–840.

Mannucci, C., Tedesco, M., Bellomo, M., Caputi, A. P., & Calapai, G. (2006). Long-term effects of nicotine on the forced swimming test in mice: an experimental model for the study of depression caused by smoke. *Neurochemistry International*, *49*(5), 481–486. http://dx.doi.org/10.1016/j.neuint.2006.03.010.

Marcinkiewcz, C. A., Prado, M. M., Isaac, S. K., Marshall, A., Rylkova, D., & Bruijnzeel, A. W. (2009). Corticotropin-releasing factor within the central nucleus of the amygdala and the nucleus accumbens shell mediates the negative affective state of nicotine withdrawal in rats. *Neuropsychopharmacology*, *34*(7), 1743–1752.

McEwen, B. S. (2000). The neurobiology of stress: from serendipity to clinical relevance. *Brain Research, 886*(1–2), 172–189.

Moore, R. Y., & Card, J. P. (1984). Noradrenaline-containing neuron systems. In A. Bjorklund, & T. Hokfelt (Eds.), *Handbook of chemical neuroanatomy* (pp. 123–156). Amsterdam: Elsevier.

Myers, W. D., Ng, K. T., & Singer, G. (1982). Intravenous self-administration of acetaldehyde in the rat as a function of schedule, food deprivation and photoperiod. *Pharmacology Biochemistry and Behavior, 17*(4), 807–811.

Nesil, T., Kanit, L., Ugur, M., & Pogun, S. (2015). Nicotine withdrawal in selectively bred high and low nicotine preferring rat lines. *Pharmacology, Biochemistry, and Behavior, 131c*, 91–97. http://dx.doi.org/10.1016/j.pbb.2015.02.009.

Nestler, E. J., & Hyman, S. E. (2010). Animal models of neuropsychiatric disorders. *Nature Neuroscience, 13*(10), 1161–1169. http://dx.doi.org/10.1038/nn.2647.

Nijsen, M. J., Croiset, G., Diamant, M., De Wied, D., & Wiegant, V. M. (2001). CRH signalling in the bed nucleus of the stria terminalis is involved in stress-induced cardiac vagal activation in conscious rats. *Neuropsychopharmacology, 24*(1), 1–10.

O'Dell, L. E., Bruijnzeel, A. W., Smith, R. T., Parsons, L. H., Merves, M. L., Goldberger, B. A., … Markou, A. (2006). Diminished nicotine withdrawal in adolescent rats: implications for vulnerability to addiction. *Psychopharmacology (Berlin), 186*(4), 612–619.

O'Dell, L. E., & Torres, O. V. (2014). A mechanistic hypothesis of the factors that enhance vulnerability to nicotine use in females. *Neuropharmacology, 76*(Pt B), 566–580. http://dx.doi.org/10.1016/j.neuropharm.2013.04.055.

Ott, A., Slooter, A. J., Hofman, A., van Harskamp, F., Witteman, J. C., Van Broeckhoven, C., … Breteler, M. M. (1998). Smoking and risk of dementia and Alzheimer's disease in a population-based cohort study: the Rotterdam study. *Lancet, 351*(9119), 1840–1843.

Pellegrino, R. M., Tinghino, B., Mangiaracina, G., Marani, A., Vitali, M., Protano, C., & Catta-ruzza, M. S. (2012). Electronic cigarettes: an evaluation of exposure to chemicals and fine particulate matter (PM). *Annali di igiene: medicina preventiva e di comunita, 24*(4), 279–288.

Perrin, M. H., Donaldson, C. J., Chen, R., Lewis, K. A., & Vale, W. W. (1993). Cloning and functional expression of a rat brain corticotropin releasing factor (CRF) receptor. *Endocrinology, 133*(6), 3058–3061.

Pirie, K., Peto, R., Reeves, G. K., Green, J., & Beral, V. (2013). The 21st century hazards of smoking and benefits of stopping: a prospective study of one million women in the UK. *Lancet, 381*(9861), 133–141. http://dx.doi.org/10.1016/s0140-6736(12)61720-6.

Postma, D. S., Bush, A., & van den Berge, M. (2014). Risk factors and early origins of chronic obstructive pulmonary disease. *Lancet.* http://dx.doi.org/10.1016/s0140-6736(14)60446-3.

Qi, X., Shan, Z., Ji, Y., Guerra, V., Alexander, J. C., Ormerod, B. K., & Bruijnzeel, A. W. (2014). Sustained AAV-mediated overexpression of CRF in the central amygdala diminishes the depressive-like state associated with nicotine withdrawal. *Translational Psychiatry, 4*, e385.

Roni, M. A., & Rahman, S. (2014). The effects of lobeline on nicotine withdrawal-induced depression-like behavior in mice. *Psychopharmacology (Berlin), 231*(15), 2989–2998. http://dx.doi.org/10.1007/s00213-014-3472-y.

Sapolsky, R. M. (1992). Do glucocorticoid concentrations rise with age in the rat? *Neurobiology of Aging, 13*(1), 171–174.

Shiffman, S., Ferguson, S. G., Gwaltney, C. J., Balabanis, M. H., & Shadel, W. G. (2006). Reduction of abstinence-induced withdrawal and craving using high-dose nicotine replacement therapy. *Psychopharmacology (Berlin), 184*(3–4), 637–644. http://dx.doi.org/10.1007/s00213-005-0184-3.

Smith, B. R., Amit, Z., & Splawinsky, J. (1984). Conditioned place preference induced by intraventricular infusions of acetaldehyde. *Alcohol, 1*(3), 193–195.

Steckler, T., & Holsboer, F. (1999). Corticotropin-releasing hormone receptor subtypes and emotion. *Biological Psychiatry, 46*(11), 1480–1508.

Stolerman, I. P., & Jarvis, M. J. (1995). The scientific case that nicotine is addictive. *Psychopharmacology (Berlin)*, *117*(1), 2–10.

Sutton, R. E., Koob, G. F., Le Moal, M., Rivier, J., & Vale, W. (1982). Corticotropin releasing factor produces behavioural activation in rats. *Nature*, *297*(5864), 331–333.

Suzuki, T., Ise, Y., Tsuda, M., Maeda, J., & Misawa, M. (1996). Mecamylamine-precipitated nicotine-withdrawal aversion in rats. *European Journal of Pharmacology*, *314*(3), 281–284.

Swanson, L. W., Sawchenko, P. E., Rivier, J., & Vale, W. W. (1983). Organization of ovine corticotropin-releasing factor immunoreactive cells and fibers in the rat brain: an immunohistochemical study. *Neuroendocrinology*, *36*, 165–186.

Tanaka, M., & Telegdy, G. (2008). Antidepressant-like effects of the CRF family peptides, urocortin 1, urocortin 2 and urocortin 3 in a modified forced swimming test in mice. *Brain Research Bulletin*, *75*(5), 509–512.

Thun, M. J., Carter, B. D., Feskanich, D., Freedman, N. D., Prentice, R., Lopez, A. D., … Gapstur, S. M. (2013). 50-year trends in smoking-related mortality in the United States. *The New England Journal of Medicine*, *368*(4), 351–364. http://dx.doi.org/10.1056/NEJMsa1211127.

Tzschentke, T. M. (1998). Measuring reward with the conditioned place preference paradigm: a comprehensive review of drug effects, recent progress and new issues. *Progress in Neurobiology*, *56*(6), 613–672.

Vale, W., Spiess, J., Rivier, C., & Rivier, J. (1981). Characterization of a 41-residue ovine hypothalamic peptide that stimulates secretion of corticotropin and beta-endorphin. *Science*, *213*(4514), 1394–1397.

Wesnes, K., & Warburton, D. M. (1983). Smoking, nicotine and human performance. *Pharmacology & Therapeutics*, *21*(2), 189–208.

WHO. (2011). *Systematic review of the link between tobacco and poverty*.

The Habenulo-Interpeduncular Pathway and Nicotine Withdrawal

C.D. Fowler
University of California Irvine, Irvine, CA, United States

The habenula is classified as part of the epithalamus, a subregion of the diencephalon, and is located bilaterally on the midline, dorsal to the thalamus. This structure was first identified by Serres in 1824 and later described in more anatomical detail by Ramon y Cajal (1911). The habenula is relatively highly conserved across species and serves as a connection between the limbic forebrain and midbrain. Animals with a photoreceptive pineal, such as fish, amphibians, and reptiles, exhibit asymmetrical development between the right and left habenula with regard to size, molecular properties, and connectivity, whereas the habenula is bilaterally symmetrical in mammals. The main afferent pathway of the habenula, the stria medullaris, comprises axons originating from the septum, basal ganglia, nucleus of the diagonal band, nucleus basalis, lateral hypothalamus, and lateral preoptic area. Efferents from the habenula extend along the fasciculus retroflexus (RF) to innervate midbrain and hindbrain structures. Interestingly, the fasciculus retroflexus has recently been shown to be among the first fiber tracts that form in the developing human fetal brain (Cho et al., 2014). The habenula has been implicated in a variety of functions, including sleep, reward, pain, and sexual behaviors. However, many of these prior studies have resulted in conflicting findings based on limitations of the experimental approaches utilized, and as such, the specific function has remained unclear until recently (see review in Klemm, 2004; Sutherland, 1982). Advances in genetic research approaches have permitted more detailed and sophisticated investigations into habenular function. As such, the habenula has now become recognized as an essential

Negative Affective States and Cognitive Impairments in Nicotine Dependence
http://dx.doi.org/10.1016/B978-0-12-802574-1.00011-9

regulator of aversive motivational states and negative feedback process-ing. In this chapter, an overview of the habenula nuclei and recent find-ings demonstrating the importance of this structure in mediating aspects of nicotine withdrawal and self-administration will be discussed.

CHARACTERIZATION OF THE HABENULAR NUCLEI

Anatomical Structure and Discrete Expression Patterns

The habenula has been traditionally divided into the medial and lateral nuclei based on cellular morphology, gene expression, and afferent and efferent projections. The medial nucleus (MHb) is composed of densely packed, smaller cells with complex dendrites (Kim & Chang, 2005). Two types of neurons have been described: piriform neurons with two to five primary dendrites with many spines, and fusiform neurons with one to three primary dendrites and fewer spines. In the lateral nucleus (LHb), the majority of neurons are larger in size with long dendritic branches extending throughout the lateral region (Kim & Chang, 2005). These larger neurons have been subdivided into three types based on their rela-tive size and primary dendrite number (Iwahori, 1977). In addition to the large cells of the LHb, dispersed smaller neurons with short axons have also been identified and are thought to mediate local signaling (Iwahori, 1977). Gene and protein expression differ among the various subdivisions of the habenula. In mammals, the transcription factor Brn3a has been shown to regulate neuronal development of the MHb, as well as a subset of LHb neurons, in part through its actions on the orphan nuclear receptor Nurr1 (Quina, Wang, Ng, & Turner, 2009). During adulthood, restricted expression profiles further define the subregions. For instance, the dorsal MHb (dMHb) exhibits selective enrichment of certain genes, such as *Tacr1* (tachykinin receptor 1), *Oprm* (μ opioid receptor), *Il18* (interleukin-18), *Gpr151, Nhlh2, Adcyap1, Cubn, Wif1,* and *Tac1* (Aizawa, Kobayashi, Tanaka, Fukai, & Okamoto, 2012; Sugama et al., 2002; Wagner, French, & Veh, 2014). *Tac1* encodes two of the main signaling mechanisms of the dMHb, neurokinin1 and substance P. Of further interest, the presence of inter-leukin-18 signifies the only known neuron-specific expression site in the brain. The ventral MHb (vMHb) exhibits selectively higher expression of cholinergic-associated genes (*Chat, Slc18a3,* and *VAChT*), *Sstr4,* and *Myo16* (Contestabile et al., 1987; Wagner et al., 2014). Such subregion distinctions are not as evident in the LHb, in which a more heterogeneous expres-sion pattern is found. Genes enriched selectively throughout this region include *Prokr2, Kcnab2, Htr2c,* and *Chrm2* (Wagner et al., 2014). LHb neu-rons are mainly glutamatergic projection neurons intermingled with sparse GABAergic local interneurons.

Efferent Projections of the Habenular Nuclei

The vast majority of MHb axons project ventrolaterally and exit the region as part of the fasciculus retroflexus tract. MHb terminals preferentially innervate the interpeduncular nucleus (IPN), resulting in the formation of the habenulo-interpeduncular (MHb–IPN) pathway. MHb fibers are cholinergic, glutamatergic, and/or express substance P and project to innervate all subnuclei of the IPN. Substance P and glutamatergic fibers from the dMHb preferentially innervate the lateral subnuclei of the IPN, whereas the vMHb cholinergic and glutamatergic co-expressing fibers primarily innervate the central and intermediate nuclei of the IPN (Contestabile et al., 1987; Kawaja, Flumerfelt, & Hrycyshyn, 1988; Ren et al., 2011). Interestingly, the fibers innervating the central region appear to zigzag throughout the structure and likely form *en passant* synaptic connections (Kawaja et al., 1988). In the intermediate subregion, MHb axons have additionally been noted to form crest synapses in conjunction with disc-shaped IPN dendrites; at these terminal sites, input appears to be integrated from both left and right MHb (Lenn, Wong, & Hamill, 1983). In addition to innervating the IPN, axonal collaterals also appear to extend connections to neighboring MHb cells (Ramon y Cajal, 1911), and further, a minor number of MHb fibers have been found to project to the LHb (Kim & Chang, 2005). This minor pathway between the habenular nuclei is asymmetric, as axons from the LHb have not been found to reciprocally innervate the MHb, although a few projections from the LHb to the IPN have been described and thus integration may occur at this downstream site. The majority of neurons in the MHb have been shown to fire tonic spontaneous action potentials at baseline levels in vitro, suggesting sustained release of acetylcholine in the IPN (Gorlich et al., 2013; McCormick & Prince, 1987; Ren et al., 2011). In cholinergic neurons, hyperpolarization-activated cyclic nucleotide-gated (HCN) pacemaker channels are thought to maintain the spontaneous tonic firing rate at 2–10 Hz (Gorlich et al., 2013). In addition to a variety of neuronal nicotinic acetylcholine receptors (nAChRs; see discussion below), other receptors localized on MHb neurons or at their terminals include adenosine triphosphate (ATP), GABA, α-amino-3-hydroxy-5-methyl-4-isoxazolepropionic acid (AMPA), N-methyl-D-aspartate (NMDA), mu opioid, neurokinin, and phosphodiesterase 2A receptors. Interestingly, atrial natriuretic peptide has been shown to inhibit glutamate release in the central region of the IPN through phosphodiesterase 2A-mediated mechanisms localized on MHb terminals (Hu, Ren, Zhang, Zhong, & Luo, 2012). However, it is unclear whether the source of atrial natriuretic peptide is derived from circulating levels entering the brain, or whether MHb neurons themselves produce the peptide and release directly into the IPN (Hu et al., 2012; Skofitsch, Jacobowitz, Eskay, & Zamir, 1985).

Similar to the MHb, the vast majority of LHb glutamatergic axons extend along the FR, but in contrast, these projections exhibit diversity in their innervation of a variety of structures, which include the raphe, central gray, substantia nigra pars compacta, reticular formation, and rostral medial tegmental area (RMTg). These neurons display a heterogeneous pattern of activity with tonic, burst oscillation, or silent profiles at rest (Kim & Chang, 2005). The LHb has been shown to regulate negative reward-related processing, motivation, and depression-related states. With specific regard to drugs of abuse, the LHb has been implicated in cocaine-mediated avoidance behaviors through its connections to the RMTg and VTA (Jhou et al., 2013). Stimulation of the LHb results in excitation of the RMTg and subsequent inhibition of dopaminergic neurons in the VTA (Hong, Jhou, Smith, Saleem, & Hikosaka, 2011). The LHb also receives input from GABAergic and glutamatergic projections of the VTA (Root et al., 2014). In addition to GABA, NMDA, and AMPA receptors in the LHb, dopamine, serotonin, and muscarinic acetylcholine receptors are also found in this region. Interestingly, injection of a dopamine D3 receptor antagonist into the LHb was found to attenuate cue-induced reinstatement of nicotine seeking (Khaled, Pushparaj, Di Ciano, Diaz, & Le Foll, 2014). However, given that nAChRs are selectively localized in the MHb, the vast majority of evidence thus far has specifically implicated nicotinic signaling mechanisms in the MHb in nicotine-mediated negative affective states.

THE HABENULO-INTERPEDUNCULAR PATHWAY AND NICOTINE

Nicotinic Signaling Mechanisms

Acetylcholine, the endogenous ligand of nAChRs, is expressed in high density in the vMHb along with multiple nAChR subunits, including $\alpha2$, $\alpha3$, $\alpha4$, $\alpha5$, $\alpha6$, $\beta2$, $\beta3$, and $\beta4$ (Grady et al., 2009). Upon further delineation of the vMHb into the lateral, central, and medial subregions, differential nAChR subunit expression patterns and physiological properties can be localized. In the lateral vMHb, $\alpha3$, $\alpha4$, $\beta2$, $\beta3$, and $\beta4$ nAChR subunits appear to be preferentially expressed, whereas in the central and medial vMHb, $\alpha3$, $\beta2$, $\beta3$, and $\beta4$ nAChR subunits are found (Shih et al., 2014). The $\alpha6$ nAChR subunit exhibits the most selective profile with expression only in the medial vMHb. Interestingly, while most nAChRs are expressed in cholinergic neurons, $\alpha6$ and $\alpha4$ nAChR subunits are localized in noncholinergic neurons as well (Shih et al., 2014). In consideration of the variety of nAChR subunits selectively expressed and the pharmacokinetics of nAChR subtypes, the functional characteristics of MHb neurons expectedly vary among the subregions. In cholinergic neurons of the vMHb, nicotine enhances intrinsic neuronal excitability through α5β2- or α3β4-containing nAChRs, and this excitability may be modulated by local neurokinin signaling mechanisms (Dao, Perez, Teng, Dani, & De Biasi, 2014; Gorlich et al., 2013). Furthermore, the lateral vMHb neurons appear to be more highly excitable and responsive to nicotine compared to the central vMHb (Shih et al., 2014). Interestingly, the medial vMHb cholinergic neurons are more sensitive to the neurotoxic effects of high doses of nicotine following chronic administration (Ciani, Severi, Bartesaghi, & Contestabile, 2005). In the IPN, preterminal nAChRs on MHb axons have been shown to regulate firing of postsynaptic GABAergic neurons (Lena, Changeux, & Mulle, 1993), and these GABAergic neurons have also been found to express α4β2α5- and α3β4α5-containing nAChRs (Hsu et al., 2013). Of the nAChRs present in the IPN, it has been estimated that ~50% of the nicotinic binding sites are presynaptic (Clarke, Hamill, Nadi, Jacobowitz, & Pert, 1986). Importantly, acetylcholine release is modulated at the terminal region specifically by α3β4- and α3β3β4-containing nAChR subtypes (Grady et al., 2009) and appears to occur via volume transmission, as opposed to the more direct "wired" transmission demonstrated with glutamate (Ren et al., 2011). Together, these findings suggest that a main function of acetylcholine in the IPN is to mediate presynaptic release of glutamate and GABA from axonal terminals.

Nicotine Withdrawal

Cessation of tobacco use results in an aversive withdrawal syndrome, which can persist from weeks to months in humans (Shiffman & Jarvik, 1976). The duration and severity of withdrawal symptoms have both been strongly correlated with the likelihood to relapse (Piasecki et al., 2000). As such, the aversive physical and affective symptoms of withdrawal induced during abstinence are thought to promote re-consumption of the drug in an individual's attempt to alleviate the negative affective state, thereby prompting relapse and sustaining drug dependence. Nicotinic signaling mechanisms have been shown to play an essential role in these processes. In a recent genome-wide association study, allelic variation in the α4 nAChR subunit gene, CHRNA4, has been associated with intense withdrawal symptoms in humans (Lazary et al., 2014). Another genetic locus, chromosome 15q24, contains the CHRNA5–CHRNA3–CHRNB4 gene cluster that encodes the α5, α3, and β4 nAChR subunits, respectively. Two single nucleotide polymorphisms (SNPs), rs16969968 in CHRNA5 and rs1051730 in CHRNA3, have been strongly and repeatedly correlated with an increased vulnerability for tobacco dependence (Bierut et al., 2008; Thorgeirsson et al., 2008). Most notably, the α5 nAChR risk variant was specifically associated with early onset of smoking behavior, a self-reported "pleasurable buzz" during smoking, heavy smoking, and smoking-associated diseases, such as chronic obstructive pulmonary disease and lung cancer (Berrettini et al., 2008; Bierut et al., 2008; Hung et al., 2008; Sherva et al., 2008; Weiss et al., 2008). Interestingly, individuals carrying the α5 nAChR risk variant are also more responsive to pharmacologic cessation therapeutics as evidenced by increased success rates with long-term abstinence (Chen et al., 2012). Furthermore, another *CHRNA3* SNP, rs8192475, is associated with increased withdrawal symptoms and self-reported levels of drug craving (Sarginson et al., 2011). Given the localized expression of these subunits in the MHb and IPN, these findings suggest that this pathway may play a significant role in addiction-related processes.

In rodent studies of withdrawal, chronic nicotine administration is most often achieved with subcutaneously implanted minipumps or via administration in the drinking water. Under chronic conditions, the overall number of nicotinic binding sites and messenger RNA (mRNA) expression levels of $\alpha2$, $\alpha3$, $\alpha4$, $\alpha5$, and $\beta2$ nAChR subunits in the MHb and IPN remain unchanged, with the exception of a moderate decrease in $\beta2$ subunit mRNA only in the lateral IPN (Marks et al., 1992). In contrast, $\beta4$-containing nAChR binding sites are found to be significantly increased in the MHb (Meyers, Loetz, & Marks, 2015), and $\beta4$ and $\beta3$ subunit mRNA are selectively increased in somatostatin neurons of the dorsal IPN (Zhao-Shea, Liu, Pang, Gardner, & Tapper, 2013). However, this increase in $\beta4$-containing nAChR sites does not appear to correlate with the expression of withdrawal-associated behaviors (Salas, Pieri, & De Biasi, 2004), and thus, the functional consequence of such receptor upregulation remains unclear. With regard to the electrophysiological properties of these neurons, the baseline level of neuronal activity does not appear to change during chronic nicotine administration (Gorlich et al., 2013; Shih et al., 2014). During the withdrawal state, however, nicotine-induced activity is dramatically decreased following shorter term nicotine administration (3 and 14 days) (Shih et al., 2014) but increased after longer periods of administration (28 days) (Gorlich et al., 2013). Induction of the withdrawal state may be achieved by removal of the nicotine source for a more gradual spontaneous withdrawal, or alternatively, a nAChR antagonist may be administered to immediately block nicotine's direct actions on nAChRs and thereby precipitate withdrawal. In rodents, the somatic signs of withdrawal are often observed as shaking, scratching, head nods, chewing, and increased grooming, whereas the affective signs of withdrawal may include assessments of anxiety-related behaviors, conditioned place aversion, or elevated brain reward thresholds. Although the general nicotinic receptor antagonist, mecamylamine, is commonly used to precipitate withdrawal, other antagonists selective for $\alpha3\beta4$-, $\alpha4\beta2$-, or $\alpha7$-containing nAChRs are also highly effective (Damaj, Kao, & Martin, 2003). This finding highlights all of the potential receptor subtypes that likely mediate the withdrawal state. Interestingly, administration of an antagonist selective for the $\alpha6$-containing nAChR exerts an opposing effect as evidenced by a reduction in the expression of a withdrawal-induced conditioned place aversion (Jackson, McIntosh, Brunzell, Sanjakdar, & Damaj, 2009).

Initial insight into the MHb–IPN pathway's importance in nicotine-mediated negative affective states is derived from studies of mice containing null mutation in specific nAChR subunits (knockout mice). Mice lacking the β4 nAChR subunit exhibit an attenuation of somatic signs and hyperalgesia following mecamylamine-precipitated withdrawal (Salas et al., 2004). Furthermore, during spontaneous, but not precipitated, withdrawal, β4 knockout mice fail to exhibit elevated brain reward thresholds during the first 3–6h (Stoker, Olivier, & Markou, 2012b). These findings indicate that β4-containing nAChRs are involved in the somatic signs of withdrawal, hyperalgesia, and initial anhedonia induced with nicotine cessation. In mice lacking the α2 or α5 nAChR subunit, the somatic signs of precipitated withdrawal are also significantly attenuated (Salas, Sturm, Boulter, & De Biasi, 2009). Interestingly, the effects of the α2 nAChR subunit, which is expressed in the IPN but not the MHb, appear to be environment dependent. In a familiar environment, α2 knockout mice display decreased somatic signs of withdrawal (Salas et al., 2009), whereas in a novel environment, the knockout mice exhibit an increase in the number of somatic and affective signs of withdrawal, as assessed by a cued fear-conditioning paradigm (Lotfipour et al., 2013). Differences in the affective signs of withdrawal are also found in β2 knockout mice as evidenced by decreased anxiety-related behaviors and withdrawal-induced conditioned place aversion (Jackson, Martin, Changeux, & Damaj, 2008). Furthermore, while the β2-containing nAChR may mediate affective components, it does not appear to modulate somatic behaviors during withdrawal (Jackson et al., 2008; Salas et al., 2004). Finally, although the presence of the α7 nAChR in the MHb–IPN pathway has not been as well documented as other nAChR subunits (Sheffield, Quick, & Lester, 2000), α7 knockout mice do exhibit reduced somatic signs induced by mecamylamine-precipitated withdrawal (Salas, Main, Gangitano, & De Biasi, 2007). In addition to nAChRs enriched in the habenula, alternate signaling mechanisms expressed in high density in the MHb–IPN further support the involvement of habenular function in mediating withdrawal. Mu opioid receptor knockout mice demonstrate an attenuation of somatic signs during precipitated withdrawal (Berrendero, Kieffer, & Maldonado, 2002), and decreased anhedonia and somatic signs are found in metabotropic glutamate 5 receptor knockout mice during spontaneous withdrawal (Stoker, Olivier, & Markou, 2012a). Given the constitutive gene knockout in these mouse models for both the central and peripheral systems, more site-specific investigations are required to clearly parse out the contribution of MHb–IPN-specific signaling mechanisms. As an example, increased brain reward thresholds are found with peripheral mecamylamine administration in both saline and nicotine-treated α5 knockout mice (Fowler, Tuesta, & Kenny, 2013), suggesting that the α5 deletion may render these mice more sensitive to the aversive effects of mecamylamine in general. Furthermore, injection of the β4-selective antagonist, SR16584, into the IPN increases somatic signs of withdrawal in both saline- and nicotine-treated wild-type mice (Zhao-Shea et al., 2013). These unexpected findings may suggest that administration of an antagonist can alter nicotinic signaling in the MHb–IPN pathway to induce an aversive state similar to the withdrawal syndrome, even in the absence of nicotine.

Importantly, direct manipulation of the MHb–IPN pathway has provided more direct validation of the importance of this brain structure in the various aspects of nicotine withdrawal. Injection of mecamylamine directly into the MHb or IPN, but not in the cortex, hippocampus, or ventral tegmental area, is sufficient to elicit an increase in somatic withdrawal signs in nicotine-treated mice (Salas et al., 2009). Disruption of HCN pacemaker activity in cholinergic MHb neurons can precipitate both the somatic and affective signs of withdrawal (Gorlich et al., 2013). Furthermore, administration of the substance P receptor neurokinin 1 antagonist or neurokinin B receptor antagonist directly into the MHb results in a precipitation of somatic signs withdrawal (Dao et al., 2014). Within the IPN, infusion of SR16584, a β4-containing nAChR selective antagonist, increases somatic withdrawal signs (Zhao-Shea et al., 2013). These β4-containing nAChR-mediated effects are likely due to presynaptic receptors, as glutamatergic signaling from MHb terminals has been shown to enhance GABAergic neuronal activity during mecamylamine-precipitated withdrawal and optogenetic-mediated activation of GABAergic neurons is sufficient to induce somatic withdrawal signs (Zhao-Shea et al., 2013).

MHb signaling mechanisms have also been implicated in other psychological states, which may directly or indirectly alter the expression of withdrawal signs. For instance, substance P, mu opioid receptors, and phosphodiesterase 2A have all been implicated in stress and pain-related behavioral responses. Postnatal ablation of GPR151-expressing cells, which compose a subset of MHb neurons, results in impulsive and compulsive behavior, hyperactivity, environmental maladaptation, and learning deficits (Kobayashi et al., 2013). In contrast, fear-related processing appears to involve a circuit from the medial amygdala to the bed nucleus of the anterior commissure and subsequently to the substance P-expressing neurons of the dMHb (Yamaguchi, Danjo, Pastan, Hikida, & Nakanishi, 2013). Finally, anxiolytic effects of nicotine can be modified by a circuit originating in the hippocampus and projecting to the triangular septum and then to cholinergic neurons of the vMHb, which subsequently terminates in the central IPN (Yamaguchi et al., 2013). Indeed, given that α4-, β3-, and β4-containing nAChRs are expressed in the vMHb cholinergic neurons, it is not surprising that these subunits have also been implicated in anxiety-related behaviors (Booker, Butt, Wehner, Heinemann, & Collins, 2007; Ross et al., 2000; Salas, Pieri, Fung, Dani, & De Biasi, 2003).

Nicotine Reinforcement, Reward, and Aversion

Similar neurobiological mechanisms may be expected to regulate the aversive properties of nicotine during both the dependence and withdrawal phases. For instance, α5-containing nAChRs and the MHb–IPN pathway have both been implicated in regulating nicotine consumption at high doses of the drug (Fowler, Lu, Johnson, Marks, & Kenny, 2011), as well as the somatic signs of nicotine withdrawal (Salas et al., 2009; Zhao-Shea et al., 2013). With chronic nicotine use, brain regions regulating the aversive response to nicotine could become modified to lessen the negative reaction to the drug and thus promote further drug intake leading to dependence. Given that variation in the *CHRNA5* gene diminishes α5-containing nAChR activity (Bierut et al., 2008; Wang et al., 2009), investigations of α5 knockout mice have provided insight into certain mechanisms mediating the dependent state. Interestingly, α5 knockout mice do not differ in intravenous nicotine self-administration at moderately rewarding doses, but rather exhibit an increased level of responding at higher doses that attenuate responding in wild-type mice (Fowler et al., 2011). These findings suggest that α5-containing nAChRs do not regulate the reinforcing properties of the drug, but rather mediate the aversive response to higher doses of nicotine. Indeed, rewarding doses of the drug induce similar lowering effects on brain reward thresholds in α5 knockout and wild-type mice (Fowler et al., 2013). However, as the unit dose increases, wild-type mice exhibit an attenuation of the rewarding effects, whereas the α5 knockout mice maintain lowered reward-related threshold values at these higher doses. Moreover, a high dose of nicotine maintains a rewarding value in α5 knockout mice, but not wild-type mice, as assessed in a conditioned place preference procedure (Jackson et al., 2010). In addition to the α5 nAChR subunit, the β4 nAChR subunit has also been implicated in mediating the aversive effects of nicotine. Mice with transgenic overexpression of the β4 nAChR subunit demonstrate an enhanced aversive response to nicotine, as evidenced by a decrease in nicotine-drinking behavior (Frahm et al., 2011). These data provide evidence that the α5 and β4 nAChR subunits play specific roles in regulating nicotine-mediated aversion. Further investigations have more discretely localized these aversive effects to the MHb–IPN pathway. Re-expression of α5 nAChR subunits in the MHb–IPN pathway of α5 knockout mice results in a "rescued" behavioral phenotype, as nicotine intake becomes normalized to wild-type levels (Fowler et al., 2011). Conversely, in rats, knockdown of α5 nAChR subunits in the MHb–IPN pathway via RNA-mediated interference results in an increased nicotine intake at higher doses of the drug and a decreased sensitivity to the negative effects of high-dose nicotine on brain reward function (Fowler et al., 2011). These data provide further evidence that α5-containing nAChRs specifically in the MHb–IPN pathway regulate the aversive processing of nicotine that serves to limit behavioral intake. In a further study, injections of the ibo-gaine derivative, 18-MC, increased or decreased nicotine self-adminis-tration when injected directly into the IPN or MHb, respectively, in rats (Glick, Sell, McCallum, & Maisonneuve, 2011). Although 18-MC induces a number of effects, the influence on nicotine intake is likely through its actions as an antagonist at α3β4-containing nAChRs. Finally, in addition to the nAChR-expressing circuits in the MHb–IPN, the dMHb also appears to mediate general aversive states, as optogenetic-mediated inhibition of the dMHb is sufficient to induce an acute place aversion (Hsu et al., 2014).

CONCLUSIONS

Converging lines of evidence have begun to define the importance of the MHb–IPN pathway in negative affective states during nicotine dependence and withdrawal. However, one must also acknowledge the contribution of other brain regions, including the prefrontal cortex, ven-tral tegmental area, and nucleus accumbens, in these processes. As such, signals from several addiction-related brain regions likely differentially contribute to aspects of withdrawal response. Moreover, brain regions and/or signaling mechanisms mediating drug dependence may simi-larly modulate various components of the negative affective state, thus serving to promote relapse and re-consumption of the drug. By attaining a more comprehensive understanding of the neurobiological underpin-nings of the various facets mediating nicotine dependence, withdrawal, and relapse, further research will likely lead to the development of novel pharmacotherapeutics to alleviate negative withdrawal symptoms and thus promote long-term abstinence.

References

Aizawa, H., Kobayashi, M., Tanaka, S., Fukai, T., & Okamoto, H. (2012). Molecular charac-terization of the subnuclei in rat habenula. *The Journal of Comparative Neurology, 520*(18), 4051–4066.

Berrendero, F., Kieffer, B. L., & Maldonado, R. (2002). Attenuation of nicotine-induced antinoci-ception, rewarding effects, and dependence in mu-opioid receptor knock-out mice. *The Jour-nal of Neuroscience: the Official Journal of the Society for Neuroscience, 22*(24), 10935–10940.

Berrettini, W., Yuan, X., Tozzi, F., Song, K., Francks, C., Chilcoat, H., … Mooser, V. (2008). Alpha-5/alpha-3 nicotinic receptor subunit alleles increase risk for heavy smoking. *Molecular Psychiatry, 13*(4), 368–373.

Bierut, L. J., Stitzel, J. A., Wang, J. C., Hinrichs, A. L., Grucza, R. A., Xuei, X., … Goate, A. M. (2008). Variants in nicotinic receptors and risk for nicotine dependence. *The American Journal of Psychiatry, 165*(9), 1163–1171.

Booker, T. K., Butt, C. M., Wehner, J. M., Heinemann, S. F., & Collins, A. C. (2007). Decreased anxiety-like behavior in beta3 nicotinic receptor subunit knockout mice. *Pharmacology, Biochemistry, and Behavior, 87*(1), 146–157.

Chen, L. S., Baker, T. B., Piper, M. E., Breslau, N., Cannon, D. S., Doheny, K. F., ... Bierut, L. J. (2012). Interplay of genetic risk factors (CHRNA5-CHRNA3-CHRNB4) and cessation treatments in smoking cessation success. *The American Journal of Psychiatry, 169*(7), 735–742.

Cho, K. H., Mori, S., Jang, H. S., Kim, J. H., Abe, H., Rodriguez-Vazquez, J. F., & Murakami, G. (2014). The habenulo-interpeduncular and mammillothalamic tracts: early developed fiber tracts in the human fetal diencephalon. *Child's Nervous System, 30*(9), 1477–1484.

Ciani, E., Severi, S., Bartesaghi, R., & Contestabile, A. (2005). Neurochemical correlates of nicotine neurotoxicity on rat habenulo-interpeduncular cholinergic neurons. *Neurotoxicology, 26*(3), 467–474.

Clarke, P. B., Hamill, G. S., Nadi, N. S., Jacobowitz, D. M., & Pert, A. (1986). 3H-nicotine- and 125I-alpha-bungarotoxin-labeled nicotinic receptors in the interpeduncular nucleus of rats. II. Effects of habenular deafferentation. *The Journal of Comparative Neurology, 251*(3), 407–413.

Contestabile, A., Villani, L., Fasolo, A., Franzoni, M. F., Gribaudo, L., Oktedalen, O., & Fonnum, F. (1987). Topography of cholinergic and substance P pathways in the habenulo-interpeduncular system of the rat. An immunocytochemical and microchemical approach. *Neuroscience, 21*(1), 253–270.

Damaj, M. I., Kao, W., & Martin, B. R. (2003). Characterization of spontaneous and precipitated nicotine withdrawal in the mouse. *The Journal of Pharmacology and Experimental Therapeutics, 307*(2), 526–534.

Dao, D. Q., Perez, E. E., Teng, Y., Dani, J. A., & De Biasi, M. (2014). Nicotine enhances excitability of medial habenular neurons via facilitation of neurokinin signaling. *The Journal of Neuroscience: the Official Journal of the Society for Neuroscience, 34*(12), 4273–4284.

Fowler, C. D., Lu, Q., Johnson, P. M., Marks, M. J., & Kenny, P. J. (2011). Habenular alpha5 nicotinic receptor subunit signalling controls nicotine intake. *Nature, 471*(7340), 597–601.

Fowler, C. D., Tuesta, L., & Kenny, P. J. (2013). Role of alpha5* nicotinic acetylcholine receptors in the effects of acute and chronic nicotine treatment on brain reward function in mice. *Psychopharmacology, 229*(3), 503–513.

Frahm, S., Slimak, M. A., Ferrarese, L., Santos-Torres, J., Antolin-Fontes, B., Auer, S., ... Ibanez-Tallon, I. (2011). Aversion to nicotine is regulated by the balanced activity of beta4 and alpha5 nicotinic receptor subunits in the medial habenula. *Neuron, 70*(3), 522–535. http://dx.doi.org/10.1016/j.neuron.2011.04.013.

Glick, S. D., Sell, E. M., McCallum, S. E., & Maisonneuve, I. M. (2011). Brain regions mediating alpha3beta4 nicotinic antagonist effects of 18-MC on nicotine self-administration. *European Journal of Pharmacology, 669*(1–3), 71–75.

Gorlich, A., Antolin-Fontes, B., Ables, J. L., Frahm, S., Slimak, M. A., Dougherty, J. D., & Ibanez-Tallon, I. (2013). Reexposure to nicotine during withdrawal increases the pacemaking activity of cholinergic habenular neurons. *Proceedings of the National Academy of Sciences of the United States of America, 110*(42), 17077–17082.

Grady, S. R., Moretti, M., Zoli, M., Marks, M. J., Zanardi, A., Pucci, L., ... Gotti, C. (2009). Rodent habenulo-interpeduncular pathway expresses a large variety of uncommon nAChR subtypes, but only the alpha3beta4* and alpha3beta3beta4* subtypes mediate acetylcholine release. *The Journal of Neuroscience: the Official Journal of the Society for Neuroscience, 29*(7), 2272–2282.

Hong, S., Jhou, T. C., Smith, M., Saleem, K. S., & Hikosaka, O. (2011). Negative reward signals from the lateral habenula to dopamine neurons are mediated by rostromedial tegmental nucleus in primates. *The Journal of Neuroscience: the Official Journal of the Society for Neuroscience, 31*(32), 11457–11471.

Hsu, Y. W., Tempest, L., Quina, L. A., Wei, A. D., Zeng, H., & Turner, E. E. (2013). Medial habenula output circuit mediated by alpha5 nicotinic receptor-expressing GABAergic neurons in the interpeduncular nucleus. *The Journal of Neuroscience: the Official Journal of the Society for Neuroscience, 33*(46), 18022–18035.

Hsu, Y. W., Wang, S. D., Wang, S., Morton, G., Zariwala, H. A., de la Iglesia, H. O., & Turner, E. E. (2014). Role of the dorsal medial habenula in the regulation of voluntary activity, motor function, hedonic state, and primary reinforcement. *The Journal of Neuroscience: the Official Journal of the Society for Neuroscience*, 34(34), 11366–11384.

Hu, F., Ren, J., Zhang, J. E., Zhong, W., & Luo, M. (2012). Natriuretic peptides block synaptic transmission by activating phosphodiesterase 2A and reducing presynaptic PKA activity. *Proceedings of the National Academy of Sciences of the United States of America*, 109(43), 17681–17686.

Hung, R. J., McKay, J. D., Gaborieau, V., Boffetta, P., Hashibe, M., Zaridze, D., … Brennan, P. (2008). A susceptibility locus for lung cancer maps to nicotinic acetylcholine receptor subunit genes on 15q25. *Nature*, 452(7187), 633–637.

Iwahori, N. (1977). A Golgi study on the habenular nucleus of the cat. *The Journal of Comparative Neurology*, 72(3), 319–344.

Jackson, K. J., Marks, M. J., Vann, R. E., Chen, X., Gamage, T. F., Warner, J. A., & Damaj, M. I. (2010). Role of alpha5 nicotinic acetylcholine receptors in pharmacological and behavioral effects of nicotine in mice. *The Journal of Pharmacology and Experimental Therapeutics*, 334(1), 137–146.

Jackson, K. J., Martin, B. R., Changeux, J. P., & Damaj, M. I. (2008). Differential role of nicotinic acetylcholine receptor subunits in physical and affective nicotine withdrawal signs. *The Journal of Pharmacology and Experimental Therapeutics*, 325(1), 302–312.

Jackson, K. J., McIntosh, J. M., Brunzell, D. H., Sanjakdar, S. S., & Damaj, M. I. (2009). The role of alpha6-containing nicotinic acetylcholine receptors in nicotine reward and withdrawal. *The Journal of Pharmacology and Experimental Therapeutics*, 331(2), 547–554.

Jhou, T. C., Good, C. H., Rowley, C. S., Xu, S. P., Wang, H., Burnham, N. W., … Ikemoto, S. (2013). Cocaine drives aversive conditioning via delayed activation of dopamine-responsive habenular and midbrain pathways. *The Journal of Neuroscience: the Official Journal of the Society for Neuroscience*, 33(17), 7501–7512.

Kawaja, M. D., Flumerfelt, B. A., & Hrycyshyn, A. W. (1988). Topographical and ultrastructural investigation of the habenulo-interpeduncular pathway in the rat: a wheat germ agglutinin-horseradish peroxidase anterograde study. *The Journal of Comparative Neurology*, 275(1), 117–127.

Khaled, M. A., Pushparaj, A., Di Ciano, P., Diaz, J., & Le Foll, B. (2014). Dopamine D3 receptors in the basolateral amygdala and the lateral habenula modulate cue-induced reinstatement of nicotine seeking. *Neuropsychopharmacology: Official Publication of the American College of Neuropsychopharmacology*, 39(13), 3049–3058.

Kim, U., & Chang, S. Y. (2005). Dendritic morphology, local circuitry, and intrinsic electrophysiology of neurons in the rat medial and lateral habenular nuclei of the epithalamus. *The Journal of Comparative Neurology*, 483(2), 236–250.

Klemm, W. R. (2004). Habenular and interpeduncularis nuclei: shared components in multiple-function networks. *Medical Science Monitor: International Medical Journal of Experimental and Clinical Research*, 10(11), RA261–273.

Kobayashi, Y., Sano, Y., Vannoni, E., Goto, H., Suzuki, H., Oba, A., … Itohara, S. (2013). Genetic dissection of medial habenula-interpeduncular nucleus pathway function in mice. *Frontiers in Behavioral Neuroscience*, 7, 17.

Lazary, J., Dome, P., Csala, I., Kovacs, G., Faludi, G., Kaunisto, M., & Dome, B. (2014). Massive withdrawal symptoms and affective vulnerability are associated with variants of the CHRNA4 gene in a subgroup of smokers. *PLoS One*, 9(1), e87141.

Lena, C., Changeux, J. P., & Mulle, C. (1993). Evidence for "preterminal" nicotinic receptors on GABAergic axons in the rat interpeduncular nucleus. *The Journal of Neuroscience: the Official Journal of the Society for Neuroscience*, 13(6), 2680–2688.

Lenn, N. J., Wong, V., & Hamill, G. S. (1983). Left-right pairing at the crest synapses of rat interpeduncular nucleus. *Neuroscience*, 9(2), 383–389.

Lotfipour, S., Byun, J. S., Leach, P., Fowler, C. D., Murphy, N. P., Kenny, P. J., … Boulter, J. (2013). Targeted deletion of the mouse alpha2 nicotinic acetylcholine receptor subunit gene (Chrna2) potentiates nicotine-modulated behaviors. *The Journal of Neuroscience: the Official Journal of the Society for Neuroscience, 33*(18), 7728–7741.

Marks, M. J., Pauly, J. R., Gross, S. D., Deneris, E. S., Hermans-Borgmeyer, I., Heinemann, S. F., & Collins, A. C. (1992). Nicotine binding and nicotinic receptor subunit RNA after chronic nicotine treatment. *The Journal of Neuroscience: the Official Journal of the Society for Neuroscience, 12*(7), 2765–2784.

McCormick, D. A., & Prince, D. A. (1987). Acetylcholine causes rapid nicotinic excitation in the medial habenular nucleus of guinea pig, in vitro. *The Journal of Neuroscience: the Official Journal of the Society for Neuroscience, 7*(3), 742–752.

Meyers, E. E., Loetz, E. C., & Marks, M. J. (2015). Differential expression of the beta4 neuronal nicotinic receptor subunit affects tolerance development and nicotinic binding sites following chronic nicotine treatment. *Pharmacology, Biochemistry, and Behavior, 130*, 1–8.

Piasecki, T. M., Niaura, R., Shadel, W. G., Abrams, D., Goldstein, M., Fiore, M. C., & Baker, T. B. (2000). Smoking withdrawal dynamics in unaided quitters. *Journal of Abnormal Psychology, 109*(1), 74–86.

Quina, L. A., Wang, S., Ng, L., & Turner, E. E. (2009). Brn3a and Nurr1 mediate a gene regulatory pathway for habenula development. *The Journal of Neuroscience: the Official Journal of the Society for Neuroscience, 29*(45), 14309–14322.

Ramon y Cajal, S. (1911). *Histologie du système nerveux de l'homme & des vertébrés* (vol. II). Paris, France: Maloine.

Ren, J., Qin, C., Hu, F., Tan, J., Qiu, L., Zhao, S., … Luo, M. (2011). Habenula "cholinergic" neurons co-release glutamate and acetylcholine and activate postsynaptic neurons via distinct transmission modes. *Neuron, 69*(3), 445–452.

Root, D. H., Mejias-Aponte, C. A., Zhang, S., Wang, H. L., Hoffman, A. F., Lupica, C. R., & Morales, M. (2014). Single rodent mesohabenular axons release glutamate and GABA. *Nature Neuroscience, 17*(11), 1543–1551.

Ross, S. A., Wong, J. Y., Clifford, J. J., Kinsella, A., Massalas, J. S., Horne, M. K., … Drago, J. (2000). Phenotypic characterization of an alpha 4 neuronal nicotinic acetylcholine receptor subunit knock-out mouse. *The Journal of Neuroscience: the Official Journal of the Society for Neuroscience, 20*(17), 6431–6441.

Salas, R., Main, A., Gangitano, D., & De Biasi, M. (2007). Decreased withdrawal symptoms but normal tolerance to nicotine in mice null for the alpha7 nicotinic acetylcholine receptor subunit. *Neuropharmacology, 53*(7), 863–869.

Salas, R., Pieri, F., & De Biasi, M. (2004). Decreased signs of nicotine withdrawal in mice null for the beta4 nicotinic acetylcholine receptor subunit. *The Journal of Neuroscience: the Official Journal of the Society for Neuroscience, 24*(45), 10035–10039.

Salas, R., Pieri, F., Fung, B., Dani, J. A., & De Biasi, M. (2003). Altered anxiety-related responses in mutant mice lacking the beta4 subunit of the nicotinic receptor. *The Journal of Neuroscience: the Official Journal of the Society for Neuroscience, 23*(15), 6255–6263.

Salas, R., Sturm, R., Boulter, J., & De Biasi, M. (2009). Nicotinic receptors in the habenulo-interpeduncular system are necessary for nicotine withdrawal in mice. *The Journal of Neuroscience: the Official Journal of the Society for Neuroscience, 29*(10), 3014–3018.

Sarginson, J. E., Killen, J. D., Lazzeroni, L. C., Fortmann, S. P., Ryan, H. S., Schatzberg, A. F., & Murphy, G. M., Jr. (2011). Markers in the 15q24 nicotinic receptor subunit gene cluster (CHRNA5-A3-B4) predict severity of nicotine addiction and response to smoking cessation therapy. *American Journal of Medical Genetics Part B: Neuropsychiatric Genetics, 156B*(3), 275–284.

Sheffield, E. B., Quick, M. W., & Lester, R. A. (2000). Nicotinic acetylcholine receptor subunit mRNA expression and channel function in medial habenula neurons. *Neuropharmacology, 39*(13), 2591–2603.

Sherva, R., Wilhelmsen, K., Pomerleau, C. S., Chasse, S. A., Rice, J. P., Snedecor, S. M., … Pomerleau, O. F. (2008). Association of a single nucleotide polymorphism in neuronal acetylcholine receptor subunit alpha 5 (CHRNA5) with smoking status and with 'pleasurable buzz' during early experimentation with smoking. *Addiction (Abingdon, England)*, 103(9), 1544–1552.

Shiffman, S. M., & Jarvik, M. E. (1976). Smoking withdrawal symptoms in two weeks of abstinence. *Psychopharmacology*, 50(1), 35–39.

Shih, P. Y., Engle, S. E., Oh, G., Deshpande, P., Puskar, N. L., Lester, H. A., & Drenan, R. M. (2014). Differential expression and function of nicotinic acetylcholine receptors in subdivisions of medial habenula. *The Journal of Neuroscience: the Official Journal of the Society for Neuroscience*, 34(29), 9789–9802.

Skofitsch, G., Jacobowitz, D. M., Eskay, R. L., & Zamir, N. (1985). Distribution of atrial natriuretic factor-like immunoreactive neurons in the rat brain. *Neuroscience*, 16(4), 917–948.

Stoker, A. K., Olivier, B., & Markou, A. (2012a). Involvement of metabotropic glutamate receptor 5 in brain reward deficits associated with cocaine and nicotine withdrawal and somatic signs of nicotine withdrawal. *Psychopharmacology*, 221(2), 317–327.

Stoker, A. K., Olivier, B., & Markou, A. (2012b). Role of alpha7- and beta4-containing nicotinic acetylcholine receptors in the affective and somatic aspects of nicotine withdrawal: studies in knockout mice. *Behavior Genetics*, 42(3), 423–436.

Sugama, S., Cho, B. P., Baker, H., Joh, T. H., Lucero, J., & Conti, B. (2002). Neurons of the superior nucleus of the medial habenula and ependymal cells express IL-18 in rat CNS. *Brain Research*, 958(1), 1–9.

Sutherland, R. J. (1982). The dorsal diencephalic conduction system: a review of the anatomy and functions of the habenular complex. *Neuroscience and Biobehavioral Reviews*, 6(1), 1–13.

Thorgeirsson, T. E., Geller, F., Sulem, P., Rafnar, T., Wiste, A., Magnusson, K. P., … Stefansson, K. (2008). A variant associated with nicotine dependence, lung cancer and peripheral arterial disease. *Nature*, 452(7187), 638–642.

Wagner, F., French, L., & Veh, R. W. (2014). Transcriptomic-anatomic analysis of the mouse habenula uncovers a high molecular heterogeneity among neurons in the lateral complex, while gene expression in the medial complex largely obeys subnuclear boundaries. *Brain Structure & Function*, 221(1), 39–58.

Wang, J. C., Grucza, R., Cruchaga, C., Hinrichs, A. L., Bertelsen, S., Budde, J. P., … Goate, A.M. (2009). Genetic variation in the CHRNA5 gene affects mRNA levels and is associated with risk for alcohol dependence. *Molecular Psychiatry*, 14(5), 501–510.

Weiss, R. B., Baker, T. B., Cannon, D. S., von Niederhausern, A., Dunn, D. M., Matsunami, N., … Leppert, M. F. (2008). A candidate gene approach identifies the CHRNA5-A3-B4 region as a risk factor for age-dependent nicotine addiction. *PLoS Genetics*, 4(7), e1000125.

Yamaguchi, T., Danjo, T., Pastan, I., Hikida, T., & Nakanishi, S. (2013). Distinct roles of segregated transmission of the septo-habenular pathway in anxiety and fear. *Neuron*, 78(3), 537–544.

Zhao-Shea, R., Liu, L., Pang, X., Gardner, P. D., & Tapper, A. R. (2013). Activation of GABAergic neurons in the interpeduncular nucleus triggers physical nicotine withdrawal symptoms. *Current Biology: CB*, 23(23), 2327–2335.

12

A Clinical Overview of Nicotine Dependence and Withdrawal

M. Frandsen¹, M. Thorpe¹, S. Shiffman², S.G. Ferguson¹

¹University of Tasmania, Hobart, TAS, Australia; ²University of Pittsburgh, Pittsburgh, PA, United States

A CLINICAL OVERVIEW OF NICOTINE DEPENDENCE AND WITHDRAWAL

Conceptualizing Nicotine Dependence

According to the World Health Organization (WHO, 2010), one person dies prematurely every 6 s as a result of their addiction to tobacco. Cigarette smoking remains the greatest modifiable cause of death and disease in the world. While having little role in disease causation, nicotine, the principal neuroactive chemical constituent of tobacco, is responsible for the highly addictive nature of tobacco smoking, and thus smokers' dependence.

Nicotine dependence is formally recognized as a medical condition by both the American Psychiatric Association's (APA, 2013) *Diagnostic and Statistical Manual of Mental Health Disorders*, fifth edition (DSM-5), and the *International Classification of Diseases*, 10th revision (WHO, 1992). Nicotine dependence describes a substance abuse disorder experienced by individuals who compulsively use tobacco products despite the known health risks. For the purposes of this chapter, dependence will be defined as a "clinical syndrome that can include physical (tolerance and/or withdrawal) and psychological (impaired control of drug/substance use) dependence" (Hughes, 2007). While definitions are debated and definitive criteria continue to evolve, general drug-dependence criteria are helpful in describing nicotine dependence and are generally agreed upon. They

Negative Affective States and Cognitive Impairments in Nicotine Dependence
http://dx.doi.org/10.1016/B978-0-12-802574-1.00012-0

include use that is highly controlled or compulsive, psychoactive effects, and drug-reinforced behavior. Additional criteria include stereotypic behaviors and patterns of use, recurrent drug craving, relapse following abstinence, and use despite evidence of harmful effects (Centers for Disease Control and Prevention, 2010).

Central to nicotine dependence is nicotine withdrawal. This manifests as a characteristic cluster of symptoms experienced when the key addictive component of tobacco, nicotine, is withheld, either during a quit attempt or during short periods of abstinence. Avoidance of nicotine withdrawal is reported by smokers to be one of the main reasons for maintaining smoking and, consequently, undermines success in quitting. The majority of the withdrawal symptoms experienced are characterized by negative affect, for example feelings of irritability, misery, tension, frustration, anger, and sadness (described in more detail later in the chapter). As such, avoidance of these symptoms and negative states is central to withdrawal-based models of dependence. In seeking to avoid these aversive experiences, and alleviate the negative feelings when they do occur, the dependent smoker re-administers the drug (nicotine) and thereby negatively reinforces continued smoking. This leads to compulsive perseverative use, and the propensity to relapse that characterizes addiction. Here, we present an overview of the clinical experience of nicotine dependence, the central role of nicotine withdrawal, and the effect of negative affect on lapse and relapse.

The Role of Nicotine

To understand how nicotine dependence develops, a pharmacological overview of the effects of tobacco, and particularly nicotine, is beneficial. Tobacco products contain in excess of 7000 chemicals (Centers for Disease Control and Prevention, 2010), and while many of these chemicals may exert psychoactive effects, there is overwhelming consensus that nicotine is *the* principal addictive component of tobacco. Nicotine is readily absorbed through the lungs and auxiliary respiratory pathways, taking just seconds to reach the brain following inhalation (Benowitz, 1996) and, depending on the delivery system used, reaching maximum concentrations in the blood in 5–20 min (Benowitz, Porchet, Sheiner, & Jaco, 1988; Fant, Owen, & Henningfield, 1999). The effects of nicotine are pervasive and pharmacologically affect most organ systems within the human body (including the central and peripheral nervous systems and the cardiovascular, peripheral vascular, respiratory, hematological, and endocrine systems). Central to its effect in mediating dependence, particularly in the establishment phase, is the activity of nicotine on the dopaminergic, reward regulatory network of the central nervous system (see Centers for Disease Control and Prevention, 2010; Shadel, Shiffman, Niaura, Nichter,

& Abrams, 2000). The hedonic—or pleasurable—sensations of arousal that are elicited act rapidly, via positive reinforcement, to entrench and reinforce smoking behaviors.

Physiological neuroadaptations are evoked by the increased exposure to nicotine that accompanies the repeated use of tobacco. These adaptations underlie the development of physiological tolerance, whereby the effects of the same dose of nicotine diminish over time, with increased doses required to achieve the same reward or effect. Regular daily cigarette smoking ensures near-complete nicotine saturation, resulting in the desensitization of specific nicotinic cholinergic neuroreceptors. These receptors remain largely desensitized as long as threshold levels of nicotine are maintained (Benowitz, 2010). When smokers abstain from smoking and nicotine levels drop, these receptors become re-sensitized and activated, resulting in the characteristic symptoms of withdrawal (depressed mood, restlessness, irritability, and craving). Research has further suggested that dependent smokers deprived of nicotine (ie, during a quit attempt) become impaired in their capacity to respond to rewards, with this responsiveness to natural rewards becoming reinstated upon restoration of nicotine levels; relapse to smoking thus further reinforces the "need" to smoke (Caggiula et al., 2009; Dawkins, Powell, West, Powell, & Pickering, 2006; Pergadia et al., 2014). Smokers are compelled to avoid or alleviate these negative affective states and other aversive withdrawal symptoms by using the most effective way they know how: re-administering nicotine. This is the key tenet of self-medication models, which contend that smokers self-administer nicotine (continue smoking) to sustain a blood nicotine level that minimizes the occurrence of craving and withdrawal symptoms. In other words, dependent smokers are rewarded by their continued smoking, as it serves, via negative reinforcement, to prevent or alleviate the experience of negative symptoms.

Development of Nicotine Dependence

Repeated exposure, or chronic regular or heavy use, of nicotine is generally considered necessary to develop nicotine dependence (cf. DiFranza, 2008). Indeed, risk of nicotine dependence increases with higher levels of use (Dierker et al., 2007; Kandel & Chen, 2000). Longitudinal studies have suggested that substantial variation exists in individual trajectories from smoking initiation to dependence (Chassin, Presson, Pitts, & Sherman, 2000; Soldz & Cui, 2002).

Many factors have been suggested that increase vulnerability to development of nicotine dependence. Risk of dependence, for example, is greater the earlier in life that smoking begins (Lynch & Bonnie, 1994), and it is further influenced by genetic and familial environmental factors (Sullivan & Kendler, 1999). Twin studies, for example, have suggested that genetic vulnerability can account for up to 80% of the likelihood of developing nicotine dependence after smoking initiation (Batra, Patkar, Berrettini, Weinstein, & Leone, 2003; Li, Cheng, Ma, & Swan, 2003). Individual variance in the gene CYP2A6, which is suggested to be largely (~90%) responsible for metabolizing nicotine, has been found to vary significantly between people (up to a fourfold difference), with this variance correlating with smoking rate (Malaiyandi, Sellers, & Tyndale, 2005). Individuals suffering from mental illness or other substance abuse disorders also have been found to be twice as likely to be dependent on nicotine, and smoke more heavily, when compared to the general population. This may be partly attributable to the pharmacological capacity of nicotine to alleviate some psychiatric symptoms (Weinberger, Desai, & McKee, 2010; Ziedonis et al., 2008). (The associations between genetics, psychiatric conditions, and nicotine dependence are addressed in other chapters in this book.) Central to the development of nicotine dependence and the difficulty in quitting—exemplified by the finding that only around 50% of ever-smokers eventually successfully quit (Centers for Disease Control and Prevention, 2010)—is the experience of nicotine withdrawal.

Nicotine Withdrawal

Symptoms

The nicotine withdrawal syndrome is characterized by a constellation of symptoms and behaviors commonly experienced by dependent smokers when abstaining from, or limiting, their consumption of tobacco (APA, 2013; Hughes & Hatsukami, 1986). Pivotal to the debilitating experience of these symptoms is their pervasive manifestation—affecting the somatic, cognitive, and, especially, affective domains—with ensuing symptomatology that is both complex and distressing. This complexity is one of the reasons why smokers find it difficult to maintain smoking abstinence. According to the DSM-5 (APA, 2013), four criteria must be met to classify/diagnose tobacco withdrawal: daily use of tobacco for at least several weeks; abrupt cessation/ reduction of tobacco use followed within 24h by four (or more) symptoms, including irritability, frustration, anger, anxiety, difficulty concentrating, increased appetite, restlessness, depressed mood, and/or insomnia; these signs/symptoms cause clinically significant distress or impairment to social, occupational, or other important areas of function; and these signs/symptoms are not attributed to another medical condition or better explained by other mental disorders (including intoxication or withdrawal from another drug). Other symptoms reported to be experienced within 2h of last tobacco use include decreased heart rate, increased appetite, lack of motivation, and impatience (Hughes, 2007). These typically peak 2–3days after last tobacco use and remit over the subsequent 3–4weeks, with severe symptoms after 1month uncommon (APA, 2013; Hughes, 2007). While the time spent experiencing these symptoms is arguably short term, the severity of the symptoms experienced by individuals abstaining from nicotine has been equated to that of individuals experiencing clinically significant episodes of psychiatric distress (Hughes, 2006), thus helping explain why smokers actively avoid experiencing withdrawal and have trouble tolerating it during cessation attempts.

Time Course and Severity of Nicotine Withdrawal

Traditionally, the time course of nicotine withdrawal (duration of symptom experience) has been regarded as relatively transient, with symptoms suggested to increase during the first week after quitting, then gradually tapering and stabilizing over the following 3–4 weeks (Hughes, Higgins, & Hatsukami, 1990). Indeed, the finding from smoking cessation trials that relapse risk is greatest during the first 5–10 days of the initial quit attempt (Hays et al., 2001; Hughes, Keely, & Naud, 2004) has fostered a recognition of the intimate relationship between the time course (and severity) of withdrawal symptomatology and quit failures (Hughes et al., 2004). This relationship, however, is conditional in nature. For example, although a positive linear relationship between craving and drug use exists at low levels of craving intensity (with increased craving linked to an increased probability of lapsing), once craving reaches a certain threshold, the association between craving and relapse risk has been found to be nonlinear, with high levels of craving not found to elicit high levels of smoking (Ferguson & Shiffman, 2013). The nature and determinants of this threshold, between and within individuals, represent a challenge for future research.

Historically, previous research has focused on the mean overall symptom experience, the different types of symptoms, and their change over time, rather than the individual's experience of these symptoms (Pergadia et al., 2010). These studies, often evaluating the efficacy of cessation treatment such as nicotine replacement therapy (NRT), have consistently shown that symptom severity typically peaks during the first week of abstinence, then returns to baseline levels within 4 weeks (eg, Shiffman et al., 2006; West, Hajek, & Belcher, 1987, 1989). Variability in the time course of symptom severity within individuals has, however, also been shown (Piasecki et al., 2000). Negative affect, mood and cognitive disturbances, and frequency of time spent with urges (craving), for example, appear to have a predictable natural history, with return to baseline levels within 30 days. Conversely, hunger, intensity of urge (West et al., 1987, 1989), deregulated arousal, and sleep disturbances (Shiffman et al., 2006) often persist beyond 3 weeks. These findings point to the multifaceted and complex nature of the withdrawal syndrome and underscore the difficulty faced by smokers in attempting to overcome them.

Individuals' unique experiences of overall symptom severity have been the focus of extensive research in recent years, with many clinical studies and trials indicating that substantial variability exists in individual experiences of withdrawal (eg, Gilbert et al., 2002; Piasecki, Jorenby, Smith, Fiore, & Baker, 2002), and furthermore, that these differences are not attributable to the mode of nicotine consumption, the duration of tobacco use, or premorbid psychological and genetic vulnerabilities (Lazary et al., 2014; Saccone et al., 2007). Individual differences, for example, have been found in the pattern of symptom experience over time, with some individuals experiencing a gradual increase, rather than decrease, in symptom frequency and/or intensity during the withdrawal phase. Fluctuations (volatility) in symptomatology during the time course of withdrawal, or in symptom remission during smoking cessation lapse (eg, some abstainers do not have their withdrawal symptoms relieved during initial cigarette lapse), have also been demonstrated (Ferguson, Shiffman, & Gwaltney, 2006; Piasecki et al., 2002; Piasecki, Jorenby, Smith, Fiore, & Baker, 2003; Piper et al., 2009). Smokers most likely to lapse, for example, have been found to have greater symptom severity, smaller linear decreases in symptoms over time, and higher volatility scores across 8 weeks, reflecting greater symptom fluctuations during the period of abstinence (Piasecki et al., 2003). These authors also demonstrated that smoking lapses post cessation do not always reduce symptoms, with small amounts of smoking increasing withdrawal symptoms post quit, through priming mechanisms, in some individuals (Piasecki et al., 2003). Attempting quitters who reported diminished attenuation of withdrawal symptoms during a smoking lapse (negative cigarette coefficients; Piasecki et al., 2003) were found to engage in more smoking occasions post quit, more total cigarettes, and increased cigarette consumption when they did smoke. These data point to the need for caution in assuming that aggregate time course patterns and withdrawal symptom experience of smokers is applicable to all individuals.

Craving

Often defined as a strong desire, urge, or intense need to use a substance or engage in a behavior, craving has been reported by smokers as an experience characterized by an overwhelming feeling of loss of control over one's behavior and reactions (Ferguson & Shiffman, 2013). Craving, now recognized by the latest revision of the DSM as one of 11 criteria used to diagnose tobacco use disorder, can also be conceptualized as a neurophysiologically derived effect elicited by withdrawal from nicotine. The natural history of abstinence-induced craving mirrors the trajectory of the abstinence–withdrawal curve, with an acute increase in intensity following smoking cessation, followed by a return to baseline levels within a few weeks, therefore supporting the notion that it has a central role in hindering quit attempts and maintaining smokers' dependence (Ferguson & Shiffman, 2013).

The finding, however, that craving can trigger relapse long after initial abstinence (Ferguson & Shiffman, 2013; Ussher, Beard, Abikoye, Hajek,

& West, 2013), and be reliably provoked even when smokers are sated (Carter & Tiffany, 1999; Hogarth, Dickinson, & Duka, 2010), suggests that craving is not induced by drug abstinence alone. Indeed, as explained by social learning and cognitive models, craving can also be triggered through the process of classical conditioning and the pairing of a stimulus (smoking) with external (environmental, situational) and internal (emotional, thoughts) cues. While initial pairing of substance use and cues is necessary, through the process of learning, the associated cues are eventually sufficient to trigger the urge or craving. As such, craving can be conceptualized in two ways depending on how it is induced. Abstinence-induced craving (also known as background or tonic craving) is linked to nicotine levels and can be categorized as a withdrawal symptom with a relatively predictable time course. Cue-induced craving, in contrast, is characterized by fluctuations that depend on the individual's immediate environment and internal states.

Recognition of the role of cue-induced craving and its clinical manifestations can help explain relapse that occurs long after acute withdrawal has subsided, and explain why craving to smoke remains pervasive and powerful for an extended duration, even if the frequency of the urge and time spent with the urge diminish over time (Shiffman et al., 1996; West et al., 1987, 1989). It also helps to explain why many smokers who attempt to quit using only pharmacotherapy eventually fail. While pharmacotherapies are efficacious in reducing background tonic craving and may buffer some of the effects from smoking cues (Ferguson & Shiffman, 2009), they do not alleviate the day-to-day fluctuations of symptoms (eg, negative affect, craving) caused by stressors and cues (at least for some smokers; Ferguson & Shiffman, 2014; cf. Shiffman et al., 2003, and Hogarth, 2012, for discussion of the effects of fast-acting NRT on cue-induced craving).

Studies exploring antecedents of smoking lapses have further emphasized the important role of craving and negative affect states in triggering relapse (Allen, Bade, Hatsukami, & Center, 2008; Ferguson & Shiffman, 2014; Shiffman & Waters, 2004). Utilizing smoking diaries (either paper and pen, or electronic), these studies have demonstrated uniform increases in negative affect and craving in the days leading up to a lapse, and marked escalations in the preceding hours immediately before a lapse. These rapid increases, or peaks, in negative affect (compared to day-to-day average fluctuations) appear especially important in influencing relapse (Ferguson & Shiffman, 2014; Shiffman & Waters, 2004) and thus represent a particular challenge for developing effective smoking cessation treatments.

Negative Affect and Self-Control

One explanation for this intensification of negative affect prior to smoking lapse is that the chronicity of negative affective episodes serves to erode, progressively, the individual's coping (psychological) reserves. Self-control requires constant attention, resources, and energy to maintain, and, analogous to a muscle, it is believed to grow weak from exertion (Baumeister, Vohs, & Tice, 2007). As such, over time, the repeated experience of negative affective episodes may "exhaust" the attempting quitter's self-control resources, compromising the effectiveness of coping strategies and eventually leading to them "giving up, giving up" (Ferguson & Shiffman, 2014). Providing attempting quitters with self-control training has been shown to increase the duration of abstinence compared to a control group of quitters (eg, Muraven, 2010), and offers a direction for future research and treatment development.

SUMMARY

Tobacco smoking is the leading modifiable cause of mortality worldwide, and while research has helped clarify the nature of this dependence phenomenon, the fact that (based on current treatment strategies) half of all ever-smokers will never be able to successfully quit highlights the fact that much remains unclear. Significant research attention has historically been applied to understanding and informing treatments for abstinence-induced withdrawal symptoms. The recognition of the significant influence of both tonic and cue-induced craving has provided greater insight into the difficulty of maintaining abstinence and the importance of not treating smokers with pharmacotherapy alone. Novel techniques have further advanced understanding of individual differences in not only vulnerability to nicotine dependence, but also the individual experience of nicotine dependence and withdrawal. Central to understanding nicotine dependence is negative reinforcement and the avoidance of withdrawal symptoms. While much has been uncovered regarding the important role of negative affect states and the part they play in smoking maintenance and relapse, substantial knowledge gaps still exist. Future research now faces the challenge of finding ways to ameliorate these states and negate their deleterious impact on the psychological reserves that mediate coping and self-control in individuals attempting to quit. Perhaps then, more effective treatments can be developed to offer cessation-seeking smokers better hope.

References

Allen, S. S., Bade, T., Hatsukami, D., & Center, B. (2008). Craving, withdrawal, and smoking urges on days immediately prior to smoking relapse. *Nicotine & Tobacco Research: Official Journal of the Society for Research on Nicotine and Tobacco*, 10(1), 35–45. http://dx.doi.org/10.1080/14622200701705076.
American Psychiatric Association. (2013). *American Psychiatric Association: Diagnostic and Statistical Manual of Mental Health Disorders* (5th ed.). Arlington, VA: American Psychiatric Association.

Batra, V., Patkar, A. A., Berrettini, W. H., Weinstein, S. P., & Leone, F. T. (2003). The genetic determinants of smoking. *Chest, 123*(5), 1730–1739.

Baumeister, R. F., Vohs, K. D., & Tice, D. M. (2007). The strength model of self-control. *Current Directions in Psychological Science, 16*(6), 351–355. http://dx.doi.org/10.1111/j.1467-8721.2007.00534.x.

Benowitz, N. L. (1996). Pharmacology of nicotine: addiction and therapeutics. *Annual Review of Pharmacology and Toxicology, 36*, 597–613. http://dx.doi.org/10.1146/annurev.pa.36.040196.003121.

Benowitz, N. L. (2010). Nicotine addiction. *The New England Journal of Medicine, 362*(24), 2295–2303. http://dx.doi.org/10.1056/NEJMra0809890.

Benowitz, N. L., Porchet, H., Sheiner, L., & Jaco, P. (1988). Nicotine absorption and cardiovascular effects with smokeless tobacco use: comparison with cigarettes and nicotine gum. *Clinical Pharmacology and Therapeutics, 44*, 23–28.

Caggiula, A. R., Donny, E. C., Palmatier, M. I., Liu, X., Chaudhri, N., & Sved, A. F. (2009). The role of nicotine in smoking: a dual-reinforcement model. *Nebraska Symposium on Motivation, 55*, 91–109.

Carter, B. L., & Tiffany, S. T. (1999). Meta-analysis of cue-reactivity in addiction research. *Addiction (Abingdon, England), 94*(3), 327–340.

Centers for Disease Control and Prevention (CDCP). (2010). *Publications and Reports of the Surgeon General. How tobacco smoke causes disease: The biology and behavioral basis for smoking-attributable disease: A report of the Surgeon General.* Atlanta, GA: Centers for Disease Control and Prevention (US).

Chassin, L., Presson, C. C., Pitts, S. C., & Sherman, S. J. (2000). The natural history of cigarette smoking from adolescence to adulthood in a midwestern community sample: multiple trajectories and their psychosocial correlates. *Health Psychology: Official Journal of the Division of Health Psychology, American Psychological Association, 19*(3), 223–231.

Dawkins, L., Powell, J. H., West, R., Powell, J., & Pickering, A. (2006). A double-blind placebo controlled experimental study of nicotine: I–effects on incentive motivation. *Psychopharmacology (Berlin), 189*(3), 355–367. http://dx.doi.org/10.1007/s00213-006-0588-8.

Dierker, L. C., Donny, E., Tiffany, S., Colby, S. M., Perrine, N., & Clayton, R. R. (2007). The association between cigarette smoking and DSM-IV nicotine dependence among first year college students. *Drug and Alcohol Dependence, 86*(2–3), 106–114. http://dx.doi.org/10.1016/j.drugalcdep.2006.05.025.

DiFranza, J. R. (2008). Hooked from the first cigarette. *Scientific American, 298*(5), 82–87.

Fant, R. V., Owen, L. L., & Henningfield, J. E. (1999). Nicotine replacement therapy. *Primary Care, 26*(3), 633–652.

Ferguson, S. G., & Shiffman, S. (2009). The relevance and treatment of cue-induced cravings in tobacco dependence. *Journal of Substance Abuse Treatment, 36*(3), 235–243. http://dx.doi.org/10.1016/j.jsat.2008.06.005.

Ferguson, S. G., & Shiffman, S. (2013). Relation of craving and appetitive behavior. *Principles of Addiction*, 473–479.

Ferguson, S. G., & Shiffman, S. (2014). Effect of high-dose nicotine patch on craving and negative affect leading up to lapse episodes. *Psychopharmacology (Berlin), 231*(13), 2595–2602. http://dx.doi.org/10.1007/s00213-013-3429-6.

Ferguson, S. G., Shiffman, S., & Gwaltney, C. J. (2006). Does reducing withdrawal severity mediate nicotine patch efficacy? A randomized clinical trial. *Journal of Consulting and Clinical Psychology, 74*(6), 1153–1161. http://dx.doi.org/10.1037/0022-006x.74.6.1153.

Gilbert, D. G., McClernon, F. J., Rabinovich, N. E., Plath, L. C., Masson, C. L., Anderson, A. E., et al. (2002). Mood disturbance fails to resolve across 31 days of cigarette abstinence in women. *Journal of Consulting and Clinical Psychology, 70*(1), 142–152.

Hays, J. T., Hurt, R. D., Rigotti, N. A., Niaura, R., Gonzalez, D., Durcan, M. J., et al. (2001). Sustained-release bupropion for pharmacologic relapse prevention after smoking cessation. *Annals of Internal Medicine, 135*, 423–433.

Hogarth, L. (2012). Goal-directed and transfer-cue-elicited drug-seeking are dissociated by pharmacotherapy: evidence for independent additive controllers. *Journal of Experimental Psychology. Animal Behavior Processes, 38*(3), 266–278. http://dx.doi.org/10.1037/a0028914.

Hogarth, L., Dickinson, A., & Duka, T. (2010). The associative basis of cue-elicited drug taking in humans. *Psychopharmacology, 208*(3), 337–351. http://dx.doi.org/10.1007/s00213-009-1735-9.

Hughes, J. R. (2006). Clinical significance of tobacco withdrawal. *Nicotine & Tobacco Research: Official Journal of the Society for Research on Nicotine and Tobacco, 8*(2), 153–156. http://dx.doi.org/10.1080/14622200500494856.

Hughes, J. R. (2007). Effects of abstinence from tobacco: valid symptoms and time course. *Nicotine & Tobacco Research, 9*(3), 315–327. http://dx.doi.org/10.1080/14622200701188919.

Hughes, J. R., & Hatsukami, D. (1986). Signs and symptoms of tobacco withdrawal. *Archives of General Psychiatry, 43*(3), 289–294.

Hughes, J. R., Higgins, S. T., & Hatsukami, D. K. (1990). Effects of abstinence from tobacco: a critical review. In L. T. Kozlowski, H. Annis, H. D. Cappell, F. Glaser, M. Goodstadt, Y. Isreal, et al. (Eds.), *Research advances in alcohol and drug problems* (pp. 317–398). New York: Plenum Press.

Hughes, J. R., Keely, J., & Naud, S. (2004). Shape of the relapse curve and long-term abstinence among untreated smokers. *Addiction (Abingdon, England), 99*(1), 29–38.

Kandel, D. B., & Chen, K. (2000). Extent of smoking and nicotine dependence in the United States: 1991–1993. *Nicotine & Tobacco Research, 2*(3), 263–274. http://dx.doi.org/10.1080/14622200050147538.

Lazary, J., Dome, P., Csala, I., Kovacs, G., Faludi, G., Kaunisto, M., et al. (2014). Massive withdrawal symptoms and affective vulnerability are associated with variants of the CHRNA4 gene in a subgroup of smokers. *PLoS One, 9*(1), e87141. http://dx.doi.org/10.1371/journal.pone.0087141.

Li, M. D., Cheng, R., Ma, J. Z., & Swan, G. E. (2003). A meta-analysis of estimated genetic and environmental effects on smoking behavior in male and female adult twins. *Addiction (Abingdon, England), 98*(1), 23–31.

The nature of nicotine addiction. In B. S. Lynch, & R. J. Bonnie (Eds.), (1994). *Growing up tobacco free: Preventing nicotine addiction in children and youths.* Washington, DC: National Academies Press.

Malaiyandi, V., Sellers, E. M., & Tyndale, R. F. (2005). Implications of CYP2A6 genetic variation for smoking behaviors and nicotine dependence. *Clinical Pharmacology and Therapeutics, 77*(3), 145–158. http://dx.doi.org/10.1016/j.clpt.2004.10.011.

Muraven, M. (2010). Practicing self-control lowers the risk of smoking lapse. *Psychology of Addictive Behaviors: Journal of the Society of Psychologists in Addictive Behaviors, 24*(3), 446–452. http://dx.doi.org/10.1037/a0018545.

Pergadia, M. L., Agrawal, A., Heath, A. C., Martin, N. G., Bucholz, K. K., & Madden, P. A. (2010). Nicotine withdrawal symptoms in adolescent and adult twins. *Twin Research and Human Genetics: the Official Journal of the International Society for Twin Studies, 13*(4), 359–369. http://dx.doi.org/10.1375/twin.13.4.359.

Pergadia, M. L., Der-Avakian, A., D'Souza, M. S., Madden, P. A., Heath, A. C., Shiffman, S., et al. (2014). Association between nicotine withdrawal and reward responsiveness in humans and rats. *JAMA Psychiatry, 71*(11), 1238–1245. http://dx.doi.org/10.1001/jamapsychiatry.2014.1016.

Piasecki, T. M., Jorenby, D. E., Smith, S. S., Fiore, M. C., & Baker, T. B. (2002). Smoking withdrawal dynamics: II. Improved tests of withdrawal-relapse relations. *Journal of Abnormal Psychology, 112*(1), 14–27.

Piasecki, T. M., Jorenby, D. E., Smith, S. S., Fiore, M. C., & Baker, T. B. (2003). Smoking withdrawal dynamics: I. Abstinence distress in lapsers and abstainers. *Journal of Abnormal Psychology, 112*(1), 3–13.

Piasecki, T. M., Niaura, R., Shadel, W. G., Abrams, D., Goldstein, M., Fiore, M. C., et al. (2000). Smoking withdrawal dynamics in unaided quitters. *Journal of Abnormal Psychology*, *109*(1), 74–86.

Piper, M. E., Smith, S. S., Schlam, T. R., Fiore, M. C., Jorenby, D. E., Fraser, D., et al. (2009). A randomized placebo-controlled clinical trial of five smoking cessation pharmacotherapies. *Archives of General Psychiatry*, *66*(11), 1253–1262. http://dx.doi.org/10.1001/archgenpsychiatry.2009.142.

Saccone, S. F., Pergadia, M. L., Loukola, A., Broms, U., Montgomery, G. W., Wang, J. C., et al. (2007). Genetic linkage to chromosome 22q12 for a heavy-smoking quantitative trait in two independent samples. *American Journal of Human Genetics*, *80*(5), 856–866. http://dx.doi.org/10.1086/513703.

Shadel, W. G., Shiffman, S., Niaura, R., Nichter, M., & Abrams, D. B. (2000). Current models of nicotine dependence: what is known and what is needed to advance understanding of tobacco etiology among youth. *Drug and Alcohol Dependence*, *59*(Suppl. 1), S9–S22.

Shiffman, S., Gnys, M., Richards, T. J., Paty, J. A., Hickcox, M., & Kassel, J. D. (1996). Temptations to smoke after quitting: a comparison of lapsers and maintainers. *Health Psychology: Official Journal of the Division of Health Psychology, American Psychological Association*, *15*(6), 455–461.

Shiffman, S., Scharf, D. M., Shadel, W. G., Gwaltney, C. J., Dang, Q., Paton, S. M., et al. (2006). Analyzing milestones in smoking cessation: illustration in a nicotine patch trial in adult smokers. *Journal of Consulting and Clinical Psychology*, *74*(2), 276–285. http://dx.doi.org/10.1037/0022-006x.74.2.276.

Shiffman, S., Shadel, W. G., Niaura, R., Khayrallah, M. A., Jorenby, D. E., Ryan, C. F., et al. (2003). Efficacy of acute administration of nicotine gum in relief of cue-provoked cigarette craving. *Psychopharmacology (Berlin)*, *166*(4), 343–350. http://dx.doi.org/10.1007/s00213-002-1338-1.

Shiffman, S., & Waters, A. J. (2004). Negative affect and smoking lapses: a prospective analysis. *Journal of Consulting and Clinical Psychology*, *72*(2), 192–201. http://dx.doi.org/10.1037/0022-006x.72.2.192.

Soldz, S., & Cui, X. (2002). Pathways through adolescent smoking: a 7-year longitudinal grouping analysis. *Health Psychology: Official Journal of the Division of Health Psychology, American Psychological Association*, *21*(5), 495–504.

Sullivan, P. F., & Kendler, K. S. (1999). The genetic epidemiology of smoking. *Nicotine & Tobacco Research: Official Journal of the Society for Research on Nicotine and Tobacco*, *1*(Suppl. 2), S51–S57 discussion S69–S70.

Ussher, M., Beard, E., Abikoye, G., Hajek, P., & West, R. (2013). Urge to smoke over 52 weeks of abstinence. *Psychopharmacology (Berlin)*, *226*(1), 83–89. http://dx.doi.org/10.1007/s00213-012-2886-7.

Weinberger, A. H., Desai, R. A., & McKee, S. A. (2010). Nicotine withdrawal in U.S. smokers with current mood, anxiety, alcohol use, and substance use disorders. *Drug and Alcohol Dependence*, *108*(1–2), 7–12. http://dx.doi.org/10.1016/j.drugalcdep.2009.11.004.

West, R., Hajek, P., & Belcher, M. (1987). Time course of cigarette withdrawal symptoms during four weeks of treatment with nicotine chewing gum. *Addictive Behaviors*, *12*(2), 199–203.

West, R., Hajek, P., & Belcher, M. (1989). Time course of cigarette withdrawal symptoms while using nicotine gum. *Psychopharmacology (Berlin)*, *99*(1), 143–145.

World Health Organisation. (1992). *International statistical classification of diseases and related health problems, tenth revision*. Geneva: World Health Organisation.

World Health Organisation. (2010). In J. M. Samet, & S.-Y. Yoon (Eds.), *Gender, women, and the tobacco epidemic*. Geneva: WHO Press.

Ziedonis, D., Hitsman, B., Beckham, J. C., Zvolensky, M., Adler, L. E., Audrain-McGovern, J., et al. (2008). Tobacco use and cessation in psychiatric disorders: National Institute of Mental Health report. *Nicotine & Tobacco Research*, *10*(12), 1691–1715. http://dx.doi.org/10.1080/14622200802443569.

Epidemiologic Research on the Relationship of Nicotine Dependence to Psychiatric and Substance Use Disorders

K.S. Segal, H. Esan, A.R. Burns, A.H. Weinberger

Yeshiva University, Bronx, NY, United States

INTRODUCTION

Adults with a wide range of psychiatric and substance use disorders report higher rates of current and lifetime smoking, as well as lower rates of quitting smoking, compared to adults without these disorders (CDC, 2013; Lasser et al., 2000; Smith, Mazure, & McKee, 2014; Ziedonis et al., 2008). Further, there is a positive relationship between the number of psychiatric or substance use diagnoses and heavy smoking (Smith et al., 2014). Understanding aspects of smoking behavior (eg, nicotine dependence) in this important subgroup of smokers can help inform efforts to reduce smoking rates and hence the harmful consequences of smoking.

Not all smokers are "dependent" on nicotine. For example, when 20.9% of United States (US) adults reported current smoking (CDC, 2014), 12.8% of US adults met criteria for current nicotine dependence (ND; Grant, Hasin, Chou, Stinson, & Dawson, 2004). ND is associated with smoking persistence (Breslau, Johnson, Hiripi, & Kessler, 2001) and difficulty in quitting (Pomerleau et al., 2005; Sienkiewicz-Jarosz, Zatorski, Baranowska, & Ryglewicz, 2009). This chapter will review epidemiologic studies on ND in adults with psychiatric disorders [eg, mood disorders, anxiety disorder, personality disorders (PD)] as well as alcohol and substance use disorders.

ND has been measured in a number of ways in epidemiologic, or population-based, studies. Some epidemiologic studies assess ND diagnoses

Negative Affective States and Cognitive Impairments in Nicotine Dependence
http://dx.doi.org/10.1016/B978-0-12-802574-1.00013-2

using the Diagnostic and Statistical Manual of Mental Disorders (DSM; eg, use in larger amounts than intended, tolerance, withdrawal; APA, 2013). One example is the US-based National Epidemiologic Survey on Alcohol and Related Conditions (NESARC; Wave 1, 2001–02; Wave 2, 2004–05; Grant & Kaplan, 2005; Grant, Moore, Shepard, & Kaplan, 2003) which assessed ND using the Alcohol Use Disorders and Associated Disabilities Interview Schedule-DSM-IV (AUDADIS-IV; Grant, Dawson, & Hasin, 2001). The AUDADIS-IV demonstrated good reliability in the assessment of ND (past-year diagnosis $\kappa = 0.63$; lifetime diagnosis $\kappa = 0.60$; Grant, Dawson, et al., 2003). Other studies use self-report measures of dependence such as the Fagerström Test for Nicotine Dependence (FTND, Heatherton, Kozlowski, Frecker, & Fagerstrom, 1991) or the Heaviness of Smoking Index (HSI; Heatherton, Kozlowski, Frecker, Rickert, & Robinson, 1989). The FTND has good internal reliability ($\alpha = 0.90$; Stavem, Røgeberg, Olsen, & Boe, 2008), and the FTND and HSI are highly correlated ($\kappa = 0.70$; Pérez-Ríos et al., 2009).

NICOTINE DEPENDENCE AND PSYCHIATRIC DISORDERS

Mood Disorders

Several studies have evaluated the relationship of nicotine ND and mood disorders in US adults. Using data from Wave 1 of the NESARC, Grover, Goodwin, and Zvolensky (2012) found that past-year ND, but not former ND, was associated with increased odds of past-year major depression (MD; odds ratio (OR) = 3.05; 95% confidence interval (CI) = 2.82–3.31) and past-year mania (OR = 3.88; 95% CI = 3.34, 4.50). A second study of data from Wave 1 of the NESARC (Balk, Lynskey, & Agrawal, 2009) found that 22.5% of participants who met criteria for past-year ND had a diagnosis of major depressive disorder (MDD), three times greater than the rate of the full NESARC sample (7.1%; Grant et al., 2004). Similar results were found by John, Meyer, Rumpf, and Hapke (2004a) in a sample of 2458 daily smoking German adults where greater ND symptoms (≥ one vs. zero) and FTND score (≥ six vs. zero) were associated with an increased risk of mood disorders. Similarly, a study of 3933 young adults (ages 23 to 35; Son, Markovitz, Winders, & Smith, 1997) found an association of ND, measured as time to first cigarette, and depression symptoms, suggesting a relationship between ND and greater report of mood-related symptoms in addition to a mood disorder diagnosis.

In contrast, two studies of older adults found no relationship between ND and mood disorders. In a study of 2400 US adults who were 50 years or older who completed the National Comorbidity Survey-Replication

(NCS-R; Sachs-Ericsson, Collins, Schmidt, & Zvolensky, 2011), current smokers with past-year ND did not significantly differ from current smokers without past-year ND in the rate of past-year MD (12.1% versus 6.4%, $p = .10$; Sachs-Ericsson et al., 2011). Similarly, a NESARC study by Chou, Mackenzie, Liang, and Sareen (2011) of 8012 adults over the age of 60 found no significant association between Wave 1 ND and a new Wave 2 diagnosis of MDD (OR = 1.68; 95% CI = 0.91–3.10) or bipolar I disorder (BD; OR = 2.48; 95% CI = 0.59–10.40; Chou et al., 2011). Consequently, the relationship between ND and mood disorders appears to be stronger for younger, rather than older, adults.

While the aforementioned studies found that ND was associated with greater odds of mood disorders, other studies have found the inverse relationship: mood disorders are associated with a greater report of ND. Goodwin, Zvolensky, Keyes, and Hasin (2012), using NESARC Wave 1 data, reported increased odds of past-year ND for adults who met past-year criteria for any depressive disorder (OR = 2.28; 95% CI = 2.05–2.55), MD (OR = 1.84; 95% CI = 1.62–2.09), bipolar disorder (BD; OR = 2.37; 95% CI = 1.98–2.84), and dysthymia (OR = 2.07; 95% CI = 1.68–2.55). Similarly, young adults (ages 18–25) in the NESARC who met criteria for lifetime diagnosis of MD were more likely to report past-year ND as opposed to adults with no history of MD (OR = 2.6; 95% CI = 1.88–3.63; Dierker & Donny, 2008). Further, a study of 1905 adults with lifetime BD from the Wave 1 of the NESARC (Lev-Ran, Le Foll, McKenzie, George, & Rehm, 2013) found that adults with BD and a past-year cannabis use disorder (CUD) were at higher risk for ND than adults with BD and no past-year CUD (adjusted OR (AOR) = 3.83; 95% CI = 2.21–6.66). In a study analyzing data from 1560 US adult smokers who completed the NCS-R study (Strong et al., 2010), smokers with recurrent MDD, compared to smokers with no history of depression, reported more severe levels of ND ($p < .001$). This difference was not found for smokers with single episode MDD ($p > .11$). These data support the premise that adult smokers with depression are not just more likely to have ND but also may have more severe ND than adult smokers without depression. It should be noted that there was not a significant association between a Wave 1 diagnosis of MDD and a new Wave 2 diagnosis of ND in adults older than 60 without a previous ND diagnosis mentioned earlier (Chou et al., 2011).

Several studies examined how changes in ND status were associated with mood disorders. A study of adults who completed Wave 2 of the NESARC (Donald, Chartrand, & Bolton, 2013) found that individuals who met DSM-IV criteria for ND in the past and who had abstained from nicotine in the last year were less likely to meet criteria for past-year mood episodes or disorders (ie, MD, dysthymia, manic episodes, hypomanic episodes) than individuals who met past-year criteria for ND (AOR = 0.64; 95% CI = 0.50–0.82). While little is known about how

ND and mood disorders are associated with quit behavior, a study of 786 adult daily smokers in Germany reported that adults with no MD and no ND reported higher self-efficacy to abstain from smoking than adults with MD, adults with ND, or adults with both MD and ND (John, Meyer, Rumpf, & Hapke, 2004b).

Suicide is a serious aspect of mood disorders. In Wave 2 of NESARC, lifetime ND (AOR = 1.78; 95% CI = 1.48–2.15) and past-year ND (AOR = 1.77; 95% CI = 1.02–3.06) were independently related to suicide attempts (Yaworski, Robinson, Sareen, & Bolton, 2011). Furthermore, lifetime ND was significantly associated with three suicide-related outcomes ("felt like wanted to die," OR = 2.06; 95% CI = 1.86–2.28; "thought about committing suicide," OR = 2.22; 95% CI = 2.01–2.46; "attempted suicide," OR = 3.07; 95% CI = 2.60–3.62; Berlin, Covey, Donohue, & Agostiv, 2011). It should be noted that other studies found no relationship between ND and suicide attempts in adults with mood disorders (Kessler, Borges, Sampson, Miller, & Nock, 2009; Oquendo et al., 2010). Importantly, ND cessation was related to decreased probability of suicide attempt (AOR = 0.15; 95% CI = 0.05–0.43; Yaworski et al., 2011).

Anxiety Disorders

Similar to mood disorders, ND is associated with higher rates of a range of anxiety disorders. In a study of 5692 US adults who completed the NCS-R (Cougle, Zvolensky, Fitch, & Sachs-Ericsson, 2010), lifetime ND was associated with generalized anxiety disorder (GAD; AOR = 1.59; 95% CI = 1.28–1.98) and posttraumatic stress disorder (PTSD; AOR = 1.47; 95% CI = 1.01–2.16; Cougle et al., 2010) after adjusting for sociodemographics, alcohol or drug dependence, and depression. Similar results were found in a subsample of 2400 US adults who were 50 years and older from the NCS-R where adults with ND reported significantly elevated rates of PTSD (3.5% vs. 9.1%, $p < .04$), social phobia (5.5% vs. 12.1%, $p < 0.05$), specific phobia (9.9% vs. 18.2%, $p < .05$), and GAD (2.6% vs. 13.6%, $p < .001$; Sachs-Ericsson et al., 2011). In the NESARC, 22% of participants who met criteria for Wave 1 past-year ND reported a Wave 1 past-year anxiety disorder compared to 11.1% of the full sample (Grant et al., 2004). Wave 1 current ND was also associated with an increased likelihood of Wave 1 panic disorder (OR = 4.96; 95% CI = 3.88–6.36) and GAD (OR = 3.34; 95% CI = 2.92–3.84; Grover et al., 2012). It is worth noting that Grover et al. (2012) found no association between former dependent smoking and current anxiety disorders.

While the studies described previously reported higher rates of anxiety disorders in adults with ND, the inverse relationship has also been found. In the study described earlier by Grant et al. (2004), compared to the rate of ND in the full sample (12.8%), rates of ND were higher for participants with any past-year anxiety disorder (25.3%) and each of the specific anxiety disorders assessed (ranging from 25.6% for specific phobia to 39.8% for panic disorder). Additionally, Grover et al. (2012) reported that specific phobia and panic disorder were associated with increased odds of ND (specific phobia, OR = 1.69; 95% CI = 1.49–1.91; panic disorder, OR = 1.82; 95% CI = 1.50–2.21). An increased risk of ND among smokers with social phobia (OR = 1.69; 95% CI = 1.19–2.40) or specific phobia (OR = 1.69; 95% CI = 1.43–2.01) were also reported by Goodwin et al. (2012). Another study by Grant et al. (2005), using the NESARC Wave 1 data, found that ND was reported by 40.5% of people who met criteria for GAD alone and 59.5% of those who met criteria for both GAD and another disorder.

Regarding the transition from cigarette use to ND, Kushner, Menary, Maurer, and Thuras (2012) analyzed data from 18,013 US adults who completed the NESARC Wave 1 and smoked ≥ 100 cigarettes during their lifetime and found that individuals with one lifetime anxiety disorder reported smoking fewer packs of cigarettes in the transition from first cigarette smoked to ND than those with no lifetime anxiety disorder [hazard ratio (HR) = 1.60; 95% CI = 1.54–1.67]. Individuals who met criteria for more than one lifetime anxiety disorder reported smoking even fewer packs of cigarettes before transitioning from first cigarette smoked to ND than those with only one lifetime anxiety disorder (HR = 1.33; 95% CI = 1.27–1.40). Similarly, participants in the NCS with either pre-existing (ie, occurring before smoking onset) or current agoraphobia, simple phobia, and PTSD were significantly more likely to transition from smoking to ND than participants without the relative disorder (Breslau, Novak, & Kessler, 2004).

US adults with PTSD endorse significantly higher levels of ND compared to those without PTSD (15.7% versus 4.8%; $p < .05$; Babson, Feldner, Sachs-Ericsson, Schmidt, & Zvolensky, 2008). Interestingly, a study by Hapke et al. (2005) of 4075 German adults found that there were significantly higher rates of ND (OR = 1.52; 95% CI = 1.26–1.82) for people who experienced trauma, regardless of whether they developed PTSD. The study also found that individuals with PTSD had increased odds of ND (OR = 2.70; 95% CI = 1.57–4.65) and lower odds for remission from ND (OR = 0.18; 95% CI = 0.05–0.63; Hapke et al., 2005). Using the same data, a univariate analysis of pre-existing psychiatric disorders found that ND was a not a risk factor for increased odds of having PTSD (OR = 1.06; 95% CI = 0.47–2.41; Hapke, Schumann, Rumpf, John, & Meyer, 2006).

With regard to the link between panic disorder and ND, Babson et al. (2008) examined data from 5692 US adults who completed the NCS-R and found that a higher proportion of people with panic disorder reported ND compared to those without panic disorder (11.1% versus 5.1%; $p < .05$). Furthermore, a NESARC study by Nay, Brown, and Roberson-Nay (2013) found that a Wave 1 diagnosis of ND was related to a significantly elevated risk at Wave 2 of developing panic disorder (OR = 1.60; 95% CI = 1.31–1.94) or panic disorder with agoraphobia (OR = 1.61; 95% CI = 1.14–2.27).

Personality Disorders

Studies of ND and PDs have primarily examined US adults from the NESARC study using DSM-IV diagnostic criteria. The DSM-IV divides the 10 PDs into three clusters: Cluster A includes paranoid, schizoid, and schizotypal PDs; Cluster B includes antisocial, borderline, histrionic, and narcissistic PDs; and Cluster C includes avoidant, dependent, and obsessive-compulsive PDs (APA, 1994). Grant et al. (2004) reported that nearly 30% of US adults with past-year PDs met criteria for past-year ND, more than twice the rate of the full NESARC sample (12.8%; Grant et al., 2004). The highest rates of ND were found for dependent PD (44.0%) and antisocial PD (42.7%). Zvolensky, Jenkins, Johnson, and Goodwin (2011) similarly found that NESARC Wave 1 participants with a lifetime diagnosis of each six PDs (avoidant, dependent, obsessive-compulsive, paranoid, schizoid, and antisocial PDs) reported higher rates of current and past ND compared to adults without the PD diagnosis. The strongest associations for current ND were reported for antisocial (OR = 7.00, 95% CI = 6.10–8.03) and dependent PDs (OR = 4.27, 95% CI = 3.15–5.79), and past ND was found for antisocial PD (OR = 3.48, 95% CI = 2.83–4.28).

Chou et al. (2011) reported that individuals who had a narcissistic PD at Wave 1 were at an increased risk of a new diagnosis of ND at Wave 2 (OR = 3.60, 95% CI = 1.57–8.23). The associations between obsessive-compulsive, paranoid, borderline, and schizotypal PDs and Wave 2 ND were not significant. Hasin et al. (2011) reported that five PDs were associated with persistent ND (ie, ND at both Wave 1 and 2): antisocial (OR = 3.19, 95% CI = 1.64–6.18), borderline (OR = 2.04, 95% CI = 1.56–2.68), obsessive-compulsive (OR = 1.4, 95% CI = 1.06–1.85), schizoid (OR = 1.47, 95% CI = 1.08–2.01), and schizotypal (OR = 1.65, 95% CI = 1.19–2.28) PDs.

The research presented earlier showed that adults with PDs report higher rates of ND. As with other psychiatric disorders, the inverse relationship is also true with adults with ND reporting higher rates of PDs. Lopez-Quintero, Hasin, et al. (2011) reported that 35.9% of the NESARC Wave 1 sample who met criteria for ND also met criteria for a lifetime PD. Peters, Schwartz, Wang, O'Grady, and Blanco (2014) reported that among individuals with ND at Wave 2, the rate of any Wave 2 past-year PD was 30.9%, which is twice the rate of past-year PD reported in the general US population (14.8%; Grant et al., 2004). Pulay et al. (2010) found that ND remained significantly associated with five PDs (paranoid, schizotypal, borderline, narcissistic, and obsessive-compulsive PDs) after controlling for sociodemographics and comorbid Axis I and Axis II disorders.

Eating Disorders

John, Meyer, Rumpf, and Hapke (2005), using a sample of 4075 German adults, reported that the likelihood of being overweight (defined as a body mass index (BMI) of $\geq 25\,kg/m^2$) was higher for men who reported former ND than men with no history of ND (OR = 1.5, 95% CI = 1.1–2.1). Current ND did not differ by weight for men, and there was no association of weight to either current or former ND for women. In a second study of the same sample, adults with lifetime ND were more likely to report at least two eating disorder criteria compared to adults without lifetime ND (OR = 2.5; 95% CI = 1.5–4.2; John, Meyer, Rumpf, & Hapke, 2006). Additionally, in the study by Chou et al. (2011), discussed earlier, Wave 1 obesity (defined as a BMI of $\geq 30\,kg/m^2$) was associated with a reduced risk of Wave 2 incident ND (OR = 0.56, 95% CI = 0.32–0.99).

NICOTINE DEPENDENCE AND SUBSTANCE USE DISORDERS

Alcohol Use Disorders

Falk, Yi, and Hiller-Sturmhofel (2006) used data from Wave 1 of the NESARC to assess the prevalence of consuming alcohol and ND. The prevalence of ND among male and female lifetime alcohol abstainers was 3.8% and 2.9%, respectively, while the rates of ND among men and women with alcohol dependence was 44.6% and 47.3% (Falk et al., 2006). In a study of 4075 adults in north Germany, a lifetime ND diagnosis was more than four times more likely to co-occur with current alcohol dependence (OR = 4.69; 95% CI = 2.58–8.53; John, Meyer, Rumpf, & Hapke, 2003). In another study of the same sample, a greater number of ND symptoms were associated with a higher alcohol dependence syndrome frequency (John, Meyer, Rumpf, Schumann, et al., 2003). Goodwin, Pagura, Spiwak, Lemeshow, and Sareen (2011) compared the data between Wave 1 and Wave 2 of the NESARC and found that a diagnosis of alcohol abuse/dependence at Wave 1 was not associated with increased "persistence" of ND (ie, participants who reported ND at both Wave 1 and at Wave 2; OR = 1.00; 95% CI = 0.87–1.16).

Substance Use Disorders

High rates of ND have been found for US adults with cannabis and cocaine dependence (Agrawal & Lynskey, 2009; Lopez-Quintero, de los Cobos, et al., 2011; Lopez-Quintero, Hasin, et al., 2011) and the use of inhalants or solvents (eg, amyl nitrite, nitrous oxide, glue; Wu, Howard, & Pilowsky, 2008). Drug abuse or dependence has also been associated with significantly increased likelihood of persistent ND in several studies using

NESARC data (Goodwin et al., 2011; Hasin et al., 2011; Wagner et al., 2002). Other research has shown that ND is associated with the initiation of drug use. Young adults (ages 14–24) in Germany with prior ND had an increased risk for the development of a substance use disorder (HR = 2.6, 95% CI = 1.7–4.0; Perkonigg et al., 2006). Harrington, Robinson, Bolton, Sareen, and Bolton (2011), using data from participants in the NESARC study with no history of illicit drug use at Wave 1, reported that adults with Wave 1 ND were at a greater risk than adults without ND for Wave 2 illicit drug use (OR = 1.49; 95% CI = 1.17–1.91). Interestingly, ND was associated with remission from cocaine dependence in a study using NESARC data (HR = 1.71, 95% CI = 1.20–2.43; Lopez-Quintero, Hasin, et al., 2011). Further, NESARC Wave 2 participants with both CUD and ND were more likely to report diagnoses of BD, anxiety disorders, and PDs compared to participants with ND only (Peters et al., 2014).

Gambling Disorder

Gambling was recently added to the DSM-5 as an addictive disorder (APA, 2013). Wave 1 NESARC participants with pathological gambling (43.4%), at-risk problem gambling (ARPG; 28.3%), and low-risk gambling (17.3%) reported higher rates of ND compared to non-gamblers (10.6%; $p < .001$; Desai & Potenza, 2008). Higher rates of ND were reported by both men and women with ARPG (26.1% and 32.0%) and pathological gambling (44.0% and 42.5%) compared to men and women who did not gamble (11.5% and 9.9%; ps < 0.01; Desai & Potenza, 2008). Further, Wave 1 ARPG, compared to Wave 1 non-APRG, was significantly associated with an incident Wave 2 ND diagnosis for women (OR = 2.28, 95% CI = 1.41–3.69), but not men (OR = 1.08, 95% CI = 0.68–3.58; Pilver, Libby, Hoff, & Potenza, 2013).

SUMMARY AND CONCLUSIONS

There is a broad relationship of ND to psychiatric and substance use disorders that extends across every disorder that has been investigated using population-based data. The association between ND and psychiatric/substance use disorders has been reported more frequently for recent (eg, past year) ND rather than past ND. Further, the data support a bidirectional relationship between ND and a range of psychiatric and substance use disorders. Remission of ND appears to reduce the association; however, more research is needed. Research is also needed to examine ND in samples outside of the United States and to examine potential mediators and moderators of the relationship between ND and disorder (eg, demographics such as race, gender, and sexual orientation; symptom severity).

References

Agrawal, A., & Lynskey, M. T. (2009). Tobacco and cannabis co-occurrence: does route of administration matter? *Drug and Alcohol Dependence, 99*(1–3), 240–247. http://dx.doi. org/10.1016/j.drugalcdep.2008.08.007.

American Psychological Association. (1994). *Diagnostic and statistical manual of mental disorders, 4th ed. (DSM-IV).* Washington D.C.: American Psychiatric Association.

American Psychiatric Association. (2013). *Diagnostic and statistical manual of mental disorders* (5th ed.). Washington, DC: Author.

Babson, K. A., Feldner, M. T., Sachs-Ericsson, N., Schmidt, N. B., & Zvolensky, M. J. (2008). Nicotine dependence mediates the relations between insomnia and both panic and post-traumatic stress disorder in the NCS-R sample. *Depression and Anxiety, 25*(8), 670–679. http://dx.doi.org/10.1002/da.20374.

Balk, E., Lynskey, M. T., & Agrawal, A. (2009). The association between DSM-IV nicotine dependence and stressful life events in the national epidemiologic survey on alcohol and related conditions. *American Journal of Drug and Alcohol Abuse, 35*(2), 85–90. http://dx.doi. org/10.1080/00952990802585430.

Berlin, I., Covey, L. S., Donohue, M. C., & Agostiv, V. (2011). Duration of smoking abstinence and suicide-related outcomes. *Nicotine and Tobacco Research, 13*(10), 887–893. http:// dx.doi.org/10.1093/ntr/ntr089.

Breslau, N., Johnson, E. O., Hiripi, E., & Kessler, R. (2001). Nicotine dependence in the United States: prevalence, trends and smoking persistence. *Archives of General Psychiatry, 58*, 810–816. http://dx.doi.org/10.1001/archpsyc.58.9.810.

Breslau, N., Novak, S. P., & Kessler, R. C. (2004). Psychiatric disorders and stages of smoking. *Biological Psychiatry, 55*(1), 69–76. http://dx.doi.org/10.1016/S0006-3223(03)00317-2.

CDC. (2013). Vital signs: current cigarette smoking among adults aged ≥18 years with mental illness—United States, 2009–2011. *Morbidity and Mortality World Report (MMWR), 62*, 1–7.

CDC. (2014). Current cigarette smoking among adults – United States, 2005–2013. *Morbitity and Mortality Weekly Report, 63*(47), 1108–1112.

Chou, K. L., Mackenzie, C. S., Liang, K., & Sareen, J. (2011). Three-year incidence and predictors of first-onset of DSM-IV mood, anxiety, and substance use disorders in older adults: results from wave 2 of the epidemiologic survey on alcohol and related conditions. *The Journal of Clinical Psychiatry, 72*(2), 144–155. http://dx.doi.org/10.4088/JCP.09m05618gry.

Cougle, J. R., Zvolensky, M. J., Fitch, K. E., & Sachs-Ericsson, N. (2010). The role of comorbidity in explaining the associations between anxiety disorders and smoking. *Nicotine & Tobacco Research: Official Journal of the Society for Research on Nicotine and Tobacco, 12*(4), 355–364. http://dx.doi.org/10.1093/ntr/ntq006.

Desai, R. A., & Potenza, M. N. (2008). Gender differences in the associations between past-year gambling problems and psychiatric disorders. *Social Psychiatry and Psychiatric Epidemiology, 43*(3), 173–183. http://dx.doi.org/10.1007/s00127-007-0283-z.

Dierker, L., & Donny, E. (2008). The role of psychiatric disorders in the relationship between cigarette smoking and DSM-IV ND among young adults. *Nicotine & Tobacco Research: Official Journal of the Society for Research on Nicotine and Tobacco, 10*(3), 439–446. http://dx.doi. org/10.1080/14622200801901898.

Donald, S., Chartrand, H., & Bolton, J. M. (2013). The relationship between nicotine cessation and mental disorders in a nationally representative sample. *Journal of Psychiatric Research, 47*(11), 1673–1679. http://dx.doi.org/10.1016/j.jpsychires.2013.05.011.

Falk, D. E., Yi, H. Y., & Hiller-Sturmhofel, S. (2006). An epidemiologic analysis of co-occurring alcohol and tobacco use and disorders: findings from the national epidemiologic survey on alcohol and related conditions. *Alcohol Research & Health, 29*(3), 162–171.

Goodwin, R. D., Pagura, J., Spiwak, R., Lemeshow, A. R., & Sareen, J. (2011). Predictors of persistent nicotine dependence among adults in the United States. *Drug and Alcohol Dependence, 118*, 127–133. http://dx.doi.org/10.1016/j.drugalcdep.2011.03.010.

Goodwin, R. D., Zvolensky, M. J., Keyes, K. M., & Hasin, D. S. (2012). Mental disorders and cigarette use among adults in the United States. *American Journal on Addictions*, *21*(5), 416–423. http://dx.doi.org/10.1111/j.1521-0391.2012.00263.x.

Grant, B. F., Dawson, D. A., & Hasin, D. S. (2001). *The alcohol use disorder and associated disabilities interview schedule–DSM-IV version*. Bethesda, MD: National Institute on Alcohol Abuse and Alcoholism. http://dx.doi.org/10.1037/t04807-000.

Grant, B. F., Dawson, D. A., Stinson, F. S., Chou, P. S., Kay, W., & Pickering, R. (2003). The alcohol use disorder and associated disabilities schedule (AUDADIS): reliability of alcohol consumption, tobacco use, family history of depression, and psychiatric diagnostic modules in a general population. *Drug and Alcohol Dependence*, *71*, 7–16. http://dx.doi.org/10.1016/S0376-8716(03)00070-X.

Grant, B. F., Hasin, D. S., Chou, P., Stinson, F. S., & Dawson, D. A. (2004). Nicotine dependence and psychiatric disorders in the United States. *Archives of General Psychiatry*, *61*(11), 1107–1115. http://dx.doi.org/10.1001/archpsyc.61.11.1107.

Grant, B. F., Hasin, D. S., Stinson, F. S., Dawson, D. A., Ruan, W. J., Goldstein, R. B., … Huang, B. (2005). Prevalence, correlates, co-morbidity, and comparative disability of DSM-IV generalized anxiety disorder in the USA: results from the national epidemiologic survey on alcohol and related conditions. *Psychological Medicine*, *35*(12), 1747–1759. http://dx.doi.org/10.1017/s0033291705006069.

Grant, B. F., & Kaplan, K. D. (2005). *Source and accuracy statement: The wave 2 national epidemiologic survey on alcohol and related conditions (NESARC)*. Rockville, MD: National Institute on Alcohol Abuse and Alcoholism.

Grant, B. F., Moore, T. C., Shepard, J., & Kaplan, K. (2003). *Source and accuracy statement: Wave 1 national epidemiologic survey on alcohol and related conditions (NESARC)*. Bethesda, MD: National Institute on Alcohol Abuse and Alcoholism.

Grover, K. W., Goodwin, R. D., & Zvolensky, M. J. (2012). Does current versus former smoking play a role in the relationship between anxiety and mood disorders and ND? *Addictive Behaviors*, *37*(5), 682–685. http://dx.doi.org/10.1016/j.addbeh.2012.01.014.

Hapke, U., Schumann, A., Rumpf, H. J., John, U., Konerding, U., & Meyer, C. (2005). Association of smoking and nicotine dependence with trauma and posttraumatic stress disorder in a general population sample. *Journal of Nervous and Mental Disease*, *193*(12), 843–846. http://dx.doi.org/10.1097/01.nmd.0000188964.83476.e0.

Hapke, U., Schumann, A., Rumpf, H. J., John, U., & Meyer, C. (2006). Post-traumatic stress disorder: the role of trauma, pre-existing psychiatric disorders, and gender. *European Archives of Psychiatry and Clinical Neuroscience*, *256*(5), 299–306. http://dx.doi.org/10.1007/s00406-006-0654-6.

Harrington, M., Robinson, J., Bolton, S., Sareen, J., & Bolton, J. (2011). A longitudinal study of risk factors for incident drug use in adults: findings from a representative sample of the US population. *The Canadian Journal of Psychiatry*, *56*(11), 686–695.

Hasin, D., Fenton, M., Skodol, A., Krueger, R., Keyes, K., Geier, T., … Grant, B. (2011). Personality disorders and the 3-year course of alcohol, drug, and nicotine use disorders. *Archives of General Psychiatry*, *68*(11), 1158–1167. http://dx.doi.org/10.1001/archgenpsychiatry.2011.136.

Heatherton, T. F., Kozlowski, L. T., Frecker, R. C., & Fagerstrom, K. O. (1991). The Fagerstrom test for nicotine dependence: a revision of the Fagerstrom tolerance questionnaire. *British Journal of Addictions*, *86*, 1119–1127. http://dx.doi.org/10.1111/j.1360-0443.1991.tb01879.x.

Heatherton, T. F., Kozlowski, L. T., Frecker, R. C., Rickert, W. S., & Robinson, J. (1989). Measuring the heaviness of smoking using self-reported time to first cigarette of the day and number of cigarettes smoked per day. *British Journal of Addiction*, *86*, 1119–1127. http://dx.doi.org/10.1111/j.1360-0443.1989.tb03059.x.

John, U., Meyer, C., Rumpf, H.-J., & Hapke, U. (2003a). Probabilities of alcohol high-risk drinking, abuse, or dependence estimated on grounds of tobacco smoking and nicotine dependence. *Addiction*, *98*, 805–814. http://dx.doi.org/10.1046/j.1360-0443.2003.00381.x.

John, U., Meyer, C., Rumpf, H.-J., & Hapke, U. (2004a). Smoking, nicotine dependence and psychiatric comorbidity–a population-based study including smoking cessation after three years. *Drug and Alcohol Dependence, 76*(3), 287–295. http://dx.doi.org/10.1016/j.drugalcdep.2004.06.004.

John, U., Meyer, C., Rumpf, H.-J., & Hapke, U. (2004b). Self-efficacy to refrain from smoking predicted by major depression and nicotine dependence. *Addictive Behaviors, 29*, 857–866. http://dx.doi.org/10.1016/j.addbeh.2004.02.053.

John, U., Meyer, C., Rumpf, H.-J., & Hapke, U. (2005). Relationships of psychiatric disorders with overweight and obesity in an adult general population. *Obesity Research, 13*(1), 101–109. http://dx.doi.org/10.1038/oby.2005.13.

John, U., Meyer, C., Rumpf, H.-J., & Hapke, U. (2006). Psychiatric comorbidity including nicotine dependence among individuals with eating disorder criteria in an adult general population sample. *Psychiatry Research, 141*, 71–79. http://dx.doi.org/10.1016/j.psychres.2005.07.011.

John, U., Meyer, C., Rumpf, H. J., Schumann, A., Thyrian, J. R., & Hapke, U. (2003). Strength of the relationship between tobacco smoking, nicotine dependence and the severity of alcohol dependence syndrome criteria in a population-based sample. *Alcohol & Alcoholism, 38*(6), 606–612. http://dx.doi.org/10.1093/alcalc/agg122.

Kessler, R. C., Borges, G., Sampson, N., Miller, M., & Nock, M. K. (2009). The association between smoking and subsequent suicide-related outcomes in the national comorbidity survey panel sample. *Molecular Psychiatry, 14*(12), 1132–1142. http://dx.doi.org/10.1038/mp.2008.78.

Kushner, M. G., Menary, K. R., Maurer, E. W., & Thuras, P. (2012). Greater elevation in risk for nicotine dependence per pack of cigarettes smoked among those with an anxiety disorder. *Journal of Studies on Alcohol and Drugs, 73*(6), 920–924. http://dx.doi.org/10.15288/jsad.2012.73.920.

Lasser, K., Boyd, J. W., Woolhander, S., Himmelstein, D. U., McCormick, D., & Bor, D. H. (2000). Smoking and mental illness: a population-based prevalence study. *Journal of the American Medical Association, 284*, 2606–2610. http://dx.doi.org/10.1001/jama.284.20.2606.

Lev-Ran, S., Le Foll, B., McKenzie, K., George, T. P., & Rehm, J. (2013). Bipolar disorder and co-occurring cannabis use disorders: characteristics, co-morbidities and clinical correlates. *Psychiatry Research, 209*(3), 459–465. http://dx.doi.org/10.1016/j.psychres.2012.12.014.

Lopez-Quintero, C., de los Cobos, J. P., Hasin, D. S., Okuda, M., Wang, S., Grant, B. F., & Blanco, C. (2011). Probability and predictors of transition from first use to dependence on nicotine, alcohol, cannabis, and cocaine: results of the national epidemiologic survey on alcohol and related conditions (NESARC). *Drug and Alcohol Dependence, 115*, 120–130. http://dx.doi.org/10.1016/j.drugalcdep.2010.11.004.

Lopez-Quintero, C., Hasin, D. S., de los Cobos, J. P., Pines, A., Wang, S., Grant, B. F., & Blanco, C. (2011). Probability and predictors of remission from life-time nicotine, alcohol, cannabis or cocaine dependence: results from the national epidemiologic survey on alcohol and related conditions. *Addiction, 106*(3), 657–669. http://dx.doi.org/10.1111/j.1360-0443.2010.03194.x.

Nay, W., Brown, R., & Roberson-Nay, R. (2013). Longitudinal course of panic disorder with and without agoraphobia using the national epidemiologic survey on alcohol and related conditions (NESARC). *Psychiatry Research, 208*(1), 54–61. http://dx.doi.org/10.1016/j.psychres.2013.03.006.

Oquendo, M. A., Currier, D., Liu, S. M., Hasin, D. S., Grant, B. F., & Blanco, C. (2010). Increased risk for suicidal behavior in comorbid bipolar disorder and alcohol use disorders: results from the national epidemiologic survey on alcohol and related conditions (NESARC). *Journal of Clinical Psychiatry, 71*(7), 902–909. http://dx.doi.org/10.4088/JCP.09m05198gry.

Pérez-Ríos, M., Santiago-Pérez, M. I., Alonso, B., Malvar, A., Hervada, X., & de Leon, J. (2009). Fagerstrom test for nicotine dependence vs heavy smoking index in a general population survey. *BMC Public Health, 9*, 493. http://dx.doi.org/10.1186/1471-2458-9-493.

Perkonigg, A., Pfister, H., Hofler, M., Frohlich, C., Zimmermann, P., Lieb, R., & Wittchen, H. U. (2006). Substance use and substance use disorders in a community sample of adolescents and young adults: incidence, age effects and patterns of use. *European Addiction Research, 12*(4), 187–196. http://dx.doi.org/10.1159/000094421.

Peters, E. N., Schwartz, R. P., Wang, S., O'Grady, K. E., & Blanco, C. (2014). Psychiatric, psychosocial, and physical health correlates of co-occurring cannabis use disorders and nicotine dependence. *Drug and Alcohol Dependence, 134*, 228–234. http://dx.doi.org/10.1016/j.drugalcdep.2013.10.003.

Pilver, C. E., Libby, D. J., Hoff, R. A., & Potenza, M. N. (2013). Gender differences in the relationship between gambling problems and the incidence of substance-use disorders in a nationally representative population sample. *Drug and Alcohol Dependence, 133*(1), 204–211. http://dx.doi.org/10.1016/j.drugalcdep.2013.05.002.

Pomerleau, O. F., Pomerleau, C. S., Mehringer, A. M., Snedecor, S. M., Ninowski, R., & Sen, A. (2005). Nicotine dependence, depression, and gender: characterizing phenotypes based on withdrawal discomfort, response to smoking, and ability to abstain. *Nicotine & Tobacco Research, 7*(1), 91–102. http://dx.doi.org/10.1080/14622200412331328466.

Pulay, A. J., Stinson, F. S., Ruan, W. J., Smith, S. M., Pickering, R. P., Dawson, D. A., & Grant, B. F. (2010). The relationship of DSM-IV personality disorders to nicotine dependence: results from a national survey. *Drug and Alcohol Dependence, 108*, 141–145. http://dx.doi.org/10.1016/j.drugalcdep.2009.12.004.

Sachs-Ericsson, N., Collins, N., Schmidt, B., & Zvolensky, M. (2011). Older adults and smoking: characteristics, nicotine dependence and prevalence of DSM-IV 12-month disorders. *Aging & Mental Health, 15*(1), 132–141. http://dx.doi.org/10.1080/13607863.2010.505230.

Sienkiewicz-Jarosz, H., Zatorski, P., Baranowska, A., Ryglewicz, D., & Bienkowski, P. (2009). Predictors of smoking abstinence after first-ever ischemic stroke: a 3-month follow-up. *Stroke, 40*(7), 2592–2593. http://dx.doi.org/10.1161/strokeaha.108.542191.

Smith, P. H., Mazure, C. M., & McKee, S. A. (2014). Smoking and mental illness in the US population. *Tobacco Control, 23*, 147–153. http://dx.doi.org/10.1136/tobaccocontrol-2013-051466.

Son, B. K., Markovitz, J. H., Winders, S., & Smith, D. (1997). Smoking, nicotine dependence, and depressive symptoms in the CARDIA study. Effects of educational status. *American Journal of Epidemiology, 145*(2), 110–116. http://dx.doi.org/10.1093/oxfordjournals.aje.a009081.

Stavem, K., Røgeberg, O. J., Olsen, J. A., & Boe, J. (2008). Properties of the cigarette dependence scale and the Fagerström test of nicotine dependence in a representative sample of smokers in Norway. *Addiction, 103*, 1441–1449. http://dx.doi.org/10.1111/j.1360-0443.2008.02278.x.

Strong, D. R., Cameron, A., Feuer, S., Cohn, A., Abrantes, A. M., & Brown, R. A. (2010). Single versus recurrent depression history: differentiating risk factors among current US smokers. *Drug and Alcohol Dependence, 109*(1–3), 90–95. http://dx.doi.org/10.1016/j.drugalcdep.2009.12.020.

Wagner, F. A., & Anthony, J. C. (2002). From first drug use to drug dependence; developmental periods of risk for dependence upon marijuana, cocaine, and alcohol. *Neuropsychopharmacology: Official Publication of the American College of Neuropsychopharmacology, 26*, 479–488. http://dx.doi.org/10.1016/s0893-133x(01)00367-0.

Wu, L. T., Howard, M. O., & Pilowsky, D. J. (2008). Substance use disorders among inhalant users: results from the national epidemiologic survey on alcohol and related conditions. *Addictive Behaviors, 33*(7), 968–973. http://dx.doi.org/10.1016/j.addbeh.2008.02.019.

Yaworski, D., Robinson, J., Sareen, J., & Bolton, J. M. (2011). The relation between nicotine dependence and suicide attempts in the general population. *Canadian Journal of Psychiatry, 56*(3), 161–170.

Ziedonis, D., Hitsman, B., Beckham, J. C., Zvolensky, M., Adler, L. E., Audrain-McGovern, J., … Riley, W. T. (2008). Tobacco use and cessation in psychiatric disorders: National Institute of Mental Health report. *Nicotine & Tobacco Research, 10*(12), 1691–1715. http://dx.doi.org/10.1080/14622200802443569.

Zvolensky, M. J., Jenkins, E. F., Johnson, K. A., & Goodwin, R. D. (2011). Personality disorders and cigarette smoking among adults in the United States. *Journal of Psychiatric Research, 45*, 835–841. http://dx.doi.org/10.1016/j.jpsychires.2010.11.009.

Nicotine and Tobacco Smoking and Withdrawal in Schizophrenia

K. Kozak, T.P. George

University of Toronto, Toronto, ON, Canada

TOBACCO USE DISORDER IN SCHIZOPHRENIA

Schizophrenia (SZ) is associated with a threefold higher occurrence of cigarette smoking compared to the general population, with most studies finding prevalence rates of 70–90% (Ziedonis and George, 1997). A meta-analysis of smoking prevalence across 42 studies in 20 nations found an odds ratio of 5.9 for current smoking in SZ (de Leon and Diaz, 2005). Smoking causes a significant burden on disease outcome and is the leading cause of *avoidable* mortality (Brown, Kim, Mitchell, & Inskip, 2010). Presently, smokers with SZ have mortality rates exceeding the general population due to smoking-related fatal diseases. Studies report 3.2 and 2.2 times more risk of respiratory disease and cardiovascular mortality, respectively, both of which are highly associated with smoking (Curkendall, Mo, Glasser, Rose Stang, & Jones, 2004; Joukamaa et al., 2001). Various reasons have been proposed that may account for this increased susceptibility of the SZ population to nicotine addiction. The most commonly studied include their vulnerability to comorbidity, as well as reducing neuroleptic side effects and negative symptoms (Fig. 14.1).

Vulnerability to Comorbidity

Smoking in SZ has been suggested to be a marker of a more severe illness process (Dalack, Becks, Hill, Pomerleau, & Meador-Woodruff, 1999). A developing area of research regarding shared vulnerability

Negative Affective States and Cognitive Impairments in Nicotine Dependence
http://dx.doi.org/10.1016/B978-0-12-802574-1.00014-4

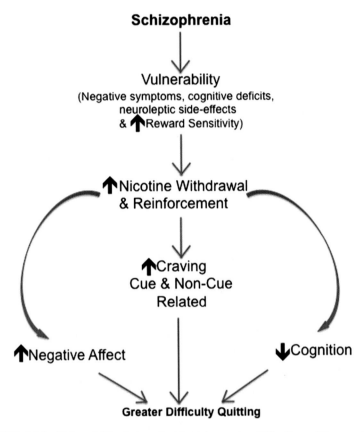

FIGURE 14.1 Vulnerability factors that lead to greater difficulty quitting smoking in schizophrenia and the relationship to nicotine withdrawal, craving, and negative affect.

of the SZ population and tobacco addiction has been centered on the putative dysregulation of nicotine acetylcholine receptor (nAChR) systems (D'Souza et al., 2012). Due to their wide distribution in the central nervous system, the pathophysiology of SZ might be mediated by mesolimbic dopamine (DA) pathway, projecting from the ventral tegmental area (VTA) to the nucleus accumbens (NAcc), as well as by the mesocortical pathway projecting from the VTA to the frontal lobes, including the prefrontal cortex (PFC) (George, Verrico, Picciotto, & Roth, 2000). Evidence suggests that nicotine, which is the main psychoactive ingredient in tobacco smoke, alters these systems by binding to nAChRs, consisting of both high-affinity β2-subunit containing, and low-affinity α7-subunit containing, which exert downstream effects on these systems (Wing, Wass, Soh, & George, 2012).

The most commonly studied nAChRs in relation to SZ and tobacco addiction are $\alpha4\beta2$ and $\alpha7$ nAChRs. It has been previously found that patients with SZ show reduced upregulation of these nAChRs, thus contributing to dysregulation of DA levels as well as other neurotransmitter systems (glutamate, GLU, and γ-aminobutyric acid, GABA) expressed in the brain (Wing, Wass, et al., 2012). Case-control postmortem studies also indicate that patients with SZ have decreased levels of nAChRs, predisposing them to nicotine dependence, among other abnormalities such as cognitive deficits (Breese et al., 2000; D'Souza et al., 2012). Further, genetic studies have found that smoking severity in SZ pertains to certain nAChR abnormalities. Single nucleotide polymorphisms in the most common gene associated as a heritability site for SZ (CHRNA7 gene) have been linked to SZ and deficits in sensory gating (Freedman et al., 1997).

Taken together the aberrant DAergic and nAChR activity in mesocorticolimbic systems may support the addiction vulnerability hypothesis, which suggests common genetic factors and brain abnormalities underlie comorbidity of SZ and tobacco addiction. High smoking rates in this population may be explained by effects of nicotine in regulating dysfunctional mesolimbic DA system by remediation of DA hypofunction associated with $\alpha4\beta2$ and $\alpha7$-containing nAChRs, however, ultimately resulting in greater nicotine dependence and consequential effects such as abstinence withdrawal (George et al., 2000).

Alleviating Neuroleptic Side Effects and Negative Symptoms

Another proposed reason for the increased predisposition of SZ patients to nicotine addiction is their benefit from nicotine by reducing side effects of antipsychotic medications used to treat their disorder. Typically, SZ patients who abstain from smoking experience nicotine withdrawal symptoms, and altered neuroleptic-induced movement disorder symptoms (Ziedonis and George, 1997). Neuroleptic medications are antidopaminergic agents that block D2 dopamine receptors producing dopaminergic hypofunction, which leads to what is known as neuroleptic-induced parkinsonism (NIP) (Decina et al., 1990; Menza, Grossman, Van Horn, Cody, & Forman, 1991). This effect is consistent with the understanding that cigarette smoking is strongly associated with reduction of NIP by increasing striatal DA function, and by lowering blood levels of antipsychotic medications (Ziedonis, Kosten, Glazer, & Frances, 1994). Hence, administration of acute nicotine releases DA lessening negative symptoms, whereas smoking abstinence would lead to decreased dorsal striatum DA release altering NIP (Zhang et al., 2012). Negative symptoms characterized by SZ, including anergia, affective blunting, amotivation, dysfunctional social relationships, and cognitive impairments, may underlie this deficiency (Ziedonis and George, 1997). Given that individuals with chronic SZ have a deficiency of DA in the PFC, it has been speculated that perhaps by augmenting cortical DA release, nicotine may reduce negative symptoms similar to clozapine and newer atypical antipsychotic agents such as risperidone (Moghaddam and Bunney, 1990).

Another neuroleptic-induced movement disorder is tardive dyskinesia (TD), a disorder characterized by involuntary movements (Ziedonis and George, 1997). TD is explained by hyperactivity of DA release, and as such, one would expect, given that smoking lowers neuroleptic serum levels thus raising DA levels acutely, this would result in increased TD (Yassa, Lal, Korpassy, & Ally, 1987). Interestingly, cross-sectional studies of neuroleptic doses in smokers versus nonsmokers have found the rate of TD has been variably reported as both lower and higher among SZ smokers (Menza et al., 1991; Yassa et al., 1987). One interpretation may be that the effects of smoking on NIP and TD are accounted for by faster metabolic clearance of neuroleptics. The mechanism of polycyclic aromatic hydrocarbon agents in smoking (non-nicotine components) inducing liver enzymes such as cytochrome P450 1A2 isoform increases metabolism of neuroleptic drugs (Bao, He, Ding, Prabhu, & Hong, 2005). In fact, clinical epidemiology studies have reported that compared to nonsmokers, SZ smokers are prescribed higher dosages of neuroleptics (Glassman, 1993). However, this mechanism of neuroleptic clearance would take days. Given that acute administration of nicotine increases striatal DA release, and conceivably that nicotine abstinence reverses this effect, the effects on TD and NIP may be more acute as well (Dalack et al., 1999). SZ is associated with hypoactivity of DA systems, specifically the dorsal striatum, which is implicated in movement disorder, thus smoking may be related to reducing side effects of administrated antipsychotic drugs by increasing release of DA. Still, given such equivocal outcomes, further research is needed to elucidate interacting mechanisms of smoking, neuroleptics, and movement disorders (Menza et al., 1991).

SMOKING ABSTINENCE AND REINSTATEMENT

Nicotine Dependence

A subjective outlook of examining the comorbidity of tobacco use disorder and SZ begins with investigating why SZ patients are nicotine dependent if both the general and SZ population smoke similar amounts of cigarettes per day. The Fagerström Test for Nicotine Dependence (FTND) is a validated standardized smoking assessment for use in smokers with SZ containing six items and closely rated to biochemical indices of smoking (Weinberger, Reutenauer, et al., 2007). Approximately half the SZ population is heavy smokers (defined as smoking > 25 cigarettes per day), with moderate to severe nicotine dependence levels (George, Vessicchio, Termine, Bergartner, et al., 2002; Lasser et al., 2000). It has been proposed that due to reduced expression of high-affinity nAChR in the brain, SZ patients are less sensitive to the effects of nicotine and compensate for this by increasing nicotine intake (Breese et al., 2000).

There is also important evidence of high nicotine dependence in this population that can be measured by nicotine and cotinine (the major proximate metabolite of nicotine) levels, shorter inter-puff intervals (Williams et al., 2011), and higher nicotine and carbon monoxide (CO) boosts, as well as other topographical measures (Tidey, Rohsenow, Kaplan, Swift, & Adolfo, 2008). Olincy, Young, and Freedman (1997) showed SZ smokers having higher urine concentration of cotinine than non-psychiatric controls despite smoking the same number of cigarettes per day. Similarly, previous work has shown comparable average baseline consumption of cigarettes and matched nicotine dependence in SZ smokers compared to controls, yet higher serum nicotine and cotinine levels (Weinberger, Sacco, et al., 2007). Accordingly, one may question whether metabolism of nicotine itself is responsible for these serum nicotine level differences. Thus, scientists conducted studies using the ratio of 3-hydroxycotinine (3HC) to cotinine (COT) as a useful biomarker of CYP2A6 metabolic activity, which is the enzyme responsible for breakdown of nicotine and cotinine (Benowitz, Pomerleau, Pomerleau, & Jacob, 2003). Surprisingly, prior work by Williams et al. (2005) found that based on the 3HC/COT ratio, there was no difference in rates of oxidative metabolism of nicotine in individuals with SZ compared to controls. In fact, studies of smokers with SZ have shown 1.3 times higher levels of plasma nicotine and cotinine, in comparison to non-psychiatric controls (Williams et al., 2005).

Another important parameter to consider when evaluating higher prevalence of smoking in SZ is nicotine boost. This nicotine boost refers to the increase in blood levels of nicotine from smoking a single cigarette (Williams et al., 2010). Given there is no difference in nicotine clearance in SZ versus non-psychiatric controls (no metabolic effect), Williams et al. (2010) conducted the first study examining nicotine intake in SZ smokers compared to controls before, during, and after smoking a single cigarette prior to a 12-h abstinence period. The authors found that SZ smokers not only had higher nicotine peak levels (as measured under a serum nicotine concentration–time curve) but also faster rates of this rise of nicotine levels (~4.8 min in patients versus 6.4 min in controls) in systemic doses of nicotine. Ultimately, non-psychiatric individuals averaged out to have a nicotine boost of 10 ng/ml compared to 28 ng/ml for SZ smokers. This finding suggested that SZ smokers smoke cigarettes more efficiently than controls, contributing to higher nicotine dependence levels in patients.

Smoking topographic assessments give detailed information on how a cigarette is smoked in real time, including puffing behaviors, rather than physical characteristics of cigarettes (Williams et al., 2011). Basic components extracted from topography studies are the number of puffs per cigarette, inter-puff intervals (IPI), and the total puff volume per cigarette, which is a function of puff number and volume per puff. Together these represent an index of "work" smokers perform when smoking a cigarette, as well as effectively examining and understanding differential toxic chemical exposures that result from smoking. Ultimately, these topographic assessments can assess cigarette reinforcement (eg, puff volumes, inter-puff intervals). Many have criticized interpretation of prior laboratory-based topography studies as the setting may influence smoking behavior, as well as the concern of the device itself being non-naturalistic (Scherer, 1999). However, technological advances have enabled smaller portable devices to become a valuable tool for assessing cigarette smoke self-administration, and in a more naturalistic environment, outside of the laboratory (Hammond, Fong, Cummings, & Hyland, 2005).

Tidey, Rohsenow, Kaplan, & Swift (2005a) compared 20 smokers with SZ to 20 non-psychiatric controls using smoking topography. After undergoing two 90-min topography assessments of *ad libitum* smoking on separate days, it was found that SZ smokers had greater CO levels, smoked significantly more total puffs, more puffs per cigarette, and shorter IPI than control smokers. Further, McKee, Weinberger, Harrison, Coppola, & George (2009) conducted a pilot study examining effects of the non-competitive antagonist of several nAChRs, mecamylamine (MEC), on *ad libitum* smoking behavior, topography across two deprivation conditions, and found no difference in smoking topography measures between two groups in the satiated session. However, following 12-h smoking abstinence, MEC was associated with increased smoking intensity in SZ smokers and overall higher nicotine levels at satiated sessions than abstinence. The authors concluded that perhaps antagonism of nAChRs might cause compensatory smoking in SZ smokers by means of intensity of smoking, highlighting the importance of topography studies.

Reports have suggested that the first cigarette of the day is a good indicator of tolerance or nicotine sensitivity in smokers, given it produces immediate effects with minimal acute tolerance due to overnight abstinence (Pillitteri, Kozlowski, Sweeney, & Heatherton, 1997). Thus, smoking behavior of the first cigarette of the day can be compared between SZ smokers and non-psychiatric smokers for nicotine dependence (Muscat, Stellman, Caraballo, & Richie, 2009). For example, morning CO levels of SZ smokers have been found to be higher than in control smokers, despite both groups having similarities in minutes to their first cigarette after awakening, similar numbers of cigarettes per day, salivary cotinine levels, and FTND scores (Tidey et al., 2008). Williams et al. (2011) used smoking topography to investigate puffing pattern and nicotine serum levels in SZ smokers as well as non-psychiatric smokers of the first cigarette of the day. The authors also compared topography measurements of both baseline characteristics, before and after a 1-h abstinence period and then afternoon, such that they measured both nicotine intake that occurs from smoking a single morning cigarette, as well as assessing smoking throughout the day. Between both groups it was found that only the topography dataset between first cigarette of the day and the pre-abstinence period was there a significant association between decreased inter-puff intervals by 1s and increased serum nicotine and cotinine levels (Williams et al., 2011). However, this effect has also been found in the general population (Bridges et al., 1990), suggesting that association between short IPI and increases in blood nicotine is not unique to SZ, but is nevertheless a mechanism associated with an intensity of cigarette smoking. The authors also found that SZ smokers not only smoked more cigarettes in 24h but also demonstrated more intensive puffing, with more frequent puffs per cigarette, waiting less time between puffs, shorter time to peak (measuring time to maximum puff velocity) and faster peak flow rate. These findings suggest smokers with SZ smoke more intensely than matched non-psychiatric smokers and that their smoking behavior is reliable when assessed under laboratory conditions.

Overall, this body of research illustrates greater nicotine dependence in SZ smokers compared to non-psychiatric smokers. Even when matched for the same number of cigarettes, SZ smokers still have higher serum nicotine levels, which is likely due to the intensity in which they smoke cigarettes (smoking topography). Given this difference, it is no surprise that SZ smokers experience greater withdrawal and craving urges, relating to their lower cessation rates.

Nicotine Reinforcement

Nicotine exposure produces considerable reinforcement since smokers have shown higher basal levels of DA in mesolimbic regions compared to nonsmokers (Paulson, 1992). The half-life of nicotine is 1–2h, and that may explain the outcome of strong cravings seen in SZ smokers, along with continuous usage in heavy smokers (Hukkanen, Jacob, & Benowitz, 2005). Reward-related disturbances after withdrawal and craving from nicotine during a nicotine-deprived state are correlated with a negative reinforcement factor derived from the Questionnaire for Smoking Urges (QSU) (Willner, Hardman, & Eaton, 1995; Ziedonis and George, 1997). In contrast, positive reinforcement is prevalent during the non-deprived state (Willner et al., 1995). Nicotine may be particularly reinforcing in SZ smokers as it stimulates the PFC and subcortical reward system, both of which appear to be hypofunctional in SZ (Watkins, Koob, & Markou, 2000). Thus, individuals with SZ may smoke more due to alterations in brain dopaminergic systems, increasing their sensitivity to positive reinforcement (Chambers, Krystal, & Self, 2001).

Spring, Pingitore, and McChargue (2003) conducted a study to determine if perception of reinforcement and value of cigarette smoking differed in SZ smokers compared to controls. They concluded that reward value of cigarette smoking in SZ heavy smokers is based on the rationale of bias decisional balance perceiving that smoking has more advantages ("pros") and fewer disadvantages ("cons") (Spring, Pingitore, McChargue, 2003). Greater pros are perceived as smoking serving as potent negative reinforcers by dispelling troublesome psychiatric symptoms, such as neuroleptic side effects and negative symptoms. Fewer perceived cons are rationalized by cognitive deficits that are present in the SZ population, such that learning and fully appreciating negative consequences of smoking are less established.

MacKillop and Tidey examined delayed reward discounting to understand smoking prevalence in SZ (MacKillop and Tidey, 2011). Delay discounting is an index of impulsivity as it refers to the rate at which the value of a reward is discounted as it is delayed in time of retrieval (Odum, 2011). The authors also decided to use demand curve analysis, which yields several topographical factors reflecting different dimensions of the relative value of cigarettes. It was found that SZ smokers exhibited higher intensity of demand for cigarettes, demonstrating unconstrained consumption, as well as greater expenditure for cigarettes compared to control smokers, in spite of no differences in craving or withdrawal. Therefore, perhaps to avoid greater withdrawal symptoms, SZ smokers allocate larger portions of their income to smoking as they find greater reward value of cigarettes such as decreased craving and withdrawal (Spring et al., 2003; Steinberg, Williams, & Ziedonis, 2004). Furthermore, no differences were evident for delay discounting between both diagnostic groups. One thing to consider is that smokers in this study were satiated, and it has been previously shown that acute withdrawal affects discounting. Thus, perhaps the initial state to which decisions are made may alter choices. Tidey et al. (2008) found that smokers with SZ exhibited larger rebound in smoking following a period of abstinence. Overall, domains of withdrawal and craving symptoms may represent plausible explanations for the difference between SZ and non-psychiatric smokers.

Another study conducted by Wing and colleagues (Wing, Moss, Rabin, & George, 2012) investigated the effect of smoking on delay discounting in SZ and control smokers. Similarly, they found no differences in delay discounting between psychiatric groups. Notably, smokers with SZ exhibited more delay discounting than nonsmokers, and within the SZ group, former smokers discount rates were similar to current smokers. The authors suggested that deficits in delay discounting in patients appears to be a trait rather than a state-dependent phenomenon. This deficit may be associated with how drug-dependent individuals typically relieve transient withdrawal symptoms by their preference for immediate rewards and impulsivity.

Moreover, Tidey, Colby, and Xavier (2014) demonstrated that SZ smokers had stronger reinforcing effects of nicotine after a 72-h abstinence period, and they resumed smoking significantly sooner after abstinence than control smokers. The authors suggested that a plausible contributor to early relapse is that SZ smokers make more hypothetical choices for smoking versus alternative reinforcers. However, they found that effects of nicotine reinforcement and abstinence on craving did not drive the relationship between SZ and lapse latency, rather on baseline depression and withdrawal levels. This suggests the two behaviors may not be correlated as expected, but rather highlight as key contributors to poor cessation outcomes by negative affect.

Overall, poor smoking cessation outcomes in SZ smokers may be due to stronger reinforcing effects of nicotine after abstinence, as the majority of studies have shown. Clinical studies suggest that beneficial effects may reinforce smoking behavior due to abnormalities in neurotransmission associated with SZ and related withdrawal reward disturbance, such that SZ smokers overvalue smoking compared to non-psychiatric smokers. This overvaluation is reflected in their impulsive discounting as found in decision-making studies. However, recently it has been found that another contributor to withdrawal symptoms and high smoking prevalence may be due to the prominence of negative affect in SZ.

Nicotine Withdrawal and Craving

During quit attempts, cigarette craving and nicotine withdrawal symptoms are important predictors of continuing smoking and relapse (Tidey et al., 2014). Signs associated with nicotine withdrawal include insomnia, anxiety, irritability, depressed mood, restlessness, increased appetite, decreased heart rate, and difficulty concentrating (Hughes and Hutsukami, 1986). Cigarette craving, on the other hand, is described as a subjective experience of strong motivation to smoke (Brown et al., 2013). Smokers who temporarily abstain in naturalistic settings experience a linear emergence of craving and withdrawal symptoms over the first 6 h of abstinence (Brown et al., 2013). Specifically, changes in craving and several mood symptoms can be detected within the first 3 h, while nicotine withdrawal manifests within the first 24–36 h of smoking cessation (Brown et al., 2013; Ziedonis and George, 1997). It is vital to characterize individual differences associated with withdrawal symptoms for a number of reasons. For example, it may reveal why some populations, such as those with SZ, are more likely to relapse, and it may lead to a better understanding of withdrawal's causal determinants, as well as why some treatments are more effective than others.

Studies have used questionnaires to assess nicotine withdrawal as well as to examine effects of cigarette smoking, while undergoing acute abstinence and reinstatement in controlled human lab settings. Recent evidence has demonstrated reliability of administrating smoking measures for smokers with SZ (Weinberger, Reutenauer, et al., 2007). Commonly the Minnesota Nicotine Withdrawal Scale (M-NWS) is administered to determine DSM-IV symptoms of tobacco withdrawal, including craving for nicotine, anxiety, and irritability, with higher scores indicating greater nicotine withdrawal (Hughes, Hatsukami, Mitchell, & Dahlgren, 1986). Furthermore, the Tiffany Questionnaire for Smoking Urges (T-QSU) is commonly used to assess urging responses to smoking in reaction to two affective systems: positive affect related to expectancy of reinforcement, and second, negative affect related to expectancy of reduced withdrawal (Tiffany and Drobes, 1991). Together, cigarette craving and withdrawal symptoms are important predictors of repeated cycles of smoking and relapse during smoker-quit attempts. Different paradigms with short-term and long-term abstinence have been used to assess effects of smoking cessation on withdrawal and craving in patients with SZ.

It has been proposed that the high prevalence of smoking and lower quit rates in the SZ population may be a result of not only neurobiological factors as mentioned previously but also due to environmental factors. Accordingly, numerous studies have demonstrated that cigarette smoking may be a form of operant behavior, and as such to be affected by environmental factors and cues (Tidey, Rohsenow, Kaplan, & Swift, 2005b).

Cue-Related Craving

The classical conditioning theory states that repeated pairing of the delivery of nicotine with smoking-related stimuli consequently causes once-neutral stimuli to become conditioned stimuli, with downstream conditioned responses such as withdrawal and craving (Carter and Tiffany, 1999). Physiologically, nicotine and smoking-like cues lead to increased release of mesolimbic DA (Balfour, Wright, Benwell, & Birrell, 2000). Since SZ is associated with intrinsically altered mesolimbic DA function, the neurobiology of this population may be particularly reactive to cue-related craving (Tidey et al., 2008).

Methodological tools such as cue exposure are useful paradigms in clinical research to investigate subjective and physiological responses of smokers with SZ (Tidey et al., 2005b). Previous studies have found that SZ smokers experience higher abstinence and cue-elicited urge levels. Fonder et al. examined the effect of smoking cue-reactivity on craving relief in SZ and control smokers by exposure to smoking images, with the effect of three doses of MEC (0, 5, and 10 mg/day) (Fonder et al., 2005). The authors found low levels of urges to smoke in the baseline condition, which was expected given both groups smoked high levels of cigarettes prior to cue-reactivity session. Interestingly, MEC was not found to alter baseline urges, implicating that nAChR antagonists do not precipitate tobacco craving. Following exposure to smoking cues, the placebo condition resulted in an increase of smoking urges in both satiated groups. Smoking urges also increased in both groups following abstinence and was accompanied by a decrease in cue-reactivity with increased abstinence duration. Notably, MEC attenuated smoking cue-reactivity in SZ smokers more robustly than in controls. The authors suggested this difference might be attributable to the decreased levels of nAChRs in SZ smokers, implicating the importance of a potential pharmacotherapeutic target for smoking cessation.

Further, Tidey and colleagues conducted a within-subjects design study examining subjective and physiological responses to smoking cues in smokers with SZ (Tidey et al., 2005b). Each participant was tested when non-abstinent (within 5 min of smoking a cigarette) and after brief abstinence (2 h). The authors wanted to use *in vivo* cues in particular as generally images are less effective at increasing urge levels, which may explain the findings of Fonder et al. (2005) of no cue-reactivity differences between groups (Shadel, Niaura, & Abrams, 2001). Neutral cues were a pencil, eraser, and small pad of paper, while smoking cues were participant's preferred brand of cigarettes, lighter, and ashtray. The main findings were that exposure to *in vivo* smoking cues increased smoking urge levels, nicotine withdrawal symptom levels, and negative affect in smokers with SZ; however, abstinence did not amplify effects of cues on urges. Similar results have been found in non-psychiatric smokers undergoing short-term abstinence (Drobes and Tiffany, 1997). The authors proposed that during abstinence, smokers with SZ are less sensitive to cues, as endogenous smoking cues such as abstinence override exogenous cues. Taken together, perhaps to illicit cue-reactivity, the smoking condition (satiated) is more effective given there is room for craving levels to increase (from baseline), whereas in abstinence conditions, measures of cue-elicited craving levels may be vulnerable to ceiling effects.

A novel approach was used to investigate effects of sensorimotor replacement for nicotine by pairing of nicotine intake and cigarettes. For example, Juliano, Donny, Houtsmuller, and Stitzer (2006) evaluated the impact of smoking lapse on relapse probability and found that those who were assigned to smoke, either nicotine-containing or de-nicotinized cigarettes, relapsed more quickly than those who were assigned to remain abstinent. Further, smoking outcomes between the two types of cigarettes did not differ, suggesting that stimulus factors play an important role in smoking and withdrawal cycles. Tidey, Rohsenow, Kaplan, Swift, and Ahnallen (2013) conducted a recent study with very low nicotine content (VLNC) cigarettes, which have less than 0.2 mg of nicotine yield, to examine that as a possible successful strategy for reducing smoking in smokers with SZ. By imitating the taste, aroma, and respiratory effects of normal nicotine content cigarettes, it has been found that VLNC cigarettes provide sensorimotor replacement for usual-brand smoking. Several studies, both laboratory and treatment, have shown in non-psychiatric smokers the

VLNC cigarettes have consistently reduced cigarette craving and negative affects (Johnson, Bickel, & Kirshenbaum, 2004; Pickworth, Fant, Nelson, Rohrer, & Henningfield, 1999). It was found that reducing nicotine content of cigarettes (VLNC) to non-addictive levels was well tolerated in terms of reduced withdrawal/craving levels in SZ smokers, and to a greater extent than in comparison to the nicotine transdermal patch (NTP).

Another study compared VLNC cigarettes versus no cigarettes and NTP (42 mg nicotine versus placebo patches). The authors showed VLNC smoking reduced cigarette craving, nicotine withdrawal, smoking habit withdrawal, and usual-brand smoking to a greater extent than the NTP during 90-min *ad libitum* smoking periods. However, compared to controls, SZ smokers found VLNC to be more effective in reducing craving rather than withdrawal symptoms, and they also smoked with greater intensity. Such persistent smoking behavior, even in the absence of nicotine, not only suggests that smoking may be associated with the ability of de-nicotinized cigarettes to suppress some aspects of craving and withdrawal but also SZ smokers' habitual learning given their insensitivity to the reward value of smoking (Donny and Jones, 2009). Overall, this reduced nicotine yield provides an effective strategy to reduce smoking in the SZ population, and it stresses the importance of cue-related craving and withdrawal in SZ smokers (Chou et al., 2014).

Taken together, the results of this series of studies provide compelling evidence that SZ smokers are sensitive to the presence of smoking-related environmental stimuli (smoking cues) by associated increased withdrawal and craving symptoms. The smoking cue exposure paradigm, as well as use of agents that antagonize high-affinity nAChRs, can be used to investigate methods of reducing nicotine withdrawal and urges in SZ.

Non-Cue-Related Craving

Alongside smoking cues, neutral cues (non-cue-related) may also be used to examine cravings in smokers. McKee et al. (2009) were the first to examine both nicotine levels and smoking topography in smokers with SZ and controls, in which they used MEC (Sacco, Bannon, & George, 2004). This study piloted the within-subject effects of MEC (0 mg/day versus 10 mg/day) and deprivation (non-nicotine deprived versus 12-hours of nicotine deprivation). The authors found that MEC increased craving for cigarettes, but only for SZ smokers under both deprivation conditions, not in controls. Interestingly, they also found that SZ smokers engaged in more intense smoking with MEC in the deprived condition, suggesting that craving in response to either positive or negative reinforcement was not relieved with increased smoking. Therefore, the authors concluded that antagonism of high-affinity nAChRs in SZ smokers might prompt compensatory smoking, thus driving more intense smoking and nicotine exposure, however, without alleviating craving.

Similarly, Weinberger, Sacco, et al. (2007) also observed this effect in their study, whereby similarities on several smoking indices at baseline and after abstinence and reinstatement were found. They found greater extraction of nicotine in patients than controls, suggesting enhanced cigarette smoking reinforcement. Further, withdrawal and craving increased due to overnight abstinence, but there was also no effect of MEC and no dose-dependent effect on craving or withdrawal. Likewise, Sacco et al. (2005) found no effect of MEC on craving in either group during abstinence and reinstatement. This finding is consistent with the notion that nicotine does not play as prominent of a role in craving, but perhaps other non-nicotine factors are involved such as tar, which MEC does not modify.

It has been shown that the tar/nicotine ratio is a key determinant of overall harshness of smoke, thus it may contribute to sensory qualities of smoking along with flavors characterizing cigarettes and their appeal to smokers (Rose, 2006). It has been found that DA transmission is also induced by non-nicotine chemicals in tobacco smoke by causing monoamine oxidase type B inhibition (Lewis, Miller, & Lea, 2007). One study even found that while reducing nicotine yield in cigarettes maintaining overall tar delivery, smokers did not compensate when smoking by taking larger or more frequent puffs (Pickworth et al., 1999). Another study gave smokers low-tar and low-nicotine cigarettes with capsaicin (the active compound of chili peppers), added to enhance sensory stimulation, and found that craving and withdrawal symptoms were reduced compared to control low-nicotine cigarettes (Behm and Jed, 1994). Therefore, other components, such as tar and respiratory tract sensations, are important in reducing craving and withdrawal symptoms for cigarette smoking and should be further studied in the SZ population.

Overall, it is clear from such studies that combining smoking and an nAChR blocker limits effects on craving and withdrawal, so it must be other non-nicotine components such as tar that likely play a critical role in addictive behaviors including tobacco use disorders in SZ. Ultimately, SZ smokers will have a more difficult time quitting if they have more severe effects of abstinence due to some of the aforementioned illness-related abnormalities or symptoms such as withdrawal.

Effects on Negative Affect

The abilities of SZ smokers to maintain smoking abstinence may be reduced by their heightened sensitivity to effects of nicotine withdrawal on negative affect (Tidey et al., 2008). Negative affect is the experience of negative emotion or feelings such as subjective distress considering a variety of aversive mood states such as anger, fear, and nervousness, and it is commonly associated with withdrawal (Watson, Clark, & Tellegen, 1988). A common and reliable form of measuring negative affect is with the Positive and Negative Affect Schedule (PANAS), which is a

10-item mood scale comprised of both positive and negative affect dimensions (Watson et al., 1988). Williams and colleagues (Williams, Gandhi, Lu, Steinberg, & Benowitz, 2013) used this procedure when investigating rapid smoking in SZ and non-psychiatric smokers in a single day of *ad libitum* smoking topography. The authors found that rapid smoking in SZ smokers was associated with higher levels of negative affect and a greater anticipation that smoking would relieve negative symptoms as measured by QSU Factor-2 scores. The authors suggested that perhaps in response to the inability to tolerate negative affect from withdrawal, SZ smokers smoke more intensely by reduced IPI and more frequent puffing. Another clear finding from a large-scale study was that individuals with higher negative affect reported severe withdrawal and more likelihood of relapse (Piasecki, Jorenby, Smith, Fiore, & Baker, 2003). It is possible that prior to quitting, high negative affect scores reflect well-founded apprehension about the fate of quit attempts.

Recently, Tidey et al. (2014) compared effects of greater than 16-hr abstinence in SZ and non-psychiatric smokers, using both nicotinized (0.6 mg of nicotine and 10 mg of tar) and de-nicotinized cigarettes (< 0.05 mg of nicotine and 10 mg of tar). Their results found that over a 72-h abstinence period, nicotine withdrawal (measured using MNWS) remained higher in SZ smokers than non-psychiatric smokers. After co-varying baseline depression scores, these group differences were eliminated, suggesting an underlying group difference of nicotine withdrawal may be attributed to depression severity. Interestingly, QSU Factor-2 score differences, representing anticipation of relief of negative affect and urgent desire to smoke, remained present even after covariance. This finding again suggested a unique association of SZ with an aspect of craving that may not be due to depression, rather that negative affect is a key contributor.

Similarly, in a topography study conducted by Williams et al. (2011), baseline characteristics of SZ smokers compared to non-psychiatric smokers demonstrated that the QSU Factor-2 scale score was greater in SZ smokers, as well as having higher PANAS negative scores. The authors suggested since shortly after abstinence, negative affect of SZ smokers increased along with the intensity of smoking behaviors, this may ultimately reflect SZ smokers decreased ability to tolerate their heightened sensitivity to effects of nicotine withdrawal, thus reducing their likelihood of quitting. Future research comparing smokers with major depression and SZ is critical to clarify the extent to which mechanisms underlie smoking and importance of negative affect, as well as studies evaluating craving and nicotine withdrawal symptoms throughout long-term abstinence periods (Tidey et al., 2014).

Taken together, the importance of investigating negative affect and craving relief in SZ stems from the fact that they are the main predictors of abstinence, as well as the probability of relapse in smoking cessation

(Baker, Piper, McCarthy, Majeskie, & Fiore, 2004). However, there has been little research in SZ smokers on effects of abstinence on negative affect. Future studies should aim to examine this association, which in turn will help facilitate possible treatment options aimed to minimize these effects and maximize successful outcomes.

Effects on Negative and Depressive Symptoms

The unique pathophysiology of SZ may reflect substantially higher prevalence of smoking and effects of withdrawal. Negative symptoms, which characterize SZ, may be linked to DA deficiency and low metabolic activity (Andreasen, 1982). Given that nicotine increases firing of DA neurons in mesocorticolimbic pathways through its action on nAChRs, abstaining from smoking may consequently worsen negative symptoms (Wing, Wass, et al., 2012). However, the results of several studies have been mixed. One study found that compared to nonsmokers with SZ, smokers had higher BPRS subscale scores for both positive and negative symptoms, yet no differences in levels of depression (Goff, Henderson, & Amico, 1992). Meanwhile, Ziedonis et al. (1994) found a difference in intensity of smokers, with heavy smokers having greater positive symptoms but fewer negative symptoms. Dalack and Meador-Woodruff (1996) reported a case series that found acute nicotine withdrawal leading to an exacerbation of SZ symptoms. This exacerbation led to the suggestion that smoking in SZ represents a self-medication effort, given that during withdrawal from tobacco a common occurrence has been worsening of psychiatric symptoms (Glassman, 1993). However, this is potentially inconsistent with the observation that smoking cessation ultimately leads to a decrease in metabolism of antipsychotics. Dalack et al. (1999) conducted a study examining effects of treated and untreated 3-day smoking abstinence on psychotic symptoms and medication side effects. The active patch was predicted to reduce withdrawal, as there is still a source of nicotine. The placebo condition allowed an unhindered view of withdrawal, as there was no nicotine to alleviate withdrawal symptoms. Interestingly, the authors found no increase in psychiatric symptoms in either phase of the study. However, there was an increase in the Schedule for the Assessment of Negative Symptoms score on the first day that then returned to baseline levels. The authors suggested that if the increase were due to nicotine withdrawal, it would have been expected to persistently increase such that transient increases in negative symptoms with affective blunting and apathy was due to behavioral inactivity rather than the effect of nicotine withdrawal (Dalack et al., 1999). Another study found that reduced akathisia in SZ smokers was associated with smoking and suggested that a combination of nicotine replacement therapy (NRT) and reduced antipsychotic dose could avert worsening of symptoms as has been suggested to happen when quitting smoking (Barnes et al., 2006).

The importance of nicotine withdrawal is highlighted by another clinical measure affected by the same mechanism of nicotine augmenting DA release, which is depressed mood. Baseline clinical measures generally report higher levels of depression in smokers with SZ compared to nonpsychiatric smokers (Glassman, 1993). Several studies, such as George, Vessicchio, Termine, Sahady, et al. (2002), have not reported elevated depression symptoms in SZ versus control smokers, and no differences at baseline or during abstinence in either antipsychotic class, though smokers having greater depressive symptoms than nonsmokers. It has been suggested that perhaps a trait difference may account for this; however, further controlled evaluations are needed. Recently, Tidey et al. (2014) reported a higher BPRS-anergia factor score during abstinence, though this was not found to be related to lapse latency. However, baseline depression severity, total BPRS score, and BPRS anxiety-depression factor scores were found to be significantly associated with smoking lapse latency. After co-varying baseline depression scores, group differences of nicotine withdrawal were eliminated while urge scores were not, suggesting that an underlying group difference in nicotine withdrawal may be attributed to depression severity, not craving. This relationship has an implication that baseline depression levels and nicotine withdrawal levels after abstinence may ultimately predict the rate of successful quit attempts. Perhaps careful matching on baseline measures may clarify issues regarding the effects of withdrawal on depression as well as negative symptoms in SZ.

Taken together, there are clearly affective changes, clearly withdrawal and craving changes, but there are minimal effects on psychiatric symptoms. Nicotine withdrawal peaks over 24–48 h of abstinence; therefore these studies may be a representative evaluation of acute abstinence withdrawal effects on exacerbation of symptoms. However, study of abstinence over longer periods of time are needed. What seems to serve as a motivational or incentive role in smoking behavior is release of DA. Given that several lines of evidence suggest hypoactivity of the PFC in SZ being associated with negative symptoms and depression, minimizing nicotine withdrawal effects with smoking interventions, such as pharmacotherapeutics, may be the safest and most effective answer. Future research can examine the impact of withdrawal such that smoking interventions can be determined as to which one is more useful in SZ smokers.

Effects of Nicotine Withdrawal on Cognitive Function

Numerous studies have found that smoking is used to remediate attentional and cognitive deficits related to SZ, so not surprisingly nicotine withdrawal alters cognition. However, there do seem to be some selective effects and targets of withdrawal on cognition such as visuospatial working memory (VSWM), sustained attention, and prepulse inhibition (PPI), which is a measure of sensorimotor gating (George et al., 2006; Sacco et al., 2005). For example, George and colleagues (George, Vessichio, et al., 2002) conducted a study examining both acute (less than 1 week) and prolonged (8–10 weeks) smoking abstinence on VSWM. The authors found that both acute and long-term tobacco abstinence and withdrawal were associated with worsening of VSWM, but interestingly improved in non-psychiatric smokers. Thus, it appears that smoking may have differential effects in SZ patients and non-psychiatric individuals. Likewise, Sacco et al. (2005) found that overnight abstinence decreased VSWM in SZ smokers, but it was reversed once smoking was resumed, which was also replicated by Wing, Wass, Bacher, Rabin, and George (2013) at the 30 s delay of the VSWM task. Both animal and human studies have suggested that nicotine withdrawal leads to a decrease in central DA function. As VSWM is partially dependent on DA, these studies show how smoking abstinence may lead to alterations in such cognitive processes in SZ patients.

Evidence has also suggested that smoking improved auditory sensory gating in SZ patients, which has been previously suggested to be deficient in this population. Under normal conditions, nicotine enhances DA release inhibiting PPI, so George et al. (2006) conducted a study evaluating effects of smoking abstinence on PPI. The authors found that overnight abstinence increased tobacco craving, reduced nicotine levels, and impaired PPI, and these changes were reversed with smoking reinstatement. Therefore it can be concluded that the endogenous PPI deficit in SZ may be attenuated by smoking, and withdrawal and craving may ultimately alter this domain of cognition such that precautions should be taken in smoking cessation treatments.

GREATER DIFFICULTY QUITTING

Given that many SZ smokers attempt to quit several times before being able to stop completely, this suggests that smoking cessation is a complex behavior (de Leon and Diaz, 2005). Even more so, treatment studies of smokers with SZ indicate half the quit rates compared to the general population (Steinberg, Ziedonis, Krejci, & Brandon, 2004). There are several plausible reasons for this difference, one of which is the existing unsubstantial level of motivation to quit in the SZ population (Mann-Wrobel, Bennett, Weiner, Buchanan, & Ball, 2011). Lack of interest or inadequate support for quitting may undermine quit attempts in SZ smokers and may reduce motivation to successfully quit (Williams and Hughes, 2003). One study tested whether motivational interviewing is effective in motivating SZ smokers to seek tobacco dependent treatments to quit (Steinberg and Ziedonis, et al., 2004). Interestingly, the authors found that a greater proportion of participants receiving the motivational interviewing intervention (32%) contacted treatment providers within 1 month postintervention, compared to the other two treatments, psychoeducational counseling (11%) and minimal-control intervention (0%) (Steinberg, Zedonis, et al., 2004). These results highlight the importance of engaging patients in treatment, such that retention rates and treatment outcome would thereby improve.

Furthermore, patients have often reported experiencing substantial withdrawal symptoms during quit attempts subsequently resulting in their return to smoking. One study found that 83% of 24 patients had previously attempted to quit; however, they had failed to quit, with 71% reporting substantial withdrawal symptoms such as craving (71%), concentration problems (67%), increased appetite (62%), anxiety (52%), irritability (38%), and restlessness (14%) (Ziedonis and George, 1997). Likewise, it has been found that SZ smokers perceive reinforcement value of cigarette smoking to a higher degree than control smokers, recognizing many drawbacks associated with smoking (Kelly et al., 2012). Therefore, examining important determinants such as withdrawal and smoking urges, as well as perceived consequences and benefits of quitting, may lead to more promising smoking cessation outcomes in the SZ population.

SUMMARY AND CONCLUSIONS

During quit attempts, cigarette craving and nicotine withdrawal symptoms are important predictors of continuing smoking and relapse. Gaining knowledge from using nAChR antagonists and agonists can be used to test efficacy of treatment for smoking cessation, suggesting novel pharmacological agents, or enhancing current treatments for SZ smokers to target withdrawal related features. SZ is characterized by pathological aberrations in the nAChR system that mediates effects of nicotine in the brain (Wing, Wass, et al., 2012). Abnormalities in the regulation of nAChR systems thus may contribute to the vulnerability of the SZ population to nicotine use and dependence (George, Vessicchio, et al., 2002).

Given that an essential aspect of understanding addiction is of delivery of the drug or onset of the action of drug, topography measurements may yield important insights about drug reward and reinforcement and help to understand behaviors of nicotine addiction and withdrawal. Even when matched for number of cigarettes per day and different indices of nicotine dependence, SZ smokers had higher serum nicotine and cotinine levels. These differences are most likely associated with the intensity with which each cigarette is smoked rather than differences in nicotine metabolism or excretion. Thus greater nicotine extraction when smoking may implicate the severity of withdrawal symptoms that would have to be overcome if abstaining. Studies on smoking topography are useful in demonstrating that smokers with SZ differ in their cigarette puffing behavior and the reinforcing effect of nicotine potentially driving this comorbidity.

Correspondingly higher prevalence of addiction to smoking cigarettes coincides with less likelihood of quitting compared to non-psychiatric populations. The reduced antipsychotic blood levels caused by increased tobacco smoking may explain why SZ smokers experience reduced medication side effects such as extrapyramidal symptoms (Yang, Nelson, Kamaraju, Wilson, & McEvoy, 2002). Therefore, when psychiatrists are prescribing medications to SZ patients, smoking status should be taken into account. The ability of nicotine to alleviate negative symptoms of SZ and to improve cognition is one of main reasons patients have reported to continuously smoke.

The administration of nicotine has also been found to transiently improve many neurobiological functions such as PPI, sensory gating, antisaccade, and eye tracking, as well as cognitive functions such as sustained attention, information processing speed, and spatial information processing in SZ and schizoaffective disorder. Nicotine withdrawal leads to decreases in DA release in the reward system of the brain and may ultimately relate to its effect on decreased cognitive performance in patients. Therefore, pharmacotherapeutic treatments that selectively target these affected domains while minimizing withdrawal and craving in SZ would be ideal for developing improved treatments for comorbid nicotine addiction in SZ.

The significant role of withdrawal and craving on negative affect may also provide a novel targeted pharmacotherapy focusing on reducing related and nicotine withdrawal symptoms. Smokers with SZ have been proposed to be more efficient smokers, taking in more nicotine per cigarette than smokers without this disorder. Understanding the difference in nicotine boost in SZ from non-psychiatric smokers may explain the higher levels of nicotine addiction and low success in cessation in SZ smokers (Drobes and Tiffany, 1997; Williams et al., 2010).

Ultimately, greater experiences of severe craving and withdrawal in smokers with SZ compared to control smokers without psychiatric illnesses may contribute to poorer cessation outcomes. Targeting withdrawal symptoms and craving with novel treatments including novel nicotinic agents and brain stimulation methods (eg, Wing, Wass, et al., 2012) may produce better cessation outcomes. Differences in study design (short versus longer period of abstinence), medication dose and/or type (eg, varenicline, bupropion, NRT), patient selection (outpatient versus inpatient), motivation to quit, and criteria used to assess smoking abstinence are likely to explain some of the variability of quit rates and symptoms, and they should be addressed in future studies. Ultimately, improving cessation outcomes in schizophrenia by targeting withdrawal and craving will lead to reduced morbidity and mortality, and improved quality of life for these vulnerable patients.

References

Andreasen, N. C. (1982). Negative symptoms in schizophrenia. Definition and reliability. *Archives of General Psychiatry, 39*(7), 784–788.

Baker, T. B., Piper, M. E., McCarthy, D. E., Majeskie, M. R., & Fiore, M. C. (2004). Addiction motivation reformulated: an affective processing model of negative reinforcement. *Psychological Review, 111*(1), 33–51. http://dx.doi.org/10.1037/0033-295X.111.1.33.

Balfour, D. J., Wright, A. E., Benwell, M. E., & Birrell, C. E. (2000). The putative role of extra-synaptic mesolimbic dopamine in the neurobiology of nicotine dependence. *Behavioural Brain Research, 113*(1–2), 73–83.

Bao, Z., He, X. Y., Ding, X., Prabhu, S., & Hong, J. Y. (2005). Metabolism of nicotine and cotinine by human cytochrome P450 2A13. *Drug Metabolism and Disposition: the Biological Fate of Chemicals, 33*(2), 258–261. http://dx.doi.org/10.1124/dmd.104.002105.

Barnes, M., Lawford, B. R., Burton, S. C., Heslop, K. R., Noble, E. P., Hausdorf, K., et al. (2006). Smoking and schizophrenia: is symptom profile related to smoking and which antipsychotic medication is of benefit in reducing cigarette use? *The Australian and New Zealand Journal of Psychiatry, 40*(6–7), 575–580. http://dx.doi.org/10.1111/j.1440-1614.2006.01841.x.

Behm, F. M. R., & Jed, E. (1994). Reducing craving for cigarettes while decreasing smoke intake using capsaicin-enhanced low tar cigarettes. *Experimental and Clinical Psychopharmacology, 2*(2), 143–153. http://dx.doi.org/10.1037/1064-1297.2.2.143.

Benowitz, N. L., Pomerleau, O. F., Pomerleau, C. S., & Jacob, P., 3rd (2003). Nicotine metabolite ratio as a predictor of cigarette consumption. *Nicotine & Tobacco Research: Official Journal of the Society for Research on Nicotine and Tobacco, 5*(5), 621–624.

Breese, C. R., Lee, M. J., Adams, C. E., Sullivan, B., Logel, J., Gillen, K. M., et al. (2000). Abnormal regulation of high affinity nicotinic receptors in subjects with schizophrenia. *Neuropsychopharmacology: Official Publication of the American College of Neuropsychopharmacology, 23*(4), 351–364. http://dx.doi.org/10.1016/S0893-133X(00)00121-4.

Bridges, R. B., Combs, J. G., Humble, J. W., Turbek, J. A., Rehm, S. R., & Haley, N. J. (1990). Puffing topography as a determinant of smoke exposure. *Pharmacology, Biochemistry, and Behavior, 37*(1), 29–39.

Brown, S., Kim, M., Mitchell, C., & Inskip, H. (2010). Twenty-five year mortality of a community cohort with schizophrenia. *The British Journal of Psychiatry: the Journal of Mental Science, 196*(2), 116–121. http://dx.doi.org/10.1192/bjp.bp.109.067512.

Brown, J., Hajek, P., McRobbie, H., Locker, J., Gillison, F., McEwen, A., et al. (2013). Cigarette craving and withdrawal symptoms during temporary abstinence and the effect of nicotine gum. *Psychopharmacology, 229*(1), 209–218. http://dx.doi.org/10.1007/s00213-013-3100-2.

Carter, B. L., & Tiffany, S. T. (1999). Meta-analysis of cue-reactivity in addiction research. *Addiction, 94*(3), 327–340.

Chambers, R. A., Krystal, J. H., & Self, D. W. (2001). A neurobiological basis for substance abuse comorbidity in schizophrenia. *Biological Psychiatry, 50*(2), 71–83.

Chou, K. J., Chen, H. K., Hung, C. H., Chen, T. T., Chen, C. M., & Wu, B. J. (2014). Readiness to quit as a predictor for outcomes of smoking-reduction programme with transdermal nicotine patch or bupropion in a sample of 308 patients with schizophrenia. *European Archives of Psychiatry and Clinical Neuroscience.* http://dx.doi.org/10.1007/s00406-014-0515-7.

Curkendall, S. M., Mo, J., Glasser, D. B., Rose Stang, M., & Jones, J. K. (2004). Cardiovascular disease in patients with schizophrenia in Saskatchewan, Canada. *Journal of Clinical Psychiatry, 65*(5), 715–720.

Dalack, G. W., Becks, L., Hill, E., Pomerleau, O. F., & Meador-Woodruff, J. H. (1999). Nicotine withdrawal and psychiatric symptoms in cigarette smokers with schizophrenia. *Neuropsychopharmacology: Official Publication of the American College of Neuropsychopharmacology, 21*(2), 195–202. http://dx.doi.org/10.1016/S0893-133X(98)00121-3.

Dalack, G. W., & Meador-Woodruff, J. H. (1996). Smoking, smoking withdrawal and schizophrenia: case reports and a review of the literature. *Schizophrenia Research, 22*(2), 133–141.

de Leon, J., & Diaz, F. J. (2005). A meta-analysis of worldwide studies demonstrates an association between schizophrenia and tobacco smoking behaviors. *Schizophrenia Research, 76*(2–3), 135–157. http://dx.doi.org/10.1016/j.schres.2005.02.010.

Decina, P., Caracci, G., Sandik, R., Berman, W., Mukherjee, S., & Scapicchio, P. (1990). Cigarette smoking and neuroleptic-induced parkinsonism. *Biological Psychiatry, 28*(6), 502–508.

Donny, E. C., & Jones, M. (2009). Prolonged exposure to denicotinized cigarettes with or without transdermal nicotine. *Drug and Alcohol Dependence, 104*(1–2), 23–33. http://dx.doi.org/10.1016/j.drugalcdep.2009.01.021.

Drobes, D. J., & Tiffany, S. T. (1997). Induction of smoking urge through imaginal and in vivo procedures: physiological and self-report manifestations. *Journal of Abnormal Psychology, 106*(1), 15–25.

D'Souza, D. C., Esterlis, I., Carbuto, M., Krasenics, M., Seibyl, J., Bois, F., et al. (2012). Lower ss2*-nicotinic acetylcholine receptor availability in smokers with schizophrenia. *The American Journal of Psychiatry, 169*(3), 326–334. http://dx.doi.org/10.1176/appi.ajp.2011.11020189.

Fonder, M. A., Sacco, K. A., Termine, A., Boland, B. S., Seyal, A. A., Dudas, M. M., et al. (2005). Smoking cue reactivity in schizophrenia: effects of a nicotinic receptor antagonist. *Biological Psychiatry, 57*(7), 802–808. http://dx.doi.org/10.1016/j.biopsych.2004.12.027.

Freedman, R., Coon, H., Myles-Worsley, M., Orr-Urtreger, A., Olincy, A., Davis, A., et al. (1997). Linkage of a neurophysiological deficit in schizophrenia to a chromosome 15 locus. *Proceedings of the National Academy of Science USA, 94*(2), 587–592.

George, T. P., Verrico, C. D., Picciotto, M. R., & Roth, R. H. (2000). Nicotinic modulation of mesoprefrontal dopamine neurons: pharmacologic and neuroanatomic characterization. *The Journal of Pharmacology and Experimental Therapeutics, 295*(1), 58–66.

George, T. P., Vessicchio, J. C., Termine, A., Bregartner, T. A., Feingold, A., Rounsaville, B. J., et al. (2002a). A placebo controlled trial of bupropion for smoking cessation in schizophrenia. *Biological Psychiatry, 52*(1), 53–61.

George, T. P., Vessicchio, J. C., Termine, A., Sahady, D. M., Head, C. A., Pepper, W. T., et al. (2002b). Effects of smoking abstinence on visuospatial working memory function in schizophrenia. *Neuropsychopharmacology: Official Publication of the American College of Neuropsychopharmacology, 26*(1), 75–85. http://dx.doi.org/10.1016/S0893-133X(01)00296-2.

George, T. P., Termine, A., Sacco, K. A., Allen, T. M., Reutenauer, E., Vessicchio, J. C., et al. (2006). A preliminary study of the effects of cigarette smoking on prepulse inhibition in schizophrenia: involvement of nicotinic receptor mechanisms. *Schizophrenia Research, 87*(1–3), 307–315. http://dx.doi.org/10.1016/j.schres.2006.05.022.

Glassman, A. H. (1993). Cigarette smoking: implications for psychiatric illness. *The American Journal of Psychiatry, 150*(4), 546–553.

Goff, D. C., Henderson, D. C., & Amico, E. (1992). Cigarette smoking in schizophrenia: relationship to psychopathology and medication side effects. *The American Journal of Psychiatry, 149*(9), 1189–1194.

Hammond, D., Fong, G. T., Cummings, K. M., & Hyland, A. (2005). Smoking topography, brand switching, and nicotine delivery: results from an in vivo study. *Cancer Epidemiology, Biomarkers & Prevention: a Publication of the American Association for Cancer Research, Cosponsored By the American Society of Preventive Oncology, 14*(6), 1370–1375. http://dx.doi.org/10.1158/1055-9965.EPI-04-0498.

Hughes, J. R., & Hatsukami, D. (1986). Signs and symptoms of tobacco withdrawal. *Archives of General Psychiatry, 43*(3), 289–294.

Hughes, J. R., Hatsukami, D. K., Mitchell, J. E., & Dahlgren, L. A. (1986). Prevalence of smoking among psychiatric outpatients. *The American Journal of Psychiatry, 143*(8), 993–997.

Hukkanen, J., Jacob, P., 3rd, & Benowitz, N. L. (2005). Metabolism and disposition kinetics of nicotine. *Pharmacological Reviews, 57*(1), 79–115. http://dx.doi.org/10.1124/pr.57.1.3.

Johnson, M. W., Bickel, W. K., & Kirshenbaum, A. P. (2004). Substitutes for tobacco smoking: a behavioral economic analysis of nicotine gum, denicotinized cigarettes, and nicotine-containing cigarettes. *Drug and Alcohol Dependence, 74*(3), 253–264. http://dx.doi.org/10.1016/j.drugalcdep.2003.12.012.

Joukamaa, M., Heliovaara, M., Knekt, P., Aromaa, A., Raitasalo, R., & Lehtinen, V. (2001). Mental disorders and cause-specific mortality. *The British Journal of Psychiatry: the Journal of Mental Science, 179*, 498–502.

Juliano, L. M., Donny, E. C., Houtsmuller, E. J., & Stitzer, M. L. (2006). Experimental evidence for a causal relationship between smoking lapse and relapse. *Journal of Abnormal Psychology, 115*(1), 166–173. http://dx.doi.org/10.1037/0021-843X.115.1.166.

Kelly, D. L., Raley, H. G., Lo, S., Wright, K., Liu, F., McMahon, R. P., et al. (2012). Perception of smoking risks and motivation to quit among nontreatment-seeking smokers with and without schizophrenia. *Schizophrenia Bulletin, 38*(3), 543–551. http://dx.doi.org/10.1093/schbul/sbq124.

Lasser, K., Boyd, J. W., Woolhandler, S., Himmelstein, D. U., McCormick, D., & Bor, D. H. (2000). Smoking and mental illness: a population-based prevalence study. *JAMA, 284*(20), 2606–2610.

Lewis, A., Miller, J. H., & Lea, R. A. (2007). Monoamine oxidase and tobacco dependence. *Neurotoxicology, 28*(1), 182–195. http://dx.doi.org/10.1016/j.neuro.2006.05.019.

MacKillop, J., & Tidey, J. W. (2011). Cigarette demand and delayed reward discounting in nicotine-dependent individuals with schizophrenia and controls: an initial study. *Psychopharmacology, 216*(1), 91–99. http://dx.doi.org/10.1007/s00213-011-2185-8.

Mann-Wrobel, M. C., Bennett, M. E., Weiner, E. E., Buchanan, R. W., & Ball, M. P. (2011). Smoking history and motivation to quit in smokers with schizophrenia in a smoking cessation program. *Schizophrenia Research, 126*(1–3), 277–283. http://dx.doi.org/10.1016/j.schres.2010.10.030.

McKee, S. A., Weinberger, A. H., Harrison, E. L., Coppola, S., & George, T. P. (2009). Effects of the nicotinic receptor antagonist mecamylamine on ad-lib smoking behavior, topography, and nicotine levels in smokers with and without schizophrenia: a preliminary study. *Schizophrenia Research, 115*(2–3), 317–324. http://dx.doi.org/10.1016/j.schres.2009.07.019.

Menza, M. A., Grossman, N., Van Horn, M., Cody, R., & Forman, N. (1991). Smoking and movement disorders in psychiatric patients. *Biological Psychiatry, 30*(2), 109–115.

Moghaddam, B., & Bunney, B. S. (1990). Acute effects of typical and atypical antipsychotic drugs on the release of dopamine from prefrontal cortex, nucleus accumbens, and striatum of the rat: an in vivo microdialysis study. *Journal of Neurochemistry, 54*(5), 1755–1760.

Muscat, J. E., Stellman, S. D., Caraballo, R. S., & Richie, J. P., Jr. (2009). Time to first cigarette after waking predicts cotinine levels. *Cancer Epidemiology, Biomarkers & Prevention: a Publication of the American Association for Cancer Research, Cosponsored By the American Society of Preventive Oncology, 18*(12), 3415–3420. http://dx.doi.org/10.1158/1055-9965.EPI-09-0737.

Odum, A. L. (2011). Delay discounting: I'm a k, you're a k. *Journal of the Experimental Analysis of Behavior, 96*(3), 427–439. http://dx.doi.org/10.1901/jeab.2011.96-423.

Olincy, A., Young, D. A., & Freedman, R. (1997). Increased levels of the nicotine metabolite cotinine in schizophrenic smokers compared to other smokers. *Biological Psychiatry, 42*(1), 1–5. http://dx.doi.org/10.1016/S0006-3223(96)00302-2.

Paulson, G. W. (1992). Addiction to nicotine is due to high intrinsic levels of dopamine. *Medical Hypotheses, 38*(3), 206–207.

Piasecki, T. M., Jorenby, D. E., Smith, S. S., Fiore, M. C., & Baker, T. B. (2003). Smoking withdrawal dynamics: III. Correlates of withdrawal heterogeneity. *Experimental and Clinical Psychopharmacology, 11*(4), 276–285. http://dx.doi.org/10.1037/1064-1297.11.4.276.

Pickworth, W. B., Fant, R. V., Nelson, R. A., Rohrer, M. S., & Henningfield, J. E. (1999). Pharmacodynamic effects of new de-nicotinized cigarettes. *Nicotine & Tobacco Research: Official Journal of the Society for Research on Nicotine and Tobacco, 1*(4), 357–364.

Pillitteri, J. L., Kozlowski, L. T., Sweeney, C. T., & Heatherton, T. F. (1997). Individual differences in the subjective effects of the first cigarette of the day: a self-report method for studying tolerance. *Experimental and Clinical Psychopharmacology, 5*(1), 83–90.

Rose, J. E. (2006). Nicotine and nonnicotine factors in cigarette addiction. *Psychopharmacology*, *184*(3–4), 274–285. http://dx.doi.org/10.1007/s00213-005-0250-x.

Sacco, K. A., Bannon, K. L., & George, T. P. (2004). Nicotinic receptor mechanisms and cognition in normal states and neuropsychiatric disorders. *Journal of Psychopharmacology*, *18*(4), 457–474. http://dx.doi.org/10.1177/0269881104047273.

Sacco, K. A., Termine, A., Seyal, A., Dudas, M. M., Vessicchio, J. C., Krishnan-Sarin, S., et al. (2005). Effects of cigarette smoking on spatial working memory and attentional deficits in schizophrenia: involvement of nicotinic receptor mechanisms. *Archives of General Psychiatry*, *62*(6), 649–659. http://dx.doi.org/10.1001/archpsyc.62.6.649.

Scherer, G. (1999). Smoking behaviour and compensation: a review of the literature. *Psychopharmacology*, *145*(1), 1–20.

Shadel, W. G., Niaura, R., & Abrams, D. B. (2001). Effect of different cue stimulus delivery channels on craving reactivity: comparing in vivo and video cues in regular cigarette smokers. *Journal of Behavior Therapy and Exprimental Psychiatry*, *32*(4), 203–209.

Spring, B., Pingitore, R., & McChargue, D. E. (2003). Reward value of cigarette smoking for comparably heavy smoking schizophrenic, depressed, and nonpatient smokers. *The American Journal of Psychiatry*, *160*(2), 316–322.

Steinberg, M. L., Williams, J. M., & Ziedonis, D. M. (2004). Financial implications of cigarette smoking among individuals with schizophrenia. *Tobacco Control*, *13*(2), 206.

Steinberg, M. L., Ziedonis, D. M., Krejci, J. A., & Brandon, T. H. (2004). Motivational interviewing with personalized feedback: a brief intervention for motivating smokers with schizophrenia to seek treatment for tobacco dependence. *Journal of Consulting and Clinical Psychology*, *72*(4), 723–728. http://dx.doi.org/10.1037/0022-006X.72.4.723.

Tidey, J. W., Rohsenow, D. J., Kaplan, G. B., & Swift, R. M. (2005a). Cigarette smoking topography in smokers with schizophrenia and matched non-psychiatric controls. *Drug and Alcohol Dependence*, *80*(2), 259–265. http://dx.doi.org/10.1016/j.drugalcdep.2005.04.002.

Tidey, J. W., Rohsenow, D. J., Kaplan, G. B., & Swift, R. M. (2005b). Subjective and physiological responses to smoking cues in smokers with schizophrenia. *Nicotine & Tobacco Research: Official Journal of the Society for Research on Nicotine and Tobacco*, *7*(3), 421–429. http://dx.doi.org/10.1080/14622200500125724.

Tidey, J. W., Rohsenow, D. J., Kaplan, G. B., Swift, R. M., & Adolfo, A. B. (2008). Effects of smoking abstinence, smoking cues and nicotine replacement in smokers with schizophrenia and controls. *Nicotine & Tobacco Research: Official Journal of the Society for Research on Nicotine and Tobacco*, *10*(6), 1047–1056. http://dx.doi.org/10.1080/14622200802097373.

Tidey, J. W., Rohsenow, D. J., Kaplan, G. B., Swift, R. M., & Ahnallen, C. G. (2013). Separate and combined effects of very low nicotine cigarettes and nicotine replacement in smokers with schizophrenia and controls. *Nicotine & Tobacco Research: Official Journal of the Society for Research on Nicotine and Tobacco*, *15*(1), 121–129. http://dx.doi.org/10.1093/ntr/nts098.

Tidey, J. W., Colby, S. M., & Xavier, E. M. (2014). Effects of smoking abstinence on cigarette craving, nicotine withdrawal, and nicotine reinforcement in smokers with and without schizophrenia. *Nicotine & Tobacco Research: Official Journal of the Society for Research on Nicotine and Tobacco*, *16*(3), 326–334. http://dx.doi.org/10.1093/ntr/ntt152.

Tiffany, S. T., & Drobes, D. J. (1991). The development and initial validation of a questionnaire on smoking urges. *British Journal of Addiction*, *86*(11), 1467–1476.

Watkins, S. S., Koob, G. F., & Markou, A. (2000). Neural mechanisms underlying nicotine addiction: acute positive reinforcement and withdrawal. *Nicotine & Tobacco Research: Official Journal of the Society for Research on Nicotine and Tobacco*, *2*(1), 19–37.

Watson, D., Clark, L. A., & Tellegen, A. (1988). Development and validation of brief measures of positive and negative affect: the PANAS scales. *Journal of Personality and Social Psychology*, *54*(6), 1063–1070.

Weinberger, A. H., Reutenauer, E. L., Allen, T. M., Termine, A., Vessicchio, J. C., Sacco, K. A., et al. (2007). Reliability of the Fagerstrom test for nicotine dependence, Minnesota nicotine withdrawal scale, and Tiffany questionnaire for smoking urges in smokers with and without schizophrenia. *Drug and Alcohol Dependence*, *86*(2–3), 278–282. http://dx.doi.org/10.1016/j.drugalcdep.2006.06.005.

Weinberger, A. H., Sacco, K. A., Creeden, C. L., Vessicchio, J. C., Jatlow, P. I., & George, T. P. (2007d). Effects of acute abstinence, reinstatement, and mecamylamine on biochemical and behavioral measures of cigarette smoking in schizophrenia. *Schizophrenia Research*, *91*(1–3), 217–225. http://dx.doi.org/10.1016/j.schres.2006.12.007.

Williams, J. M., & Hughes, J. R. (2003). Pharmacotherapy treatments for tobacco dependence among smokers with mental illness or addiction. *Psychiatric Annals*, *33*, 457–466.

Williams, J. M., Ziedonis, D. M., Abanyie, F., Steinberg, M. L., Foulds, J., & Benowitz, N. L. (2005). Increased nicotine and cotinine levels in smokers with schizophrenia and schizoaffective disorder is not a metabolic effect. *Schizophrenia Research*, *79*(2–3), 323–335. http://dx.doi.org/10.1016/j.schres.2005.04.016.

Williams, J. M., Gandhi, K. K., Lu, S. E., Kumar, S., Shen, J., Foulds, J., et al. (2010). Higher nicotine levels in schizophrenia compared with controls after smoking a single cigarette. *Nicotine & Tobacco Research: Official Journal of the Society for Research on Nicotine and Tobacco*, *12*(8), 855–859. http://dx.doi.org/10.1093/ntr/ntq102.

Williams, J. M., Gandhi, K. K., Lu, S. E., Kumar, S., Steinberg, M. L., Cottler, B., et al. (2011). Shorter interpuff interval is associated with higher nicotine intake in smokers with schizophrenia. *Drug and Alcohol Dependence*, *118*(2–3), 313–319. http://dx.doi.org/10.1016/j.drugalcdep.2011.04.009.

Williams, J. M., Gandhi, K. K., Lu, S. E., Steinberg, M. L., & Benowitz, N. L. (2013). Rapid smoking may not be aversive in schizophrenia. *Nicotine & Tobacco Research: Official Journal of the Society for Research on Nicotine and Tobacco*, *15*(1), 262–266. http://dx.doi.org/10.1093/ntr/ntr314.

Willner, P., Hardman, S., & Eaton, G. (1995). Subjective and behavioural evaluation of cigarette cravings. *Psychopharmacology*, *118*(2), 171–177.

Wing, V. C., Moss, T. G., Rabin, R. A., & George, T. P. (2012). Effects of cigarette smoking status on delay discounting in schizophrenia and healthy controls. *Addictive Behaviors*, *37*(1), 67–72. http://dx.doi.org/10.1016/j.addbeh.2011.08.012.

Wing, V. C., Wass, C. E., Bacher, I., Rabin, R. A., & George, T. P. (2013). Varenicline modulates spatial working memory deficits in smokers with schizophrenia. *Schizophrenia Research*, *149*(1–3), 190–191. http://dx.doi.org/10.1016/j.schres.2013.06.032.

Wing, V. C., Wass, C. E., Soh, D. W., & George, T. P. (2012). A review of neurobiological vulnerability factors and treatment implications for comorbid tobacco dependence in schizophrenia. *Annals of New York Academy of Sciences*, *1248*, 89–106. http://dx.doi.org/10.1111/j.1749-6632.2011.06261.x.

Yang, Y. K., Nelson, L., Kamaraju, L., Wilson, W., & McEvoy, J. P. (2002). Nicotine decreases bradykinesia-rigidity in haloperidol-treated patients with schizophrenia. *Neuropsychopharmacology: Official Publication of the American College of Neuropsychopharmacology*, *27*(4), 684–686. http://dx.doi.org/10.1016/S0893-133X(02)00325-1.

Yassa, R., Lal, S., Korpassy, A., & Ally, J. (1987). Nicotine exposure and tardive dyskinesia. *Biological Psychiatry*, *22*(1), 67–72.

Zhang, X. Y., Chen da, C., Xiu, M. H., Haile, C. N., Sun, H., Lu, L., et al. (2012). Cigarette smoking and cognitive function in Chinese male schizophrenia: a case-control study. *PLoS One*, *7*(5), e36563. http://dx.doi.org/10.1371/journal.pone.0036563.

Ziedonis, D. M., & George, T. P. (1997). Schizophrenia and nicotine use: report of a pilot smoking cessation program and review of neurobiological and clinical issues. *Schizophrenia Bulletin*, *23*(2), 247–254.

Ziedonis, D. M., Kosten, T. R., Glazer, W. M., & Frances, R. J. (1994). Nicotine dependence and schizophrenia. *Hospital and Community Psychiatry*, *45*(3), 204–206.

15

Emergent Cognitive Impairment During Early Nicotine Withdrawal*

R.M. Schuster, A.E. Evins

Massachusetts General Hospital, Boston, MA, United States

INTRODUCTION

Despite growing public awareness of the negative health consequences of tobacco smoking, the relapse rate among smokers who attempt to quit remains high. Approximately 5–25% of smokers who attempt to quit without pharmacotherapeutic cessation aids remain abstinent after 6 months (Clinical Practice Guideline Treating Tobacco Dependence Update Panel & Staff, 2008), while those who use such aids (eg, nicotine replacement therapies (NRTs), varenicline, bupropion) achieve significantly higher initial abstinence rates while on treatment but only slightly higher abstinence rates after 6 months (17–32%; Cahill, Stevens, & Lancaster, 2014). This low rate of longer term abstinence highlights the need to define relapse risk factors to develop effective smoking cessation treatments that lead to sustained abstinence.

*This publication was made possible by the National Institute on Drug Abuse (NIDA; K24 DA030443, PI: Evins) as well as the following fellowships from Massachusetts General Hospital and Harvard Medical School (PI: Schuster): Norman E. Zinberg Fellowship in Addiction Psychiatry, Livingston Fellowship, and Louis V. Gerstner III Research Scholar Award. Its contents are solely the responsibility of the authors and do not necessarily represent the official views of NIDA, the National Institutes of Health, Massachusetts General Hospital, or Harvard Medical School. Dr. Schuster declares no conflicts of interest. Dr. Evins has received research grant support from Pfizer Inc, Forum Pharmaceuticals, and GSK.

Negative Affective States and Cognitive Impairments in Nicotine Dependence
http://dx.doi.org/10.1016/B978-0-12-802574-1.00015-6

Disrupted cognition, particularly in the domains of attention, working memory, and response inhibition, is a core phenotype of nicotine withdrawal (Hughes, 2007a, 2007b) and is clinically significant with respect to risk for relapse (Powell, Pickering, Dawkins, West, & Powell, 2004; Rukstalis, Jepson, Patterson, & Lerman, 2005). Deficits across cortically and subcortically mediated domains of cognition can emerge within 30 min of last use (Hendricks, Ditre, Drobes, & Brandon, 2006), peak in intensity within a few days (Hughes, 2007b), and may persist for four weeks or longer (Gilbert et al., 2004). Given this time course of withdrawal-related cognitive deficits, it is not surprising that most smokers relapse within the first week of abstinence (Hughes, 2004), and that first week abstinence following a cessation attempt predicts smoking outcomes six months later (Ashare, Wileyto, Perkins, & Schnoll, 2013). As recently abstinent smokers may be motivated to resume use to alleviate withdrawal-emergent cognitive dysfunction (Heishman, Kleykamp, & Singleton, 2010), a priority has been to identify pharmacological treatments that can attenuate abstinence-associated cognitive deficits during withdrawal and thereby reduce risk for subsequent relapse (Myers, Taylor, Moolchan, & Heishman, 2008; Patterson et al., 2010).

The goal of this chapter is to review what is known and what remains unknown regarding the domain-specific cognitive manifestations of nicotine withdrawal as well as the neurophysiological underpinnings of these deficits. We also focus on implications for treatment by exploring individual difference factors that may moderate how cognitive impairments are expressed during withdrawal. We conclude with recommendations for future scientific study.

NEUROPHYSIOLOGICAL MECHANISMS OF COGNITIVE EFFECTS OF NICOTINE WITHDRAWAL

Nicotine, the main addictive constituent in tobacco, binds to and stimulates nicotinic acetylcholine receptors (nAChRs), pentameric, ligand-gated ion channels that are distributed widely in the brain (Albuquerque, Pereira, Alkondon, & Rogers, 2009). A central role of nAChRs is neuromodulation, as most of these receptors are located presynaptically (Wonnacott, 1997) and regulate the release of other neurotransmitters. The nAChR subtypes most abundant in brain are $\alpha 7$ and $\alpha 4\beta 2$. $\alpha 4\beta 2$ receptors, in particular, have high affinity for nicotine. SPECT studies have demonstrated that cigarette smoking results in nearly complete occupancy of $\alpha 4\beta 2$ nAChRs, with daily smokers exhibiting near complete $\alpha 4\beta 2$ receptor binding throughout the day (Brody et al., 2006). Substantial receptor occupancy is even achieved via secondhand cigarette smoke exposure (Brody et al., 2009). Substantial $\alpha 4\beta 2$ receptor occupancy is also achieved with use of varenicline, a full α4β2 nAChR agonist and partial α7 nAChR agonist (Lotfipour, Mandelkern, Alvarez-Estrada, & Brody, 2012).

nAChR stimulation by both endogenous (ie, acetylcholine) and exogenous (ie, nicotine) ligands results in release of multiple neurotransmitters including dopamine, GABA, and glutamate (Livingstone & Wonnacott, 2009), all of which influence cognitive function (Levin, McClernon, & Rezvani, 2006; Loughead et al., 2009; Wonnacott, 1997). For example, executive function is related to α4β2 stimulation in the ventral tegmental area, the midbrain region that houses dopamine cell bodies that project to the ventral striatum (Nisell, Nomikos, & Svensson, 1994). Stimulation of these receptors triggers dopamine release in various brain regions including the prefrontal cortex, which is central to higher order executive functioning (Arnsten & Jin, 2014; Croxson, Kyriazis, & Baxter, 2011; Livingstone & Wonnacott, 2009; Nocente et al., 2013). Spatial working memory is also impacted by nAChR activity. Spatial memory deficits induced by cortical dopamine depletion were reversed in monkeys following administration of an α7 nAChR agonist (Brozoski, Brown, Rosvold, & Goldman, 1979). Together, converging lines of research suggest that nicotine targets endogenous receptors with alpha and beta subunits that have clear associations with cognition (Bancroft & Levin, 2000; Felix & Levin, 1997; Levin, 2013; Levin, Bradley, Addy, & Sigurani, 2002) through downstream release of multiple neurotransmitters in the brain (Levin et al., 2006).

The precise neural mechanisms that underlie nicotine withdrawal-emergent deficits are not fully understood, but mounting evidence implicates altered nAChR availability as a plausible aberrant pathophysiological mediator. Chronic nicotine administration results in dose-dependent upregulation of nAChRs and desensitization in multiple areas of the brain (Lester & Dani, 1994; Wooltorton, Pidoplichko, Broide, & Dani, 2003) via enhanced induction of long-term potentiation (Welsby, Rowan, & Anwyl, 2006), which has been shown in both humans and rodents (Gentry & Lukas, 2002; Marks et al., 2011; Pauly, Stitzel, Marks, & Collins, 1989; Shoaib, Schindler, Goldberg, & Pauly, 1997; Yates, Bencherif, Fluhler, & Lippiello, 1995). For example, chronic smokers show elevated levels α4β2 nAChRs compared to nonusers in post-mortem pathology analysis in various brain regions such as the cortex and striatum (Benwell, Balfour, & Anderson, 1988; Breese et al., 1997; Cosgrove et al., 2012; Staley et al., 2006). Typically, this upregulation normalizes within as little as one week of abstinence (Breese et al., 1997; Cosgrove et al., 2009; Mamede et al., 2007), yet the degree and persistence of upregulation varies with interindividual factors (eg, more pronounced in men, Cosgrove et al., 2012; more pronounced in menthol cigarette smokers, Brody et al., 2013). Additionally, the extent of upregulation is linked to craving and withdrawal symptoms (Cosgrove et al., 2009; Staley et al., 2006), and the duration of abstinence-associated nAChR upregulation is associated with persistence of cognitive deficits in rodents (Gould et al., 2012). Taken together, this suggests that one potential neurophysiological mediator of nicotine withdrawal may be the high level of unbound α4β2 nAChRs during early abstinence (eg, the first week) that downregulate to relatively normal levels of expression over approximately 30 days of abstinence. Reduced nAChR availability has been linked with the degree of cognitive compromise in Alzheimer disease (Kendziorra et al., 2011; Sabri, Kendziorra, Wolf, Gertz, & Brust, 2008), but nAChR availability in relation to changes in cognition during withdrawal and early abstinence has not been evaluated in humans as of 2016 to our knowledge.

Altered withdrawal-related neural activity and irregular functional network patterns suggest inefficient processing during nicotine deprivation. A consistent finding is a withdrawal-associated diminished inhibition of the default mode network during cognitive tasks (Falcone et al., 2014; Loughead et al., 2010), which is suggestive of a shift in cognitive resources away from the executive control network (Sutherland, McHugh, Pariyadath, & Stein, 2012). For example, Lerman et al. (2014) reported that individuals with 24h of nicotine abstinence exhibited dysregulated inter-network connectivity and reduced suppression of default mode activity in the ventromedial prefrontal and posterior cingulate cortices during a working memory task compared to those who were nicotine satiated. Diminished inhibition of the default mode network has also been associated with reduced accuracy on various cognitive tasks (Eichele et al., 2008; Prado, Carp, & Weissman, 2011). Resumption of smoking and pharmacotherapeutic cessation aids have been reported to downregulate default mode activity (Hahn et al., 2007, 2009), with tighter negative coupling between executive control and default mode networks linearly associated with improved cognitive performance (Cole et al., 2010). These data support the premise that poor cognitive functioning during nicotine withdrawal may be driven by inefficient inhibition of regions and networks typically active in rest and insufficient neural activity in regions and circuits that guide task-related or goal-directed activity.

BENCH TO BEDSIDE MODELS OF COGNITION DURING NICOTINE WITHDRAWAL

Attention

Nicotine enhances performance on tasks involving attentional processing (Barr et al., 2008; Koelega, 1993; Levin et al., 2006; Rezvani & Levin, 2001). Nicotine withdrawal is associated with attentional performance deficits that are accompanied by aberrant task activation including increased BOLD signaling in the parietal cortex, caudate, and thalamus during sustained attention tasks and reduced BOLD in the parahippocampal gyrus, insula, and right frontal regions (Kozink, Lutz, Rose, Froeliger, & McClernon, 2010; Lawrence, Ross, & Stein, 2002), many of which are reversed with nicotine exposure (Beaver et al., 2011). These findings converge with patient reports of difficulty concentrating during nicotine withdrawal (Hughes, 2007b). Preclinical models have shown associations between spontaneous nicotine withdrawal in rats and performance deficits on a 5-choice serial reaction time task, a widely used rodent model of attention (Robbins, 2002). Nicotine withdrawal in the 5-choice serial reaction time task yields an overall decline in the number of correct responses and an increase in the number of omission errors after 10–16h of withdrawal without effect on response accuracy and response latencies (Semenova, Stolerman, & Markou, 2007; Shoaib & Bizarro, 2005). Similar associations have been reported in humans with withdrawal (and with use of nicotinic receptor antagonists), including decreased task accuracy, slower reaction times, greater variability, and increased inhibitory control failures (Harrison, Coppola, & McKee, 2009; Heishman et al., 2010; Kozink et al., 2010; Roh et al., 2014; Wesnes, Edgar, Kezic, Salih, & de Boer, 2013). Generally speaking, attention deficits tend to emerge as soon as 30 min following nicotine discontinuation (Hendricks et al., 2006), but they are short-lasting, with progressive and complete recovery of abilities after a few hours to days of nonuse (Harrison et al., 2009; Kozink et al., 2010; Semenova et al., 2007). Yet, other studies show more rapid resolution of deficits (Ashare & Hawk, 2012; Ashare & McKee, 2012; Jacobsen, Slotkin, Westerveld, Mencl, & Pugh, 2006).

Various pharmacologic treatments attenuate withdrawal-emergent attention deficits. NRTs improve target identification on continuous performance tests compared to placebo after overnight abstinence (Atzori, Lemmonds, Kotler, Durcan, & Boyle, 2008; Beaver et al., 2011; Dawkins, Powell, West, Powell, & Pickering, 2007; Myers et al., 2008). Similarly, varenicline but not bupropion increases correct responding and reduces reaction times following up to 72h of abstinence in some studies (Ashare & McKee, 2012; Patterson et al., 2009). Bupropion has been associated with improved sustained attention during early abstinence in at risk populations with schizophrenia, however (Evins et al., 2005). Although numerous studies have found that poor baseline attention confers risk for relapse, particularly in high risk groups such as those with ADHD and schizophrenia (Culhane et al., 2008; Humfleet et al., 2005; Pomerleau et al., 2003), there have been no studies to date linking attention deficits that specifically emerge during withdrawal to risk for relapse.

Learning and Memory

Nicotine modulation of learning processes has been well documented (Heishman et al., 2010; Jubelt et al., 2008). Animal models show impaired contextual and trace fear conditioning as well as impaired incidental spatial learning, but intact cued fear conditioning and novel object recognition during nicotine withdrawal (Davis, James, Siegel, & Gould, 2005; Kenney, Adoff, Wilkinson, & Gould, 2011; Raybuck & Gould, 2009). These deficits are present following administration of nAChR antagonists (Davis et al., 2005) and are ameliorated by bupropion and varenicline (Portugal & Gould, 2007; Raybuck, Portugal, Lerman, & Gould, 2008). Variability in the nature and extent of deficits has been associated with individual-level factors such as age (Portugal, Wilkinson, Kenney, Sullivan, & Gould, 2012; Portugal, Wilkinson, Turner, Blendy, & Gould, 2012). Additionally, inconsistencies arise with respect to the specific memory processes that are worsened with nicotine withdrawal. Some animal studies implicate compromised encoding and consolidation with spared retrieval capabilities (Davis & Gould, 2009; Kenney & Gould, 2008a, 2008b), whereas human models clearly demonstrate worsened delayed recall accuracy and recognition memory (Hirshman, Rhodes, Zinser, & Merritt, 2004; Wesnes et al., 2013) that is not simply an artifact of diminished attention at the time of encoding (Merritt, Cobb, Moissinac, & Hirshman, 2010). Chronic nicotine exposure may result in neural adaptation in the hippocampus and subsequent desensitization of hippocampal $\beta2$ nAChR subunits (eg, $\alpha4\beta2$ nAChRs) as well as altered downstream cell-signaling processes (eg, long-term potentiation) in the hippocampus (Davis & Gould, 2008, 2009; Gentry & Lukas, 2002). This neural adaptation could account for deficits in learning processes that may be experienced during withdrawal among smokers.

Working Memory

Nicotine withdrawal is associated with working memory deficits that predict subsequent relapse. Animal models reveal deficits on the radial-arm maze (Levin et al., 1990; LevinMcClernon, & Rezvani, 2006) during nicotine withdrawal and reversal of these decrements with the re-introduction of nicotine (Bettany & Levin, 2001; Levin, Christopher, Briggs, & Rose, 1993). Further, nAChR antagonist infusions reduce working memory performance, but only when these infusions are targeted to the hippocampus or mesencephalic structures (eg, substantia nigra, ventral tegmental area) that serve as inputs to circuits central to reward, addiction, and cognition (Bancroft & Levin, 2000; Bettany & Levin, 2001; Cannady et al., 2009; Kim & Levin, 1996; Levin, Briggs, Christopher, & Auman, 1994). Many studies similarly find less accurate and slower reaction times on working memory tasks (eg, N-back) among smokers following overnight abstinence (Falcone et al., 2014; Jacobsen et al., 2005; Mendrek et al., 2006; Myers et al., 2008) (but see Greenstein & Kassel, 2009; Jacobsen, Pugh, Constable, Westerveld, & Mencl, 2007; Sweet et al.,

2010; Wesnes et al., 2013; Xu et al., 2005). Working memory deficits during abstinence are amplified as task demands increase (Jacobsen et al., 2007; Loughead et al., 2009, 2010; Mendrek et al., 2006). One of the greatest difficulties for examining mechanisms of withdrawal-induced working memory deficits across species is the differences in assessment between rodents and humans, especially comparing to classic human tests such as the N-back task (Dudchenko, Talpos, Young, & Baxter, 2013).

Functional imaging studies suggest insufficient neural activation to meet the cognitive demands necessary for effective working memory during early withdrawal, with insufficient deactivation of the default mode network. For example, nicotine withdrawal is associated with reduced working memory activation in the dorsolateral prefrontal cortex and medial frontal and anterior cingulate gyrus (Falcone et al., 2014; Loughead et al., 2010; Xu et al., 2005, 2006), decreased suppression of default mode network nodes, posterior cingulate cortex and ventromedial prefrontal cortex (Beaver et al., 2011; Falcone et al., 2014; Loughead et al., 2010), as well as disrupted internetwork connectivity (Jacobsen et al., 2007; Lerman et al., 2014; Sutherland, Carroll, Salmeron, Ross, & Stein, 2013). Few differences in hippocampal function following withdrawal in humans further highlight rodent to human differences in mechanisms (Dudchenko et al., 2013). Withdrawal-emergent behavioral and neural working memory deficits are mitigated by treatments such as NRT, varenicline, and bupropion (Ashare & McKee, 2012; Atzori et al., 2008; Loughead et al., 2010; Patterson et al., 2009; Perkins, Karelitz, Jao, Gur, & Lerman, 2013). Importantly, working memory deficits and related neural activation patterns predict relapse liability (Loughead et al., 2015; Patterson et al., 2010), perhaps due to the central role of working memory in maintaining mental representations of goal-related information (Barr et al., 2008; Evins et al., 2005; Jubelt et al., 2008). However, to the best of our knowledge, studies have only shown these effects at a group level, but yet not translated to an individual level to determine whether working memory deficits and associated functional activation during abstinence is associated with interindividual variability in cessation success rates.

Response Inhibition

Spontaneous and antagonist-induced nicotine withdrawal has been associated with poor response inhibition in both animal (Day et al., 2007; Kirshenbaum et al., 2011; Shoaib & Bizarro, 2005) as well as human investigations using stop signal tasks (Ashare & Hawk, 2012), go/no-go tasks (Harrison et al., 2009; Sofuoglu, Herman, Li, & Waters, 2012), continuous performance tests (Harrison et al., 2009), and inhibitory control tasks (Tsaur, Strasser, Souprountchouk, Evans, & Ashare, 2015). These deficits, evidenced by premature responding and failed inhibitions, are mitigated by re-exposure to nicotine (Dawkins et al., 2007). Functional neuroimaging studies, though limited to date, have implicated exaggerated task-related activation in regions of the executive control network such as the anterior cingulate cortex and right inferior and middle frontal cortex, which may suggest inefficient executive function processing during nicotine withdrawal (Azizian et al., 2010; Froeliger, Modlin, Wang, Kozink, & McClernon, 2012; Kozink et al., 2010). The clinical relevance of these deficits have been clearly established because although they do not necessarily occur in parallel to peak craving (Tsaur et al., 2015), they have been reported to predict relapse to smoking up to 3 months after quitting (Krishnan-Sarin et al., 2007; Powell, Dawkins, West, Powell, & Pickering, 2010). These findings suggest that diminished response inhibition may be reflected in an inability to suppress prepotent responses such as habitual smoking (Janes, Pizzagalli, Richardt, Frederick Bde, Chuzi, et al., 2010; Janes, Pizzagalli, Richardt, Frederick Bde, Holmes, et al., 2010).

SUMMARY AND CONCLUSIONS

Cognitive disruption represents a central feature of the nicotine withdrawal syndrome: it is both commonly endorsed among treatment seekers (Covey, Manubay, Jiang, Nortick, & Palumbo, 2008; Hughes, 2007b; Rukstalis et al., 2005) as well as frequently exhibited on a variety of objective neurocognitive paradigms across domains of attention, learning and memory, working memory, and response inhibition. The emergence of cognitive deficits during withdrawal are generally thought to be associated with time-limited continued upregulation of nAChRs during a period in which nicotine is no longer present, altered neuronal plasticity as well as alterations in regional and network functional activity. Neuroimaging and neurocognitive studies together point to overall ineffective cognitive processing during nicotine withdrawal, evidenced primarily by insufficient recruitment in task-dependent regions, inefficient deactivation of task-independent regions, and altered regional connectivity. However, the precise physiological mechanisms that subserve cognitive deficits during withdrawal remain largely unknown, and the expression of these deficits may vary according to several interindividual factors such as genetics (Herman & Sofuoglu, 2010), gender (Jacobsen et al., 2005; McClernon, Kozink, & Rose, 2008; Merritt, Cobb, & Cook, 2012), age (Falcone et al., 2014), and psychiatric comorbidity (eg, schizophrenia and ADHD; AhnAllen, Nestor, Shenton, McCarley, & Niznikiewicz, 2008; Barr et al., 2008; George et al., 2002; Jubelt et al., 2008; Kollins, McClernon, & Epstein, 2009; Sacco et al., 2005).

The time course of cognitive symptoms relative to smoking cessation, involving an onset of symptoms within 30–120 min of abstinence (Hendricks et al., 2006) and peak of intensity with 7 days abstinence (Hughes, 2007b), overlaps with the time when the vast majority of recently quit smokers resume using (Ashare et al., 2013), and the extent of deficits during withdrawal predict relapse. The suggestion that diminished cognitive capacity during withdrawal may serve as a critical trigger for risk to relapse is theoretically plausible given that cognitive deficits may manifest in increased difficulties maintaining goal-directed behavior and motivation as well as resisting smoking urges and engaging in effective, efficient, and flexible decision-making. However, future studies need to translate group-level findings to the individual. For example, are those for whom varenicline or NRT do not reverse or ameliorate withdrawal-related cognitive deficits more likely to relapse, and if so, how early does this occur?

Given that cognitive deficits emerge early during withdrawal and follow a parallel time course as the reinstatement of normal neuronal activity and risk for relapse, much work has been done developing pharmacotherapies that enhance cognition in hopes that this will reduce the risk for early relapse (Brady, Gray, & Tolliver, 2011; Sofuoglu, DeVito, Waters, & Carroll, 2013). Preliminary animal and human studies have found that nAChR agonists do, indeed, reduce cognitive deficits and reduce relapse rates (Loughead et al., 2010; Raybuck et al., 2008). However, given that relapse rates remain high even when agents such as varenicline or bupropion are used, alternative agents and strategies should be explored, as reviewed by Ashare and Schmidt (2014). Additionally, only correlations between cognition and risk for relapse have been established, and future translational studies are critically needed that empirically examine cognition as a mediator between withdrawal and relapse.

References

AhnAllen, C. G., Nestor, P. G., Shenton, M. E., McCarley, R. W., & Niznikiewicz, M. A. (2008). Early nicotine withdrawal and transdermal nicotine effects on neurocognitive performance in schizophrenia. Schizophrenia Research, 100(1–3), 261–269. http://dx.doi.org/10.1016/j.schres.2007.07.030.

Albuquerque, E. X., Pereira, E. F., Alkondon, M., & Rogers, S. W. (2009). Mammalian nicotinic acetylcholine receptors: from structure to function. Physiological Reviews, 89(1), 73–120. http://dx.doi.org/10.1152/physrev.00015.2008.

Arnsten, A. F., & Jin, L. E. (2014). Molecular influences on working memory circuits in dorsolateral prefrontal cortex. Progress in Molecular Biology and Translational Science, 122, 211–231. http://dx.doi.org/10.1016/B978-0-12-420170-5.00008-8.

Ashare, R. L., & Hawk, L. W., Jr. (2012). Effects of smoking abstinence on impulsive behavior among smokers high and low in ADHD-like symptoms. Psychopharmacology, 219(2), 537–547. http://dx.doi.org/10.1007/s00213-011-2324-2.

Ashare, R. L., & McKee, S. A. (2012). Effects of varenicline and bupropion on cognitive processes among nicotine-deprived smokers. Experimental and Clinical Psychopharmacology, 20(1), 63–70. http://dx.doi.org/10.1037/a0025594.

Ashare, R. L., & Schmidt, H. D. (2014). Optimizing treatments for nicotine dependence by increasing cognitive performance during withdrawal. *Expert Opinion on Drug Discovery, 9*(6), 579–594. http://dx.doi.org/10.1517/17460441.2014.908180.

Ashare, R. L., Wileyto, E. P., Perkins, K. A., & Schnoll, R. A. (2013). The first 7 days of a quit attempt predicts relapse: validation of a measure for screening medications for nicotine dependence. *Journal of Addictive Medicine, 7*(4), 249–254. http://dx.doi.org/10.1097/ADM.0b013e31829363e1.

Atzori, G., Lemmonds, C. A., Kotler, M. L., Durcan, M. J., & Boyle, J. (2008). Efficacy of a nicotine (4 mg)-containing lozenge on the cognitive impairment of nicotine withdrawal. *Journal of Clinical Psychopharmacology, 28*(6), 667–674. http://dx.doi.org/10.1097/JCP.0b013e31818c9bb8.

Azizian, A., Nestor, L. J., Payer, D., Monterosso, J. R., Brody, A. L., & London, E. D. (2010). Smoking reduces conflict-related anterior cingulate activity in abstinent cigarette smokers performing a stroop task. *Neuropsychopharmacology: Official Publication of the American College of Neuropsychopharmacology, 35*(3), 775–782. http://dx.doi.org/10.1038/npp.2009.186.

Bancroft, A., & Levin, E. D. (2000). Ventral hippocampal alpha4beta2 nicotinic receptors and chronic nicotine effects on memory. *Neuropharmacology, 39*(13), 2770–2778.

Barr, R. S., Culhane, M. A., Jubelt, L. E., Mufti, R. S., Dyer, M. A., Weiss, A. P., ... Evins, A. E. (2008). The effects of transdermal nicotine on cognition in nonsmokers with schizophrenia and nonpsychiatric controls. *Neuropsychopharmacology: Official Publication of the American College of Neuropsychopharmacology, 33*(3), 480–490. http://dx.doi.org/10.1038/sj.npp.1301423.

Beaver, J. D., Long, C. J., Cole, D. M., Durcan, M. J., Bannon, L. C., Mishra, R. G., & Matthews, P. M. (2011). The effects of nicotine replacement on cognitive brain activity during smoking withdrawal studied with simultaneous fMRI/EEG. *Neuropsychopharmacology: Official Publication of the American College of Neuropsychopharmacology, 36*(9), 1792–1800. http://dx.doi.org/10.1038/npp.2011.53.

Benwell, M. E., Balfour, D. J., & Anderson, J. M. (1988). Evidence that tobacco smoking increases the density of (-)-[3H]nicotine binding sites in human brain. *Journal of Neurochemistry, 50*(4), 1243–1247.

Bettany, J. H., & Levin, E. D. (2001). Ventral hippocampal alpha 7 nicotinic receptor blockade and chronic nicotine effects on memory performance in the radial-arm maze. *Pharmacology, Biochemistry, and Behavior, 70*(4), 467–474.

Brady, K. T., Gray, K. M., & Tolliver, B. K. (2011). Cognitive enhancers in the treatment of substance use disorders: clinical evidence. *Pharmacology, Biochemistry, and Behavior, 99*(2), 285–294. http://dx.doi.org/10.1016/j.pbb.2011.04.017.

Breese, C. R., Marks, M. J., Logel, J., Adams, C. E., Sullivan, B., Collins, A. C., et al. (1997). Effect of smoking history on [3H]nicotine binding in human postmortem brain. *The Journal of Pharmacology and Experimental Therapeutics, 282*(1), 7–13.

Brody, A. L., Mandelkern, M. A., Costello, M. R., Abrams, A. L., Scheibal, D., Farahi, J., ... Mukhin, A. G. (2009). Brain nicotinic acetylcholine receptor occupancy: effect of smoking a denicotinized cigarette. *International Journal of Neuropsychopharmacology, 12*(3), 305–316. http://dx.doi.org/10.1017/S146114570800922X.

Brody, A. L., Mandelkern, M. A., London, E. D., Olmstead, R. E., Farahi, J., Scheibal, D., ... Mukhin, A. G. (2006). Cigarette smoking saturates brain alpha 4 beta 2 nicotinic acetylcholine receptors. *Archives of General Psychiatry, 63*(8), 907–915. http://dx.doi.org/10.1001/archpsyc.63.8.907.

Brody, A. L., Mukhin, A. G., La Charite, J., Ta, K., Farahi, J., Sugar, C. A., ... Mandelkern, M. A. (2013). Up-regulation of nicotinic acetylcholine receptors in menthol cigarette smokers. *International Journal of Neuropsychopharmacology, 16*(5), 957–966. http://dx.doi.org/10.1017/S1461145712001022.

Brozoski, T. J., Brown, R. M., Rosvold, H. E., & Goldman, P. S. (1979). Cognitive deficit caused by regional depletion of dopamine in prefrontal cortex of rhesus monkey. *Science, 205*(4409), 929–932.

Cahill, K., Stevens, S., & Lancaster, T. (2014). Pharmacological treatments for smoking cessation. *JAMA, 311*(2), 193–194. http://dx.doi.org/10.1001/jama.2013.283787.

Cannady, R., Weir, R., Wee, B., Gotschlich, E., Kolia, N., Lau, E., … Levin, E. D. (2009). Nicotinic antagonist effects in the mediodorsal thalamic nucleus: regional heterogeneity of nicotinic receptor involvement in cognitive function. *Biochemical Pharmacology, 78*(7), 788–794. http://dx.doi.org/10.1016/j.bcp.2009.05.021.

Clinical Practice Guideline Treating Tobacco, U., Dependence Update Panel, L., & Staff. (2008). A clinical practice guideline for treating tobacco use and dependence: 2008 update. A U.S. Public Health Service report. *American Journal of Preventive Medicine, 35*(2), 158–176. http://dx.doi.org/10.1016/j.amepre.2008.04.009.

Cole, D. M., Beckmann, C. F., Long, C. J., Matthews, P. M., Durcan, M. J., & Beaver, J. D. (2010). Nicotine replacement in abstinent smokers improves cognitive withdrawal symptoms with modulation of resting brain network dynamics. *Neuroimage, 52*(2), 590–599. http://dx.doi.org/10.1016/j.neuroimage.2010.04.251.

Cosgrove, K. P., Batis, J., Bois, F., Maciejewski, P. K., Esterlis, I., Kloczynski, T., … Staley, J. K. (2009). beta2-Nicotinic acetylcholine receptor availability during acute and prolonged abstinence from tobacco smoking. *Archives of General Psychiatry, 66*(6), 666–676. http://dx.doi.org/10.1001/archgenpsychiatry.2009.41.

Cosgrove, K. P., Esterlis, I., McKee, S. A., Bois, F., Seibyl, J. P., Mazure, C. M., … O'Malley, S. S. (2012). Sex differences in availability of beta2*-nicotinic acetylcholine receptors in recently abstinent tobacco smokers. *Archives of General Psychiatry, 69*(4), 418–427. http://dx.doi.org/10.1001/archgenpsychiatry.2011.1465.

Covey, L. S., Manubay, J., Jiang, H., Nortick, M., & Palumbo, D. (2008). Smoking cessation and inattention or hyperactivity/impulsivity: a post hoc analysis. *Nicotine & Tobacco Research: Official Journal of the Society for Research on Nicotine and Tobacco, 10*(12), 1717–1725. http://dx.doi.org/10.1080/14622200802443536.

Croxson, P. L., Kyriazis, D. A., & Baxter, M. G. (2011). Cholinergic modulation of a specific memory function of prefrontal cortex. *Nature Neuroscience, 14*(12), 1510–1512. http://dx.doi.org/10.1038/nn.2971.

Culhane, M. A., Schoenfeld, D. A., Barr, R. S., Cather, C., Deckersbach, T., Freudenreich, O., … & Evins, A. E. (2008). Predictors of early abstinence in smokers with schizophrenia. *Journal of Clinical Psychiatry, 69*(11), 1743–1750.

Davis, J. A., & Gould, T. J. (2008). Associative learning, the hippocampus, and nicotine addiction. *Current Drug Abuse Reviews, 1*(1), 9–19.

Davis, J. A., & Gould, T. J. (2009). Hippocampal nAChRs mediate nicotine withdrawal-related learning deficits. *European Neuropsychopharmacology: the Journal of the European College of Neuropsychopharmacology, 19*(8), 551–561. http://dx.doi.org/10.1016/j.euroneuro.2009.02.003.

Davis, J. A., James, J. R., Siegel, S. J., & Gould, T. J. (2005). Withdrawal from chronic nicotine administration impairs contextual fear conditioning in C57BL/6 mice. *The Journal of Neuroscience: the Official Journal of the Society for Neuroscience, 25*(38), 8708–8713. http://dx.doi.org/10.1523/JNEUROSCI.2853-05.2005.

Dawkins, L., Powell, J. H., West, R., Powell, J., & Pickering, A. (2007). A double-blind placebo-controlled experimental study of nicotine: II–Effects on response inhibition and executive functioning. *Psychopharmacology, 190*(4), 457–467. http://dx.doi.org/10.1007/s00213-006-0634-6.

Day, M., Pan, J. B., Buckley, M. J., Cronin, E., Hollingsworth, P. R., Hirst, W. D., … Fox, G. B. (2007). Differential effects of ciproxifan and nicotine on impulsivity and attention measures in the 5-choice serial reaction time test. *Biochemical Pharmacology, 73*(8), 1123–1134. http://dx.doi.org/10.1016/j.bcp.2006.12.004.

Dudchenko, P. A., Talpos, J., Young, J. W., & Baxter, M. G. (2013). Animal models of working memory: a review of tasks that might be useful in screening drug treatments for the memory impairments found in schizophrenia. *Neuroscience and Biobehavioral Reviews, 37*(9), 2111–2124.

Eichele, T., Debener, S., Calhoun, V. D., Specht, K., Engel, A. K., Hugdahl, K., … Ullsperger, M. (2008). Prediction of human errors by maladaptive changes in event-related brain networks. *Proceedings of the National Academy of Science USA, 105*(16), 6173–6178. http://dx.doi.org/10.1073/pnas.0708965105.

Evins, A. E., Deckersbach, T., Cather, C., Freudenreich, O., Culhane, M. A., Henderson, D. C., … Goff, D. C. (2005). Independent effects of tobacco abstinence and bupropion on cognitive function in schizophrenia. *Journal of Clinical Psychiatry, 66*(9), 1184–1190.

Falcone, M., Wileyto, E. P., Ruparel, K., Gerraty, R. T., LaPrate, L., Detre, J. A., … Lerman, C. (2014). Age-related differences in working memory deficits during nicotine withdrawal. *Addiction Biology, 19*(5), 907–917. http://dx.doi.org/10.1111/adb.12051.

Felix, R., & Levin, E. D. (1997). Nicotinic antagonist administration into the ventral hippocampus and spatial working memory in rats. *Neuroscience, 81*(4), 1009–1017.

Froeliger, B., Modlin, L., Wang, L., Kozink, R. V., & McClernon, F. J. (2012). Nicotine withdrawal modulates frontal brain function during an affective Stroop task. *Psychopharmacology, 220*(4), 707–718. http://dx.doi.org/10.1007/s00213-011-2522-y.

Gentry, C. L., & Lukas, R. J. (2002). Regulation of nicotinic acetylcholine receptor numbers and function by chronic nicotine exposure. *Current Drug Targets CNS Neurological Disorder, 1*(4), 359–385.

George, T. P., Vessicchio, J. C., Termine, A., Sahady, D. M., Head, C. A., Pepper, W. T., … Wexler, B. E. (2002). Effects of smoking abstinence on visuospatial working memory function in schizophrenia. *Neuropsychopharmacology: Official Publication of the American College of Neuropsychopharmacology, 26*(1), 75–85. http://dx.doi.org/10.1016/S0893-133X(01)00296-2.

Gilbert, D., McClernon, J., Rabinovich, N., Sugai, C., Plath, L., Asgaard, G., … Botros, N. (2004). Effects of quitting smoking on EEG activation and attention last for more than 31 days and are more severe with stress, dependence, DRD2 A1 allele, and depressive traits. *Nicotine & Tobacco Research: Official Journal of the Society for Research on Nicotine and Tobacco, 6*(2), 249–267. http://dx.doi.org/10.1080/14622200410001676305.

Gould, T. J., Portugal, G. S., Andre, J. M., Tadman, M. P., Marks, M. J., Kenney, J. W., … Adoff, M. (2012). The duration of nicotine withdrawal-associated deficits in contextual fear conditioning parallels changes in hippocampal high affinity nicotinic acetylcholine receptor upregulation. *Neuropharmacology, 62*(5–6), 2118–2125. http://dx.doi.org/10.1016/j.neuropharm.2012.01.003.

Greenstein, J. E., & Kassel, J. D. (2009). The effects of smoking and smoking abstinence on verbal and visuospatial working memory capacity. *Experimental and Clinical Psychopharmacology, 17*(2), 78–90. http://dx.doi.org/10.1037/a0015699.

Hahn, B., Ross, T. J., Wolkenberg, F. A., Shakleya, D. M., Huestis, M. A., & Stein, E. A. (2009). Performance effects of nicotine during selective attention, divided attention, and simple stimulus detection: an fMRI study. *Cerebral Cortex, 19*(9), 1990–2000. http://dx.doi.org/10.1093/cercor/bhn226.

Hahn, B., Ross, T. J., Yang, Y., Kim, I., Huestis, M. A., & Stein, E. A. (2007). Nicotine enhances visuospatial attention by deactivating areas of the resting brain default network. *The Journal of Neuroscience: the Official Journal of the Society for Neuroscience, 27*(13), 3477–3489. http://dx.doi.org/10.1523/JNEUROSCI.5129-06.2007.

Harrison, E. L., Coppola, S., & McKee, S. A. (2009). Nicotine deprivation and trait impulsivity affect smokers' performance on cognitive tasks of inhibition and attention. *Experimental and Clinical Psychopharmacology, 17*(2), 91–98. http://dx.doi.org/10.1037/a0015657.

Heishman, S. J., Kleykamp, B. A., & Singleton, E. G. (2010). Meta-analysis of the acute effects of nicotine and smoking on human performance. *Psychopharmacology, 210*(4), 453–469. http://dx.doi.org/10.1007/s00213-010-1848-1.

Hendricks, P. S., Ditre, J. W., Drobes, D. J., & Brandon, T. H. (2006). The early time course of smoking withdrawal effects. *Psychopharmacology, 187*(3), 385–396. http://dx.doi.org/10.1007/s00213-006-0429-9.

Herman, A. I., & Sofuoglu, M. (2010). Cognitive effects of nicotine: genetic moderators. *Addiction Biology, 15*(3), 250–265. http://dx.doi.org/10.1111/j.1369-1600.2010.00213.x.

Hirshman, E., Rhodes, D. K., Zinser, M., & Merritt, P. (2004). The effect of tobacco abstinence on recognition memory, digit span recall, and attentional vigilance. *Experimental and Clinical Psychopharmacology, 12*(1), 76–83. http://dx.doi.org/10.1037/1064-1297.12.1.76.

Hughes, J. R. (2004). Nicotine dependence and WHO mental health surveys. *JAMA, 292*(9), 1021–1022. http://dx.doi.org/10.1001/jama.292.9.1021-c Author reply 1022.

Hughes, J. R. (2007a). Effects of abstinence from tobacco: etiology, animal models, epidemiology, and significance: a subjective review. *Nicotine & Tobacco Research: Official Journal of the Society for Research on Nicotine and Tobacco, 9*(3), 329–339. http://dx.doi.org/10.1080/14622200701188927.

Hughes, J. R. (2007b). Effects of abstinence from tobacco: valid symptoms and time course. *Nicotine & Tobacco Research: Official Journal of the Society for Research on Nicotine and Tobacco, 9*(3), 315–327. http://dx.doi.org/10.1080/14622200701188919.

Humfleet, G. L., Prochaska, J. J., Mengis, M., Cullen, J., Munoz, R., Reus, V., et al. (2005). Preliminary evidence of the association between the history of childhood attention-deficit/hyperactivity disorder and smoking treatment failure. *Nicotine & Tobacco Research: Official Journal of the Society for Research on Nicotine and Tobacco, 7*(3), 453–460. http://dx.doi.org/10.1080/14622200500125310.

Jacobsen, L. K., Krystal, J. H., Mencl, W. E., Westerveld, M., Frost, S. J., & Pugh, K. R. (2005). Effects of smoking and smoking abstinence on cognition in adolescent tobacco smokers. *Biological Psychiatry, 57*(1), 56–66. http://dx.doi.org/10.1016/j.biopsych.2004.10.022.

Jacobsen, L. K., Pugh, K. R., Constable, R. T., Westerveld, M., & Mencl, W. E. (2007). Functional correlates of verbal memory deficits emerging during nicotine withdrawal in abstinent adolescent cannabis users. *Biological Psychiatry, 61*(1), 31–40. http://dx.doi.org/10.1016/j.biopsych.2006.02.014.

Jacobsen, L. K., Slotkin, T. A., Westerveld, M., Mencl, W. E., & Pugh, K. R. (2006). Visuospatial memory deficits emerging during nicotine withdrawal in adolescents with prenatal exposure to active maternal smoking. *Neuropsychopharmacology: Official Publication of the American College of Neuropsychopharmacology, 31*(7), 1550–1561. http://dx.doi.org/10.1038/sj.npp.1300981.

Janes, A. C., Pizzagalli, D. A., Richardt, S., Frederick Bde, B., Chuzi, S., Pachas, G., … Kaufman, M. J. (2010). Brain reactivity to smoking cues prior to smoking cessation predicts ability to maintain tobacco abstinence. *Biological Psychiatry, 67*(8), 722–729. http://dx.doi.org/10.1016/j.biopsych.2009.12.034.

Janes, A. C., Pizzagalli, D. A., Richardt, S., Frederick Bde, B., Holmes, A. J., Sousa, J., … Kaufman, M. J. (2010). Neural substrates of attentional bias for smoking-related cues: an FMRI study. *Neuropsychopharmacology: Official Publication of the American College of Neuropsychopharmacology, 35*(12), 2339–2345. http://dx.doi.org/10.1038/npp.2010.103.

Jubelt, L. E., Barr, R. S., Goff, D. C., Logvinenko, T., Weiss, A. P., & Evins, A. E. (2008). Effects of transdermal nicotine on episodic memory in non-smokers with and without schizophrenia. *Psychopharmacology, 199*(1), 89–98. http://dx.doi.org/10.1007/s00213-008-1133-8.

Kendziorra, K., Wolf, H., Meyer, P. M., Barthel, H., Hesse, S., Becker, G. A., … Sabri, O. (2011). Decreased cerebral alpha4beta2* nicotinic acetylcholine receptor availability in patients with mild cognitive impairment and Alzheimer's disease assessed with positron emission tomography. *European Journal of Nuclear Medicine and Molecular Imaging, 38*(3), 515–525. http://dx.doi.org/10.1007/s00259-010-1644-5.

Kenney, J. W., Adoff, M. D., Wilkinson, D. S., & Gould, T. J. (2011). The effects of acute, chronic, and withdrawal from chronic nicotine on novel and spatial object recognition in male C57BL/6J mice. *Psychopharmacology, 217*(3), 353–365. http://dx.doi.org/10.1007/s00213-011-2283-7.

Kenney, J. W., & Gould, T. J. (2008a). Modulation of hippocampus-dependent learning and synaptic plasticity by nicotine. *Molecular Neurobiology, 38*(1), 101–121. http://dx.doi. org/10.1007/s12035-008-8037-9.

Kenney, J. W., & Gould, T. J. (2008b). Nicotine enhances context learning but not context-shock associative learning. *Behavioral Neuroscience, 122*(5), 1158–1165. http://dx.doi. org/10.1037/a0012807.

Kim, J. S., & Levin, E. D. (1996). Nicotinic, muscarinic and dopaminergic actions in the ventral hippocampus and the nucleus accumbens: effects on spatial working memory in rats. *Brain Research, 725*(2), 231–240.

Kirshenbaum, A. P., Jackson, E. R., Brown, S. J., Fuchs, J. R., Miltner, B. C., & Doughty, A. H. (2011). Nicotine-induced impulsive action: sensitization and attenuation by mecamylamine. *Behavioural Pharmacology, 22*(3), 207–221. http://dx.doi.org/10.1097/ FBP.0b013e328345ca1c.

Koelega, H. S. (1993). Stimulant drugs and vigilance performance: a review. *Psychopharmacology, 111*(1), 1–16.

Kollins, S. H., McClernon, F. J., & Epstein, J. N. (2009). Effects of smoking abstinence on reaction time variability in smokers with and without ADHD: an ex-Gaussian analysis. *Drug and Alcohol Dependence, 100*(1–2), 169–172. http://dx.doi.org/10.1016/j. drugalcdep.2008.09.019.

Kozink, R. V., Lutz, A. M., Rose, J. E., Froeliger, B., & McClernon, F. J. (2010). Smoking withdrawal shifts the spatiotemporal dynamics of neurocognition. *Addiction Biology, 15*(4), 480–490. http://dx.doi.org/10.1111/j.1369-1600.2010.00252.x.

Krishnan-Sarin, S., Reynolds, B., Duhig, A. M., Smith, A., Liss, T., McFetridge, A., … Potenza, M. N. (2007). Behavioral impulsivity predicts treatment outcome in a smoking cessation program for adolescent smokers. *Drug and Alcohol Dependence, 88*(1), 79–82. http:// dx.doi.org/10.1016/j.drugalcdep.2006.09.006.

Lawrence, N. S., Ross, T. J., & Stein, E. A. (2002). Cognitive mechanisms of nicotine on visual attention. *Neuron, 36*(3), 539–548.

Lerman, C., Gu, H., Loughead, J., Ruparel, K., Yang, Y., & Stein, E. A. (2014). Large-scale brain network coupling predicts acute nicotine abstinence effects on craving and cognitive function. *JAMA Psychiatry, 71*(5), 523–530. http://dx.doi.org/10.1001/ jamapsychiatry.2013.4091.

Lester, R. A., & Dani, J. A. (1994). Time-dependent changes in central nicotinic acetylcholine channel kinetics in excised patches. *Neuropharmacology, 33*(1), 27–34.

Levin, E. D. (2013). Complex relationships of nicotinic receptor actions and cognitive functions. *Biochemical Pharmacology, 86*(8), 1145–1152. http://dx.doi.org/10.1016/j.bcp.2013.07.021.

Levin, E. D., Bradley, A., Addy, N., & Sigurani, N. (2002). Hippocampal alpha 7 and alpha 4 beta 2 nicotinic receptors and working memory. *Neuroscience, 109*(4), 757–765.

Levin, E. D., Briggs, S. J., Christopher, N. C., & Auman, J. T. (1994). Working memory performance and cholinergic effects in the ventral tegmental area and substantia nigra. *Brain Research, 657*(1–2), 165–170.

Levin, E. D., Christopher, N. C., Briggs, S. J., & Rose, J. E. (1993). Chronic nicotine reverses working memory deficits caused by lesions of the fimbria or medial basalocortical projection. *Brain Research Cognitive Brain Research, 1*(3), 137–143.

Levin, E. D., Lee, C., Rose, J. E., Reyes, A., Ellison, G., Jarvik, M., & Gritz, E. (1990). Chronic nicotine and withdrawal effects on radial-arm maze performance in rats. *Behavioral and Neural Biology, 53*(2), 269–276.

Levin, E. D., McClernon, F. J., & Rezvani, A. H. (2006). Nicotinic effects on cognitive function: behavioral characterization, pharmacological specification, and anatomic localization. *Psychopharmacology, 184*(3–4), 523–539. http://dx.doi.org/10.1007/s00213-005-0164-7.

Livingstone, P. D., & Wonnacott, S. (2009). Nicotinic acetylcholine receptors and the ascending dopamine pathways. *Biochemical Pharmacology, 78*(7), 744–755. http://dx.doi. org/10.1016/j.bcp.2009.06.004.

Lotfipour, S., Mandelkern, M., Alvarez-Estrada, M., & Brody, A. L. (2012). A single administration of low-dose varenicline saturates alpha4beta2* nicotinic acetylcholine receptors in the human brain. *Neuropsychopharmacology: Official Publication of the American College of Neuropsychopharmacology, 37*(7), 1738–1748. http://dx.doi.org/10.1038/npp.2012.20.

Loughead, J., Ray, R., Wileyto, E. P., Ruparel, K., Sanborn, P., Siegel, S., ... & Lerman, C. (2010). Effects of the alpha4beta2 partial agonist varenicline on brain activity and working memory in abstinent smokers. *Biological Psychiatry, 67*(8), 715–721. http://dx.doi.org/10.1016/j.biopsych.2010.01.016.

Loughead, J., Wileyto, E. P., Ruparel, K., Falcone, M., Hopson, R., Gur, R., et al. (2015). Working memory-related neural activity predicts future smoking relapse. *Neuropsychopharmacology: Official Publication of the American College of Neuropsychopharmacology, 40*(6), 1311–1320. http://dx.doi.org/10.1038/npp.2014.318.

Loughead, J., Wileyto, E. P., Valdez, J. N., Sanborn, P., Tang, K., Strasser, A. A., ... Lerman, C. (2009). Effect of abstinence challenge on brain function and cognition in smokers differs by COMT genotype. *Molecular Psychiatry, 14*(8), 820–826. http://dx.doi.org/10.1038/mp.2008.132.

Mamede, M., Ishizu, K., Ueda, M., Mukai, T., Iida, Y., Kawashima, H., ... Saji, H. (2007). Temporal change in human nicotinic acetylcholine receptor after smoking cessation: 5IA SPECT study. *Journal of Nuclear Medicine: Official Publication, Society of Nuclear Medicine, 48*(11), 1829–1835. http://dx.doi.org/10.2967/jnumed.107.043471.

Marks, M. J., McClure-Begley, T. D., Whiteaker, P., Salminen, O., Brown, R. W., Cooper, J., ... Lindstrom, J. M. (2011). Increased nicotinic acetylcholine receptor protein underlies chronic nicotine-induced up-regulation of nicotinic agonist binding sites in mouse brain. *The Journal of Pharmacology and Experimental Therapeutics, 337*(1), 187–200. http://dx.doi.org/10.1124/jpet.110.178236.

McClernon, F. J., Kozink, R. V., & Rose, J. E. (2008). Individual differences in nicotine dependence, withdrawal symptoms, and sex predict transient fMRI-BOLD responses to smoking cues. *Neuropsychopharmacology: Official Publication of the American College of Neuropsychopharmacology, 33*(9), 2148–2157. http://dx.doi.org/10.1038/sj.npp.1301618.

Mendrek, A., Monterosso, J., Simon, S. L., Jarvik, M., Brody, A., Olmstead, R., ... London, E. D. (2006). Working memory in cigarette smokers: comparison to non-smokers and effects of abstinence. *Addictive Behaviors, 31*(5), 833–844. http://dx.doi.org/10.1016/j.addbeh.2005.06.009.

Merritt, P. S., Cobb, A. R., & Cook, G. I. (2012). Sex differences in the cognitive effects of tobacco abstinence: a pilot study. *Experimental and Clinical Psychopharmacology, 20*(4), 258–263. http://dx.doi.org/10.1037/a0027414.

Merritt, P. S., Cobb, A. R., Moissinac, L., & Hirshman, E. (2010). Evidence that episodic memory impairment during tobacco abstinence is independent of attentional mechanisms. *The Journal of General Psychology, 137*(4), 331–342. http://dx.doi.org/10.1080/00221309.2010.499395.

Myers, C. S., Taylor, R. C., Moolchan, E. T., & Heishman, S. J. (2008). Dose-related enhancement of mood and cognition in smokers administered nicotine nasal spray. *Neuropsychopharmacology: Official Publication of the American College of Neuropsychopharmacology, 33*(3), 588–598. http://dx.doi.org/10.1038/sj.npp.1301425.

Nisell, M., Nomikos, G. G., & Svensson, T. H. (1994). Infusion of nicotine in the ventral tegmental area or the nucleus accumbens of the rat differentially affects accumbal dopamine release. *Pharmacology and Toxicology, 75*(6), 348–352.

Nocente, R., Vitali, M., Balducci, G., Enea, D., Kranzler, H. R., & Ceccanti, M. (2013). Varenicline and neuronal nicotinic acetylcholine receptors: a new approach to the treatment of co-occurring alcohol and nicotine addiction? *The American Journal on Addictions, 22*(5), 453–459. http://dx.doi.org/10.1111/j.1521-0391.2013.12037.x.

Patterson, F., Jepson, C., Loughead, J., Perkins, K., Strasser, A. A., Siegel, S., ... Lerman, C. (2010). Working memory deficits predict short-term smoking resumption following brief abstinence. *Drug and Alcohol Dependence, 106*(1), 61–64. http://dx.doi.org/10.1016/j.drugalcdep.2009.07.020.

Patterson, F., Jepson, C., Strasser, A. A., Loughead, J., Perkins, K. A., Gur, R. C., ... Lerman, C. (2009). Varenicline improves mood and cognition during smoking abstinence. *Biological Psychiatry, 65*(2), 144–149. http://dx.doi.org/10.1016/j.biopsych.2008.08.028.

Pauly, J. R., Stitzel, J. A., Marks, M. J., & Collins, A. C. (1989). An autoradiographic analysis of cholinergic receptors in mouse brain. *Brain Research Bulletin, 22*(2), 453–459.

Perkins, K. A., Karelitz, J. L., Jao, N. C., Gur, R. C., & Lerman, C. (2013). Effects of bupropion on cognitive performance during initial tobacco abstinence. *Drug and Alcohol Dependence, 133*(1), 283–286. http://dx.doi.org/10.1016/j.drugalcdep.2013.05.003.

Pomerleau, C. S., Downey, K. K., Snedecor, S. M., Mehringer, A. M., Marks, J. L., & Pomerleau, O. F. (2003). Smoking patterns and abstinence effects in smokers with no ADHD, childhood ADHD, and adult ADHD symptomatology. *Addictive Behaviors, 28*(6), 1149–1157.

Portugal, G. S., & Gould, T. J. (2007). Bupropion dose-dependently reverses nicotine withdrawal deficits in contextual fear conditioning. *Pharmacology, Biochemistry, and Behavior, 88*(2), 179–187. http://dx.doi.org/10.1016/j.pbb.2007.08.004.

Portugal, G. S., Wilkinson, D. S., Kenney, J. W., Sullivan, C., & Gould, T. J. (2012). Strain-dependent effects of acute, chronic, and withdrawal from chronic nicotine on fear conditioning. *Behavior Genetics, 42*(1), 133–150. http://dx.doi.org/10.1007/s10519-011-9489-7.

Portugal, G. S., Wilkinson, D. S., Turner, J. R., Blendy, J. A., & Gould, T. J. (2012). Developmental effects of acute, chronic, and withdrawal from chronic nicotine on fear conditioning. *Neurobiology of Learning and Memory, 97*(4), 482–494. http://dx.doi.org/10.1016/j.nlm.2012.04.003.

Powell, J., Dawkins, L., West, R., Powell, J., & Pickering, A. (2010). Relapse to smoking during unaided cessation: clinical, cognitive and motivational predictors. *Psychopharmacology, 212*(4), 537–549. http://dx.doi.org/10.1007/s00213-010-1975-8.

Powell, J. H., Pickering, A. D., Dawkins, L., West, R., & Powell, J. F. (2004). Cognitive and psychological correlates of smoking abstinence, and predictors of successful cessation. *Addictive Behaviors, 29*(7), 1407–1426. http://dx.doi.org/10.1016/j.addbeh.2004.06.006.

Prado, J., Carp, J., & Weissman, D. H. (2011). Variations of response time in a selective attention task are linked to variations of functional connectivity in the attentional network. *Neuroimage, 54*(1), 541–549. http://dx.doi.org/10.1016/j.neuroimage.2010.08.022.

Raybuck, J. D., & Gould, T. J. (2009). Nicotine withdrawal-induced deficits in trace fear conditioning in C57BL/6 mice–a role for high-affinity beta2 subunit-containing nicotinic acetylcholine receptors. *The European Journal of Neuroscience, 29*(2), 377–387. http://dx.doi.org/10.1111/j.1460-9568.2008.06580.x.

Raybuck, J. D., Portugal, G. S., Lerman, C., & Gould, T. J. (2008). Varenicline ameliorates nicotine withdrawal-induced learning deficits in C57BL/6 mice. *Behavioral Neuroscience, 122*(5), 1166–1171. http://dx.doi.org/10.1037/a0012601.

Rezvani, A. H., & Levin, E. D. (2001). Cognitive effects of nicotine. *Biological Psychiatry, 49*(3), 258–267.

Robbins, T. W. (2002). The 5-choice serial reaction time task: behavioural pharmacology and functional neurochemistry. *Psychopharmacology, 163*(3–4), 362–380. http://dx.doi.org/10.1007/s00213-002-1154-7.

Roh, S., Hoeppner, S. S., Schoenfeld, D., Fullerton, C. A., Stoeckel, L. E., & Evins, A. E. (2014). Acute effects of mecamylamine and varenicline on cognitive performance in non-smokers with and without schizophrenia. *Psychopharmacology, 231*(4), 765–775. http://dx.doi.org/10.1007/s00213-013-3286-3.

Rukstalis, M., Jepson, C., Patterson, F., & Lerman, C. (2005). Increases in hyperactive-impulsive symptoms predict relapse among smokers in nicotine replacement therapy. *Journal of Substance Abuse Treatment, 28*(4), 297–304. http://dx.doi.org/10.1016/j.jsat.2005.02.002.

Sabri, O., Kendziorra, K., Wolf, H., Gertz, H. J., & Brust, P. (2008). Acetylcholine receptors in dementia and mild cognitive impairment. *European Journal of Nuclear Medicine and Molecular Imaging, 35*(Suppl. 1), S30–S45. http://dx.doi.org/10.1007/s00259-007-0701-1.

Sacco, K. A., Termine, A., Seyal, A., Dudas, M. M., Vessicchio, J. C., Krishnan-Sarin, S., ... George, T. P. (2005). Effects of cigarette smoking on spatial working memory and attentional deficits in schizophrenia: involvement of nicotinic receptor mechanisms. *Archives of General Psychiatry, 62*(6), 649–659. http://dx.doi.org/10.1001/archpsyc.62.6.649.

Semenova, S., Stolerman, I. P., & Markou, A. (2007). Chronic nicotine administration improves attention while nicotine withdrawal induces performance deficits in the 5-choice serial reaction time task in rats. *Pharmacology, Biochemistry, and Behavior, 87*(3), 360–368. http://dx.doi.org/10.1016/j.pbb.2007.05.009.

Shoaib, M., & Bizarro, L. (2005). Deficits in a sustained attention task following nicotine withdrawal in rats. *Psychopharmacology, 178*(2–3), 211–222. http://dx.doi.org/10.1007/s00213-004-2004-6.

Shoaib, M., Schindler, C. W., Goldberg, S. R., & Pauly, J. R. (1997). Behavioural and biochemical adaptations to nicotine in rats: influence of MK801, an NMDA receptor antagonist. *Psychopharmacology, 134*(2), 121–130.

Sofuoglu, M., DeVito, E. E., Waters, A. J., & Carroll, K. M. (2013). Cognitive enhancement as a treatment for drug addictions. *Neuropharmacology, 64,* 452–463. http://dx.doi.org/10.1016/j.neuropharm.2012.06.021.

Sofuoglu, M., Herman, A. I., Li, Y., & Waters, A. J. (2012). Galantamine attenuates some of the subjective effects of intravenous nicotine and improves performance on a Go No-Go task in abstinent cigarette smokers: a preliminary report. *Psychopharmacology, 224*(3), 413–420. http://dx.doi.org/10.1007/s00213-012-2763-4.

Staley, J. K., Krishnan-Sarin, S., Cosgrove, K. P., Krantzler, E., Frohlich, E., Perry, E., ... van Dyck, C. H. (2006). Human tobacco smokers in early abstinence have higher levels of beta2* nicotinic acetylcholine receptors than nonsmokers. *The Journal of Neuroscience: the Official Journal of the Society for Neuroscience, 26*(34), 8707–8714. http://dx.doi.org/10.1523/JNEUROSCI.0546-06.2006.

Sutherland, M. T., Carroll, A. J., Salmeron, B. J., Ross, T. J., & Stein, E. A. (2013). Insula's functional connectivity with ventromedial prefrontal cortex mediates the impact of trait alexithymia on state tobacco craving. *Psychopharmacology, 228*(1), 143–155. http://dx.doi.org/10.1007/s00213-013-3018-8.

Sutherland, M. T., McHugh, M. J., Pariyadath, V., & Stein, E. A. (2012). Resting state functional connectivity in addiction: lessons learned and a road ahead. *Neuroimage, 62*(4), 2281–2295. http://dx.doi.org/10.1016/j.neuroimage.2012.01.117.

Sweet, L. H., Mulligan, R. C., Finnerty, C. E., Jerskey, B. A., David, S. P., Cohen, R. A., et al. (2010). Effects of nicotine withdrawal on verbal working memory and associated brain response. *Psychiatry Research, 183*(1), 69–74. http://dx.doi.org/10.1016/j.pscychresns.2010.04.014.

Tsaur, S., Strasser, A. A., Souprountchouk, V., Evans, G. C., & Ashare, R. L. (2015). Time dependency of craving and response inhibition during nicotine abstinence. *Addiction Research and Theory, 23*(3), 205–212. http://dx.doi.org/10.3109/16066359.2014.953940.

Welsby, P., Rowan, M., & Anwyl, R. (2006). Nicotinic receptor-mediated enhancement of long-term potentiation involves activation of metabotropic glutamate receptors and ryanodine-sensitive calcium stores in the dentate gyrus. *The European Journal of Neuroscience, 24*(11), 3109–3118. http://dx.doi.org/10.1111/j.1460-9568.2006.05187.x.

Wesnes, K. A., Edgar, C. J., Kezic, I., Salih, H. M., & de Boer, P. (2013). Effects of nicotine withdrawal on cognition in a clinical trial setting. *Psychopharmacology, 229*(1), 133–140. http://dx.doi.org/10.1007/s00213-013-3089-6.

Wonnacott, S. (1997). Presynaptic nicotinic ACh receptors. *Trends in Neurosciences, 20*(2), 92–98.

Wooltorton, J. R., Pidoplichko, V. I., Broide, R. S., & Dani, J. A. (2003). Differential desensitization and distribution of nicotinic acetylcholine receptor subtypes in midbrain dopamine areas. *The Journal of Neuroscience: the Official Journal of the Society for Neuroscience, 23*(8), 3176–3185.

Xu, J., Mendrek, A., Cohen, M. S., Monterosso, J., Rodriguez, P., Simon, S. L., … London, E. D. (2005). Brain activity in cigarette smokers performing a working memory task: effect of smoking abstinence. *Biological Psychiatry*, *58*(2), 143–150. http://dx.doi.org/10.1016/j. biopsych.2005.03.028.

Xu, J., Mendrek, A., Cohen, M. S., Monterosso, J., Simon, S., Brody, A. L., … London, E. D. (2006). Effects of acute smoking on brain activity vary with abstinence in smokers performing the N-Back task: a preliminary study. *Psychiatry Research*, *148*(2–3), 103–109. http://dx.doi.org/10.1016/j.pscychresns.2006.09.005.

Yates, S. L., Bencherif, M., Fluhler, E. N., & Lippiello, P. M. (1995). Up-regulation of nicotinic acetylcholine receptors following chronic exposure of rats to mainstream cigarette smoke or alpha 4 beta 2 receptors to nicotine. *Biochemical Pharmacology*, *50*(12), 2001–2008.

16

Nicotine and Posttraumatic Stress Disorder

D.T. Acheson[1,2], D.E. Glenn[1,2]

[1]University of California San Diego, La Jolla, CA, United States;
[2]VA San Diego Center for Excellence in Stress and Mental Health,
San Diego, CA, United States

INTRODUCTION

Posttraumatic stress disorder (PTSD) is a psychiatric disorder that develops following exposure to a traumatic event involving actual or threatened death, serious injury, or sexual violence. This event is commonly termed a "criterion A event," referring to the DSM-5 diagnostic criteria label (American Psychiatric Association, 2013). Traumatic exposure may occur by experiencing the event personally, witnessing the event, learning of the event happening to a close friend or family member, or experiencing repeated exposure to aversive details of the traumatic event (vicarious trauma). In DSM-5, PTSD is characterized by four symptom "clusters": (1) re-experiencing symptoms, (2) avoidance symptoms, (3) negative alterations in cognition or mood, and (4) marked alterations in arousal or reactivity. While lifetime prevalence of trauma exposure is high, with estimates up to ~80% in the United States (Breslau, 2009), only a small subset of trauma-exposed individuals subsequently develops PTSD (~10%; Kessler, Chiu, Demler, Merikangas, & Walters, 2005).

PTSD is associated with poor quality of life (Schnurr, Lunney, Bovin, & Marx, 2009), poor social and occupational functioning (Druss et al., 2008), and is a substantial financial burden for society at large (Alonso et al., 2004; Brunello et al., 2001). Further, PTSD is associated with higher risk for a wide range of negative health outcomes and health-related functional impairments (Pietrzak, Goldstein, Southwick, & Grant, 2011; Qureshi, Pyne, Magruder, Schulz, & Kunik, 2009). Medical conditions

Negative Affective States and Cognitive Impairments in Nicotine Dependence
http://dx.doi.org/10.1016/B978-0-12-802574-1.00016-8

associated with PTSD include diabetes, liver disease, cardiac conditions such as angina and tachycardia, stomach ulcers and gastritis, hypercholesterolemia, bone/joint disease, and arthritis. Effective treatments exist for PTSD, with cognitive behavioral psychotherapies such as Prolonged Exposure and Cognitive Processing Therapy having the strongest efficacy data (Institute of Medicine, 2007). However, it is still unclear how and if these treatments impact comorbid medical conditions (Rauch et al., 2009; Schnurr et al., 2003), and there is a clear need to develop more effective treatment and prevention efforts overall (Baker, Nievergelt, & Risbrough, 2009).

PTSD is associated with high rates of tobacco smoking (Breslau, Davis, & Schultz, 2003; Koenen et al., 2006; Lasser et al., 2000), and smoking contributes to numerous negative health outcomes (eg, cardiovascular and respiratory problems, multiple types of cancer), known as the leading cause of preventable death in the world (US Department of Health and Human Services, 2014; World Health Organization, 2008). Understanding the relationship between PTSD and nicotine use (the addictive chemical in tobacco) represents an important avenue toward improving health outcomes through development of more effective smoking cessation programs targeted toward this population. Further, an understanding of why individuals with PTSD use nicotine, and the role that nicotine may play in the etiology and maintenance of PTSD symptoms, may point toward novel targets for treatment and prevention of PTSD itself.

TOBACCO USE AND PTSD

Relative to the general population, smoking rates are much higher among individuals with lifetime and current psychiatric disorders. PTSD is no exception. Individuals with a lifetime history of PTSD have been found to have estimated rates of 43.5% for current smoking and 63.3% for history of smoking, in comparison with rates of 22.5% and 39.1%, respectively, for individuals with no history of mental illness (Lasser et al., 2000). Higher smoking rates in PTSD persist even when controlling for other factors related to smoking such as comorbid psychiatric disorders, race, and education (Breslau et al., 2003; Koenen et al., 2006). Further, individuals with a lifetime history of PTSD are less successful at quitting smoking (28.4% quit rate) than those with no history of mental illness (42.5% quit rate) (Lasser et al., 2000), and they have high relapse rates even following smoking cessation treatment (McFall et al., 2010).

The relationship between smoking and PTSD appears to be specific to the diagnosis of PTSD, and not simply to association with trauma exposure per se. Cross-sectional studies consistently support a stronger relationship between smoking and PTSD than with trauma exposure alone (Feldner, Babson, & Zvolensky, 2007; Fu et al., 2007; Hapke et al., 2005; Koenen et al., 2005, 2006, 2003; Shalev, Bleich, & Ursano, 1990; Solomon & Mikulincer, 1987; Thorndike, Wernicke, Pearlman, & Haaga, 2006). A 10-year prospective study found increased incidence of nicotine dependence in individuals with PTSD (31.7%) relative to trauma-exposed individuals without PTSD (19.9%) and non-trauma-exposed comparison subjects (10.5%; Breslau et al., 2003). Further, smokers with PTSD smoke at more consistent rates and with higher puff volumes than trauma-exposed smokers without PTSD (McClernon et al., 2005).

While there is a clear association between PTSD and nicotine use, the nature of this association remains unclear. It may be that PTSD predisposes one to nicotine use, that nicotine use predisposes one to PTSD, or that PTSD and nicotine use are both influenced by an unrelated third variable. Studies by Breslau et al. (2003) and Breslau, Novak, and Kessler (2004) found that PTSD was a significant risk factor for onset of daily smoking. Similarly, data from the Vietnam Era Twin Registry indicated that having active PTSD increased the risk of late-onset smoking across all levels of genetic liability toward nicotine dependence (Koenen et al., 2006). These findings suggest that PTSD might represent a risk factor for onset of nicotine use and dependence. Additional analysis of the Vietnam Era Twin Registry data estimated that shared genetic factors accounted for approximately 62% of the association between PTSD and nicotine dependence (Koenen et al., 2005). Comparing directional models of the relationship between PTSD and nicotine dependence provided strong support for a model in which prior nicotine dependence predisposes individuals toward the development of PTSD following trauma. Thus, there appears to be a strong shared genetic susceptibility for PTSD and nicotine dependence, as well as an evidence that PTSD and nicotine dependence are each risk factors for the other, suggesting a bidirectional causal relationship.

NICOTINE AND PTSD PHENOTYPES

Given the high comorbidity between nicotine use and PTSD, it is important to understand how nicotine administration interacts with symptoms of PTSD. Nicotine acts as an agonist at nicotinic acetylcholine receptors (nAChRs), which are widely distributed throughout the brain. There are numerous nAChR subtypes that produce distinct neurochemical cascades (eg, Gotti et al., 2009), so both acute and chronic nicotine administration have broad and complex neural effects. Understanding interactions between nicotine and PTSD phenotypes may help to clarify mechanisms supporting nicotine use among individuals with PTSD and also point toward novel treatment targets for alleviating PTSD symptoms. Here, we focus on the relationship between nicotine use and three PTSD-related phenotypes: heightened anxiety, impairment in attention and memory, and fear learning deficits.

Heightened Anxiety

One potential explanation for the link between PTSD and nicotine use is that individuals with PTSD use nicotine to cope with negative affective states, such as anxiety. Animal models have shown that nicotine can produce anxiolytic effects via binding to and desensitization of $\alpha4\beta2^*$ nAChRs (Anderson & Brunzell, 2012; McGranahan, Patzlaff, Grady, Heinemann, & Booker, 2011; Varani, Moutinho, Bettler, & Balerio, 2012). In humans, smokers smoke more and report increased urges to smoke during or shortly after induced stress (Gilbert, Robinson, Chamberlin, & Spielberger, 1989; Perkins & Grobe, 1992; Pomerleau & Pomerleau, 1987). However, nicotine administration can also produce anxiogenic effects in some circumstances (Benowitz, 1988; Picciotto & Corrigall, 2002), pointing to the complex role of the nAChR system in emotional behavior. Nevertheless, potential anxiolytic actions of nicotine use point to the possibility that this behavior may be maintained via negative reinforcement, or relief of aversive emotional states (Cohen et al., 2009).

A series of studies by Beckham et al. examined the relationship between smoking and negative affect in individuals with PTSD (Beckham et al., 2007; Beckham, Feldman, Vrana, Mozley, Erkanli, & Clancy, 2005; Beckham, Gerhman, McClernon, Collie, & Feldman, 2004; Beckham et al., 1996, 2008). In general, these studies indicate an increase in cravings and withdrawal symptoms in smokers with PTSD when exposed to anxiety-provoking cues, trauma reminders, and naturalistically occurring negative affect and PTSD symptoms. These findings suggest that smokers with PTSD may smoke, in part, in an attempt to relieve negative affect. This explanation is further supported by self-reported expectancy of negative affect reduction in smokers with PTSD (Carmody et al., 2012; Marshall et al., 2008).

While acute and chronic nicotine administration may help alleviate negative affect, or at least are expected to do so by individuals with PTSD, abstinence following chronic nicotine exposure elicits elevated anxiety as well as a range of other aversive withdrawal symptoms (anger, depression, impatience, insomnia, restlessness; Hughes, 2007). Results have been mixed, but some evidence indicates that for individuals with PTSD, nicotine withdrawal heightens anxiety sensitivity ("fear of fear"), leading them to be particularly distressed when experiencing symptoms of anxiety (Asnaani, Farris, Carpenter, Zandberg, & Foa, 2015; Feldner, Vujanovic, Gibson, & Zvolensky, 2008; Vujanovic, Marshall-Berenz,

Beckham, Bernstein, & Zvolensky, 2010). This model is consistent with the notion that negative reinforcement is central to chronic nicotine use and poor quit rates observed in individuals with PTSD.

Attention and Memory Deficits

Individuals with PTSD report problems with memory and attention. DSM-5 criteria for PTSD include difficulty recalling key features of the traumatic event and impairments in concentration. Studies have demonstrated impaired attention and memory for threatening and trauma-related stimuli (Bar-Haim, Lamy, Pergamin, Bakermans-Kranenburg, & van IJzendoom, 2007; Buckley, Blanchard, & Neill, 2000), but there is also evidence for an association between PTSD and neurocognitive deficits on non-trauma-related tests of attention and memory (Brewin, Kleiner, Vasterling, & Field, 2007; Horner & Hamner, 2002; Isaac, Cushway, & Jones, 2006). A review found evidence for attentional deficits in individuals with PTSD, though the authors noted that their findings should be interpreted cautiously given that psychiatric comorbidity and issues of test effort and motivation were potential confounds in nearly all studies reviewed (Horner & Hamner, 2002). A more recent review found evidence for impaired attention in individuals with PTSD on digit-span tests of attention and on more complex tests of attention (Isaac et al., 2006). There is some evidence that individuals with PTSD are more likely to have impairments in certain kinds of attention, such as sustained attention, though results have been mixed (Crowell, Kieffer, Siders, & Vanderploeg, 2002; Jenkins, Langlais, Delis, & Cohen, 2000; Stein, Kennedy, & Twamley, 2002; Vasterling, Brailey, Constans, & Sutker, 1998; Vasterling et al., 2002). A study with combat veterans found that attention deficits were associated with PTSD symptoms at one-year post-deployment but not immediately post-deployment, and they were not related to depressive symptoms, head injury, or intensity of combat exposure, suggesting that chronic PTSD is uniquely associated with impaired attention (Marx et al., 2009).

A growing body of research indicates an association between PTSD and memory impairment, though findings regarding the specific area of impairment have been inconsistent. One review found PTSD-associated deficits in immediate memory, particularly for immediate verbal memory (Horner & Hamner, 2002), while another found PTSD-associated deficits in episodic memory (Isaac et al., 2006). A meta-analysis found small to moderate memory impairments associated with PTSD, with larger deficits in verbal than visual memory, and no effect of immediate versus delayed recall (Brewin et al., 2007). Many findings of poorer memory in PTSD patients could potentially be attributed to the effect of attention deficits, though findings from a handful of studies suggest impaired memory performance are unrelated to impaired attention (Bremner et al., 1995; Gilbertson, Gurvits, Lasko, Orr, & Pitman, 2001; Jenkins, Langlais, Delis, & Cohen, 1998; Yehuda et al., 1995).

Nicotine has been found to affect numerous memory and attentional processes (Hahn, 2015; Kutlu & Gould, 2015), and administration of nicotine and other nAChR agonists have been targeted as potential means to alleviate cognitive deficits found in psychiatric disorders (Levin et al., 1996; Singh, Potter, & Newhouse, 2004; White & Levin, 1999). A recent review found that acute nicotine administration improves performance on attentional tests of vigilance and stimulus detection, and it may also improve attentional control and selective attention, though these findings have been more limited and inconsistent (Hahn, 2015). Activation of nAChRs may promote synaptic plasticity and long-term potentiation (Kenney & Gould, 2008), and acute administration of nicotine appears to generally enhance memory performance in humans and animals, though results have been somewhat mixed (Kutlu & Gould, 2015).

Chronic nicotine exposure appears to result in upregulation of nAChRs, as indicated by increased nAChR density found in post-mortem brains of smokers versus nonsmokers (Breese et al., 1997). Research suggests that nicotine-induced enhancement of hippocampal-dependent memory diminishes with the development of tolerance through chronic nicotine exposure (Kutlu & Gould, 2015). Findings have been mixed as to whether chronic nicotine administration decreases baseline attentional functioning (Rezvani et al., 2005; Snyder, Davis, & Henningfield, 1989), but nicotine-induced attentional enhancement appears to remain even after chronic exposure (Hahn, 2015). However, withdrawal following chronic nicotine exposure is associated with decrements in sustained attention, working memory, and response inhibition (Ashare, Falcone, & Lerman, 2014; McClernon, Addicott, & Sweitzer, 2015). Mechanisms of nicotine withdrawal-induced cognitive deficits are not fully understood, but one possibility is that after the upregulation of nAChRs during chronic nicotine exposure, the availability of unbound nAChRs during abstinence is associated with cognitive impairment (Ashare et al., 2014; Kendziorra et al., 2011).

Given the similarity in memory and attention decrements associated with both nicotine withdrawal and PTSD, it is notable that PTSD patients with no smoking history have been found to have higher β_2-nAChR availability than healthy controls with no smoking history (Czermak et al., 2008). This finding provides preliminary evidence that elevated rates of nicotine use in PTSD patients may be an attempt at alleviating cognitive deficits associated with PTSD-related high nAChR availability. Further, PTSD patients who consume nicotine regularly may be especially susceptible to withdrawal-induced memory and attention impairment, given high nAChR availability resulting from both PTSD state as well as nAChR upregulation. Considering the role of nAChRs in PTSD and tobacco use, comorbidity may help identify novel treatment approaches, such as the administration of cotinine (the primary metabolite of nicotine), which may have beneficial therapeutic effects without the negative consequences associated with chronic nicotine exposure (Moran, 2012).

Fear Conditioning and Extinction

Fear conditioning is the process by which an organism learns to associate a cue or context with an aversive outcome. For instance, a rodent may be trained that a tone or certain cage configuration is followed by an electrical shock to the foot. The fear then elicited by exposure to the cue or context can be measured via the freezing response in rodents (Zovkic & Sweatt, 2013) or the potentiated startle or electrodermal response in humans (Acheson, Forsyth, Prenoveau, & Bouton, 2007; Acheson et al., 2015). When the aversive outcome is associated with a discrete cue, such as a tone, this is termed *cue conditioning*. When the aversive outcome is associated with the whole environment in which it is encountered, such as a cage configuration, this is termed *context conditioning*. Fear extinction, in contrast, is the process of learning that a cue or context that once signaled threat no longer does so. Fear extinction is accomplished by presenting the organism with the cue or context over numerous trials or a long period of time without the aversive outcome. Fear extinction is not simple forgetting of the original conditioned fear response, but a new form of inhibitory learning that requires synaptic plasticity and memory consolidation (Bouton, 1993). Extinction of conditioned fear is regarded as a laboratory analog for exposure therapy used to treat PTSD and anxiety disorders (Craske & Mystkowski, 2006; Hermans, Craske, Mineka, & Lovibond, 2006).

Fear conditioning and extinction represent useful paradigms for investigating PTSD, as they allow for examination of emotional learning and memory processes associated with exposure to a traumatic event (ie, foot shock; Zovkic & Sweatt, 2013). Further, the neurobiological abnormalities associated with a diagnosis of PTSD are becoming increasingly well understood and overlap with areas known to be involved in fear conditioning and extinction (Acheson, Gresack, & Risbrough, 2012; Johnson, McGuire, Lazarus, & Palmer, 2012; Patel, Spreng, Shin, & Girard, 2012). For instance, PTSD is associated with abnormal structure and function of the limbic system, specifically hyperactivation of the amygdala, a region involved in mediating fear and stress responses and emotional memory (Garfinkel & Liberzon, 2009). The amygdala is involved in initial fear conditioning and later expression of conditioned fear (Blair, Schafe, Bauer, Rodrigues, & LeDoux, 2001). PTSD is associated with reduced volume and neuronal integrity in the hippocampus, a region involved in context conditioning and contextual gating of cued fear responses (Acheson et al., 2012). Amygdala hyperactivity and poor contextualization of fear may explain the heightened and contextually inappropriate and overgeneralized fear responses seen in PTSD.

In addition to hyperactivity in emotion-generating regions, PTSD has also been consistently associated with hypoactivation of the ventral region of the medial prefrontal cortex (mPFC; Etkin & Wager, 2007). The ventral mPFC (vmPFC) is involved in inhibition of emotional response, while the dorsal mPFC (dmPFC) is involved in emotion generation (Likhtik, Pelletier, Paz, & Pare, 2005). The vmPFC is also critical for fear extinction learning (Quirk & Mueller, 2008). Reflecting hypoactivity in the vmPFC, individuals with PTSD appear to have difficulty learning and recalling memory for fear extinction (Acheson et al., 2015; Milad et al., 2008), potentially explaining the persistence of fear responses in individuals with PTSD. The mPFC is also heavily involved in addictive behavior and drug seeking (Goldstein & Volkow, 2002; Porrino, Smith, Nader, & Beveridge, 2007).

A review of mPFC involvement in both fear and addiction proposed a model in which neural systems mediating fear response and addictive behavior overlap in the mPFC (Peters, Kalivas, & Quirk, 2009). In this model, the dmPFC is involved in the generation of both fear and drug seeking/craving, and the vmPFC is involved in both inhibition/extinction of fear and drug seeking. Most of the research supporting this model was conducted using animal models of cocaine dependence, but the model would likely apply across various addictive drugs, including nicotine. This model may suggest a common pathway for development of PTSD and nicotine dependence. Specifically, individuals with PTSD may have difficulty inhibiting both fear responses and drug seeking behavior in response to cravings, which may explain low quit rates among smokers with PTSD. As a current focus of treatment research in PTSD is enhancement of fear extinction learning (ie, Acheson et al., 2013), it is possible that such approaches may also have value for facilitating nicotine cessation for this population and preventing stress-induced relapse of use (Kaplan, Heinrichs, & Carey, 2011; Pizzimenti & Lattal, 2015).

The nAChR system is also involved in fear conditioning and extinction, though the effect of nicotine on these functions is complex (Tipps, Raybuck, & Lattal, 2014). The hippocampus, for instance, contains numerous nAChRs (Le Novere, Grutter, & Changeux, 2002). Acute nicotine administration can enhance hippocampal-dependent context conditioning via actions on $\beta2^*$ nAChRs (Davis, Porter, & Gould, 2006), though this function can become impaired at high doses of nicotine (Kenney & Gould, 2008). This enhanced fear learning can also be seen in a hippocampus-dependent type of conditioning called trace conditioning (Davis & Gould, 2007). Acute nicotine administration does not appear to have effects on cue conditioning, which is hippocampus-independent (Gould & Higgins, 2003).

Despite not affecting cue conditioning, acute nicotine has been shown to facilitate cued fear extinction when administered only during extinction training, likely through actions on β_2* nAChRs in the hippocampus and mPFC (Elias, Gurlick, Wilkenson, & Gould, 2010). Interestingly, this same study suggested that nicotine administration during extinction training disrupted contextualization of the fear extinction memory, making return of fear response in other contexts less likely. However, Kutlu and Gould (2014) found that acute nicotine administration during extinction training impaired extinction of context conditioned fear. In sum, acute nicotine administration clearly impacts fear learning processes, though these effects are complex and not fully understood.

In contrast to acute administration, chronic nicotine administration does not appear to enhance hippocampus-dependent fear learning (Portugal, Wilkinson, Turner, Blendy, & Gould, 2012), potentially because long-term nicotine exposure has desensitized nAChRs (Wilkenson & Gould, 2013). This explanation is supported by findings that withdrawal from chronic nicotine exposure creates deficits in contextual fear learning (Portugal et al., 2012), and that nicotine administration following withdrawal produces greater enhancement of fear learning than acute nicotine administration alone (Wilkenson & Gould, 2013). One study found chronic nicotine exposure to impair initial extinction of cued fear but not context fear, though subsequent memory for context fear extinction was enhanced (Tian et al., 2008). However, it was unclear if these effects were due to chronic nicotine per se or nicotine withdrawal, as there was a 2-week period between the last dose of nicotine and extinction training (Kutlu & Gould, 2015).

Fear conditioning is an important etiological model of PTSD. Given the comorbidity between PTSD and nicotine use, understanding the complex relationship between fear learning and nicotine use may provide insight into the etiology and maintenance of PTSD symptoms among nicotine users. Further, fear extinction is commonly recognized as the underlying mechanism of action in exposure-based treatments for PTSD, such as prolonged exposure. Elucidation of the role of nAChR activation in fear extinction learning and memory processes has potential to inform understanding of treatment nonresponse in these PTSD patients, such as through nicotine interference with fear extinction learning. Conversely, knowledge of the specific mechanisms by which nAChR agonists could enhance fear extinction learning and memory may provide novel pharmacological targets for facilitation of therapeutic learning in PTSD treatment (Krystal, 2007).

SUMMARY

PTSD and tobacco use are independently associated with a range of poor functional and health outcomes (Alonso et al., 2004; Brunello et al., 2001; Druss et al., 2008; Pietrzak et al., 2011; Qureshi et al., 2009; Schnurr et al., 2009; US Department of Health and Human Services, 2014; World Health Organization, 2008), which is particularly concerning given elevated rates tobacco use in individuals with PTSD (Breslau et al., 2003; Koenen et al., 2006; Lasser et al., 2000). PTSD and nicotine use are also both independently associated with alterations in affective and cognitive processes, so understanding the interaction between nicotine and PTSD phenotypes represents an important avenue toward improving treatment and prevention efforts.

Acute nicotine administration appears to have generally beneficial effects on three PTSD phenotypes: heightened anxiety, impairment in attention and memory, and altered fear learning. Acute nicotine exposure may have anxiolytic effects, or is at least expected to by individuals with PTSD, and it improves functioning in areas of attention and memory in which PTSD patients typically show deficits. Further, acute nicotine administration has been demonstrated to improve hippocampal-dependent contextual fear learning and enhance cued fear extinction, aspects of fear learning that are commonly impaired in individuals with PTSD. Chronic nicotine exposure appears to result in the upregulation and desensitization of nAChRs, and it does not afford the same benefits seen with acute administration. It is unclear if chronic nicotine exposure per se has negative consequences on PTSD phenotypes, but abstinence following chronic exposure appears to increase anxiety and anxiety sensitivity, as well as impairing memory, attention, and fear learning. In sum, these results suggest that high rates of chronic nicotine use and poor quit rates in individuals with PTSD are maintained by negative reinforcement (behavioral reinforcement through reduction in an aversive experience) of acute nicotine exposure interacting with specific PTSD phenotypes. Initially, acute nicotine administration alleviates cognitive and emotional difficulties experienced by PTSD patients. After the development of tolerance through chronic nicotine use, abstinence exacerbates affective dysregulation and impairs cognitive functioning, but subsequent acute nicotine administration relieves these aversive withdrawal symptoms.

Consider that the interaction of nicotine with PTSD phenotypes may be useful for identifying fruitful approaches to improving interventions for concurrent PTSD and smoking. First, chronic tobacco use and PTSD may be characterized by poor inhibition of drug seeking and poor inhibition of fear responding, respectively. This commonality underscores the point that further honing both behavioral and pharmacological interventions that maximize inhibitory learning (ie, Acheson et al., 2013; Craske,

Treanor, Conway, Zbozinek, & Vervliet, 2014) may be particularly valuable for PTSD patients with chronic tobacco use. Given their involvement in both the neurochemical activity of nicotine as well as a range of fear learning and memory processes, nAChRs may be a valuable target for pharmacological interventions that both alleviate negative effects of nicotine withdrawal and facilitate fear extinction (Krystal, 2007). For example, cotinine (the primary metabolite of nicotine) appears to alter nAChR sensitivity, and it may be a means of enhancing the extinction of contextual fear (Zeitlin et al., 2012) and improving cognitive performance without the addictive and negative health consequences of nicotine (Moran, 2012).

References

Acheson, D. T., Feifel, D., de Wilde, S., McKinney, R., Lohr, J., & Risbrough, V. (2013). The effect of intranasal oxytocin treatment on conditioned fear extinction and recall in healthy human subjects. *Psychopharmacology, 229*, 199–208.

Acheson, D. T., Forsyth, J. P., Prenoveau, J. M., & Bouton, M. E. (2007). Interoceptive fear conditioning as a learning model of panic disorder: an experimental evaluation using 20% CO_2-enriched air in a non-clinical sample. *Behavior Research and Therapy, 45*, 2280–2294.

Acheson, D. T., Geyer, M., Baker, D. G., Neivergelt, C., Yurgil, K., Risbrough, V. B., et al. (2015). Conditioned fear and extinction learning performance and its association with psychiatric symptoms in a sample of active duty Marines. *Psychoneuroendocrinology, 51*, 495–505.

Acheson, D. T., Gresack, J. E., & Risbrough, V. B. (2012). Hippocampal dysfunction effects on context memory: possible etiology for posttraumatic stress disorder. *Neuropharmacology, 62*, 674–685.

Alonso, J., Angermeyer, M. C., Bernert, S., Bruffaerts, R., Brugha, T. S., Bryson, H., et al. (2004). Disability and quality of life impact of mental disorders in Europe: results from the European Study of the Epidemiology of Mental Disorders (ESEMeD) project. *Acta Psychiatrica Scandinavica Supplementum, 109*, 21–27.

American Psychiatric Association. (2013). *Diagnostic and statistical manual of mental disorders* (5th ed.). Washington, DC: Author.

Anderson, S. M., & Brunzell, D. H. (2012). Low dose nicotine and antagonism of β_2 subunit containing nicotinic acetylcholine receptors have similar effects on affective behavior in mice. *PLoS One*. http://dx.doi.org/10.1371/journal.pone.0048665.

Ashare, R. L., Falcone, M., & Lerman, C. (2014). Cognitive function during nicotine withdrawal: implications for nicotine dependence treatment. *Neuropharmacology, 76*, 581–591.

Asnaani, A., Farris, S. G., Carpenter, J. K., Zandberg, L. J., & Foa, E. B. (2015). The relationship between anxiety sensitivity and posttraumatic stress disorder: what is the impact of nicotine withdrawal? *Cognitive Therapy and Research, 39*(5), 697–708. http://dx.doi.org/10.1007/s10608-015-9685-5.

Baker, D. G., Nievergelt, C. M., & Risbrough, V. B. (2009). Post-traumatic stress disorder: emerging concepts of pharmacotherapy. *Expert Opinion on Emerging Drugs, 14*, 251–272.

Bar-Haim, Y., Lamy, D., Pergamin, L., Bakermans-Kranenburg, M. J., & van IJzendoom, M. H. (2007). Threat related attention bias in anxious and nonanxious individuals: a meta-analytic study. *Psychological Bulletin, 133*, 1–12.

Beckham, J. C., Dennis, M. F., McClernon, F. J., Mozley, S. L., Collie, C. F., & Vrana, S. R. (2007). The effects of cigarette smoking on script-driven imagery in smokers with and without posttraumatic stress disorder. *Addictive Behaviors, 32*, 2900–2915.

Beckham, J. C., Feldman, M. E., Vrana, S. R., Mozley, S. L., Erkanli, A., Clancy, C. P., et al. (2005). Immediate antecedents of cigarette smoking in smokers with and without posttraumatic stress disorder: a preliminary study. *Experimental and Clinical Psychopharmacology, 13*, 219–228.

Beckham, J. C., Gerhman, P. R., McClernon, F. J., Collie, C. F., & Feldman, M. E. (2004). Cigarette smoking, ambulatory cardiovascular monitoring, and mood in Vietnam veterans with and without chronic posttraumatic stress disorder. *Addictive Behaviors, 29*, 1579–1593.

Beckham, J. C., Lytle, B. L., Vrana, S. R., Hertzberg, M. A., Feldman, M. E., & Shipley, R. H. (1996). Smoking withdrawal symptoms in response to a trauma-related stressor among Vietnam combat veterans with posttraumatic stress disorder. *Addictive Behaviors, 21*, 93–101.

Beckham, J. C., Wiley, M. T., Miller, S. C., Dennis, M. F., Wilson, S. M., McClernon, F. J., et al. (2008). Ad lib smoking in post-traumatic stress disorder: an electronic diary study. *Nicotine & Tobacco Research, 10*, 1149–1157.

Benowitz, N. L. (1988). Drug therapy. Pharmacologic aspects of cigarette smoking and nicotine addiction. *The New England Journal of Medicine, 319*, 1318–1330.

Blair, H. T., Schafe, G. E., Bauer, E. P., Rodrigues, S. M., & LeDoux, J. E. (2001). Synaptic plasticity in the lateral amygdala: a cellular hypothesis of fear conditioning. *Learning and Memory, 8*, 229–242.

Bouton, M. E. (1993). Context, time, and memory in the interference paradigms of Pavlovian learning. *Psychological Bulletin, 114*, 80–99.

Breese, C., Marks, M., Logel, J., Adams, C., Sullivan, B., Collins, A., et al. (1997). Effect of smoking history on [3H]nicotine binding in human postmortem brain. *The Journal of Pharmacology and Experimental Therapeutics, 282*, 7–13.

Bremner, J. D., Randall, P., Scott, T. M., Capelli, S., Delaney, R., McCarthy, G., et al. (1995). Deficits in short-term memory in adult survivors of childhood abuse. *Psychiatry Research, 59*, 97–107.

Breslau, N. (2009). The epidemiology of trauma, PTSD, and other posttrauma disorders. *Trauma, Violence, and Abuse, 10*, 198–210.

Breslau, N., Davis, G. C., & Schultz, L. R. (2003). Posttraumatic stress disorder and the incidence of nicotine, alcohol, and other drug disorders in persons who have experienced trauma. *Archives of General Psychiatry, 60*, 289–294.

Breslau, N., Novak, S. P., & Kessler, R. C. (2004). Psychiatric disorders and stages of smoking. *Biological Psychiatry, 55*, 69–76.

Brewin, C. R., Kleiner, J. S., Vasterling, J. J., & Field, A. P. (2007). Memory for emotionally neutral information in posttraumatic stress disorder: a meta-analytic investigation. *Journal of Abnormal Psychology, 116*, 448–463.

Brunello, N., Davidson, J. R., Deahl, M., Kessler, R. C., Mendlewicz, J., Racagni, G., et al. (2001). Posttraumatic stress disorder: diagnosis and epidemiology, comorbidity and social consequences, biology and treatment. *Neuropsychobiology, 43*, 150–162.

Buckley, T. C., Blanchard, E. B., & Neill, W. T. (2000). Information processing and PTSD: a review of the empirical literature. *Clinical Psychology Review, 28*, 1041–1065.

Carmody, T. P., McFall, M., Saxon, A. J., Malte, C. A., Chow, B., Joseph, A. M., et al. (2012). Smoking outcome expectancies in military veteran smokers with posttraumatic stress disorder. *Nicotine & Tobacco Research, 8*, 919–926.

Cohen, A., Young, R. W., Velasquez, M., Groysman, M., Noorbehesht, K., Ben-Shahar, O., et al. (2009). Anxiolytic effects of nicotine in a rodent test of approach-avoidance conflict. *Psychopharmacology, 204*, 541–549.

Craske, M. G., & Mystkowski, J. L. (2006). Exposure therapy and extinction: clinical studies. In M. G. Craske, D. Hermans, & D. Vansteenwegen (Eds.), *Fear and learning: From basic processes to clinical implications* (pp. 217–233). Washington, DC, US: American Psychological Association.

Craske, M. G., Treanor, M., Conway, C. C., Zbozinek, T., & Vervliet, B. (2014). Maximizing exposure therapy: an inhibitory learning approach. *Behaviour Research and Therapy, 58,* 10–23. http://dx.doi.org/10.1016/j.brat.2014.04.006.

Crowell, T. A., Kieffer, K. M., Siders, C. A., & Vanderploeg, R. D. (2002). Neuropsychological findings in combat-related posttraumatic stress disorder. *The Clinical Neuropsychologist, 16,* 310–321.

Czermak, C., Staley, J. K., Kasserman, S., Bois, F., Young, T., Henry, S., et al. (2008). β2 Nicotinic acetylcholine receptor availability in post-traumatic stress disorder. *The International Journal of Neuropsychopharmacology, 11,* 419–424.

Davis, J. A., & Gould, T. J. (2007). β2 subunit-containing nicotinic receptors mediate the enhancing effect of nicotine on trace cued fear conditioning in C57BL/6 mice. *Psychopharmacology, 190,* 343–352.

Davis, J. A., Porter, J., & Gould, T. J. (2006). Nicotine enhances both foreground and background contextual fear conditioning. *Neuroscience Letters, 394,* 202–205.

Druss, B. G., Hwang, I., Petukhova, M., Sampson, N. A., Wang, P. S., & Kessler, R. C. (2008). Impairment in role functioning in mental and chronic medical disorders in the United States: results from the National Comorbidity Survey Replication. *Molecular Psychiatry, 14,* 728–737.

Elias, G. A., Gurlick, D., Wilkenson, D. S., & Gould, T. J. (2010). Nicotine and extinction of fear conditioning. *Neuroscience, 165,* 1063–1073.

Etkin, A., & Wager, T. D. (2007). Functional neuroimaging of anxiety: a meta-analysis of emotional processing in PTSD, social anxiety disorder, and specific phobia. *The American Journal of Psychiatry, 164,* 1476–1488.

Feldner, M. T., Babson, K. A., & Zvolensky, M. J. (2007). Smoking, traumatic event exposure, and post-traumatic stress: a critical review of the empirical literature. *Clinical Psychology Review, 27,* 14–45.

Feldner, M. T., Vujanovic, A. A., Gibson, L. E., & Zvolensky, M. J. (2008). Posttraumatic stress disorder and anxious and fearful reactivity to bodily arousal: a test of the mediating role of nicotine withdrawal severity among daily smokers in 12-hr nicotine deprivation. *Experimental and Clinical Psychopharmacology, 16,* 144–155.

Fu, S. S., McFall, M., Saxon, A. J., Beckham, J. C., Carmody, T. P., Baker, D. G., et al. (2007). Post-traumatic stress disorder and smoking: a systematic review. *Nicotine & Tobacco Research, 9,* 1071–1084.

Garfinkel, S. N., & Liberzon, I. (2009). Neurobiology of PTSD: a review of neuroimaging findings. *Psychiatric Annals, 39,* 370–381.

Gilbert, D. G., Robinson, J. H., Chamberlin, C. L., & Spielberger, C. D. (1989). Effects of smoking/nicotine on anxiety, heart rate, and lateralization of EEG during a stressful movie. *Psychophysiology, 26,* 11–20.

Gilbertson, M. W., Gurvits, T. V., Lasko, N. B., Orr, S. P., & Pitman, R. K. (2001). Multivariate assessment of explicit memory function in combat veterans with posttraumatic stress disorder. *Journal of Traumatic Stress, 14,* 413–432.

Goldstein, R. Z., & Volkow, N. D. (2002). Drug addiction and its underlying neurobiological basis: neuroimaging evidence for the involvement of the frontal cortex. *American Journal of Psychiatry, 159,* 1642–1652.

Gotti, C., Clementi, F., Fornari, A., Gaimarri, A., Guiducci, S., Manfredi, I., et al. (2009). Structural and functional diversity of native brain neuronal nicotinic receptors. *Biochemical Pharmacology, 78,* 703–711.

Gould, T. J., & Higgins, J. S. (2003). Nicotine enhances contextual fear conditioning in C57BL/J6 mice at 1 and 7 days post-training. *Neurobiology of Learning and Memory, 107,* 108–132.

Hahn, B. (2015). Nicotinic receptors and attention. *Current Topics in Behavioral Neurosciences, 23,* 103–135.

Hapke, U., Schumann, A., Rumpf, H. J., John, U., Konerding, U., & Meyer, C. (2005). Association of smoking and nicotine dependence with trauma and posttraumatic stress disorder in a general population sample. *The Journal of Nervous and Mental Disease, 193,* 843–846.

Hermans, D., Craske, M. G., Mineka, S., & Lovibond, P. F. (2006). Extinction in human fear conditioning. *Biological Psychiatry, 60,* 361–368.

Horner, M. D., & Hamner, M. B. (2002). Neurocognitive functioning in posttraumatic stress disorder. *Neuropsychological Review, 12,* 15–30.

Hughes, J. R. (2007). Effects of abstinence from tobacco: valid symptoms and time course. *Nicotine & Tobacco Research, 9,* 315–327.

Institute of Medicine. (2007). *Treatment of posttraumatic stress disorder: An assessment of the evidence.* Washington, DC: National Academy of Sciences. Retrieved March 2009 from http://books.nap.edu/catalog.php?record_id=11955#toc.

Isaac, C. L., Cushway, D., & Jones, G. V. (2006). Is posttraumatic stress disorder associated with specific deficits in episodic memory? *Clinical Psychology Review, 26,* 939–955.

Jenkins, M. A., Langlais, P. J., Delis, D., & Cohen, R. (1998). Learning and memory in rape victims with posttraumatic stress disorder. *The American Journal of Psychiatry, 155,* 278–279.

Jenkins, M. A., Langlais, P. J., Delis, D., & Cohen, R. A. (2000). Attentional dysfunction associated with posttraumatic stress disorder among rape survivors. *The Clinical Neuropsychologist, 14,* 7–12.

Johnson, L. R., McGuire, J., Lazarus, R., & Palmer, A. A. (2012). Pavlovian fear memory circuits and phenotype models of PTSD. *Neuropharmacology, 62,* 638–646.

Kaplan, G. B., Heinrichs, S. C., & Carey, R. J. (2011). Treatment of addiction and anxiety using extinction approaches: neural mechanisms and their treatment implications. *Pharmacology, Biochemistry, and Behavior, 97,* 619–625.

Kendziorra, K., Wolf, H., Meyer, P. M., Barthel, H., Hesse, S., Becker, G. A., et al. (2011). Decreased cerebral α4β2* nicotinic acetylcholine receptor availability in patients with mild cognitive impairment and Alzheimer's disease assessed with positron emission tomography. *European Journal of Nuclear Medicine and Molecular Imaging, 38,* 515–525.

Kenney, J. W., & Gould, T. J. (2008). Modulation of hippocampus-dependent learning and synaptic plasticity by nicotine. *Molecular Neurobiology, 38,* 101–121.

Kessler, R. C., Chiu, W. T., Demler, O., Merikangas, K. R., & Walters, E. E. (2005). Prevalence, severity, and comorbidity of 12-month DSM-IV disorders in the National Comorbidity Survey Replication. *Archives of General Psychiatry, 62,* 617–627.

Koenen, K. C., Hitsman, B., Lyons, M. J., Niaura, R., McCaffery, J., Goldberg, J., et al. (2005). A twin registry study of the relationship between posttraumatic stress disorder and nicotine dependence in men. *Archives of General Psychiatry, 62,* 1258–1265.

Koenen, K. C., Hitsman, B., Lyons, M. J., Stroud, L., Niaura, R., McCaffery, J., et al. (2006). Posttraumatic stress disorder and late-onset smoking in the Vietnam era twin registry. *Journal of Consulting and Clinical Psychology, 74,* 186–190.

Koenen, K. C., Lyons, M. J., Goldberg, J., Simpson, J., Williams, W. M., Toomey, R., et al. (2003). Co-twin control study of relationships among combat exposure, combat-related PTSD, and other mental disorders. *Journal of Traumatic Stress, 16,* 433–438.

Krystal, J. H. (2007). Neuroplasticity as a target for the pharmacotherapy of psychiatric disorders: new opportunities for synergy with psychotherapy. *Biological Psychiatry, 62,* 833–834.

Kutlu, M. G., & Gould, T. J. (2014). Acute nicotine delays extinction of contextual fear in mice. *Behavioral Brain Research, 263,* 133–137.

Kutlu, M. G., & Gould, T. J. (2015). Nicotinic receptors, memory, and hippocampus. *Current Topics in Behavioral Neurosciences, 23,* 137–163.

Lasser, K., Boyd, J. W., Woolhandler, S., Himmelstein, D. U., McCormick, D., & Bor, D. H. (2000). Smoking and mental illness: a population-based prevalence study. *Journal of the American Medical Association, 284,* 2606–2610.

Le Novere, N., Grutter, T., & Changeux, J. P. (2002). Models of the extracellular domain of the nicotinic receptors and of agonist and Ca^{2+} binding sites. *Proceedings of the National Academy of Sciences of the United States of America, 99*, 3210–3215.

Levin, E. D., Conners, C. K., Sparrow, E., Hinton, S. C., Erhardt, D., Meck, W. H., et al. (1996). Nicotine effects on adults with attention-deficit/hyperactivity disorder. *Psychopharmacology, 123*, 55–63.

Likhtik, E., Pelletier, J. G., Paz, R., & Pare, D. (2005). Prefrontal control of the amygdala. *The Journal of Neuroscience, 25*, 7429–7437.

Marshall, E. C., Zvolensky, M. J., Vujanovic, A. A., Gibson, L. E., Gregor, K., & Bernstein, A. (2008). Evaluation of smoking characteristics among community-recruited daily smokers with and without posttraumatic stress disorder and panic psychopathology. *Journal of Anxiety Disorders, 22*, 1214–1226.

Marx, B. P., Brailey, K., Proctor, S. P., et al. (2009). Association of time since deployment, combat intensity, and posttraumatic stress symptoms with neuropsychological outcomes following Iraq war deployment. *Archives of General Psychiatry, 66*, 996–1004.

McClernon, F. J., Addicott, M. A., & Sweitzer, M. M. (2015). Smoking abstinence and neurocognition: implications for cessation and relapse. *Current Topics in Behavioral Neurosciences, 23*, 193–227.

McClernon, F. J., Beckham, J. C., Mozley, S. L., Feldman, M. E., Vrana, S. R., & Rose, J. E. (2005). The effects of trauma recall on smoking topography in posttraumatic stress disorder and non-posttraumatic stress disorder trauma survivors. *Addictive Behaviors, 30*, 247–257.

McFall, M., Saxon, A. J., Malte, C. A., Chow, B., Bailey, S., Baker, D. G., et al. (2010). Integrating tobacco cessation into mental health care for posttraumatic stress disorder: a randomized controlled trial. *Journal of the American Medical Association, 304*, 2485–2493.

McGranahan, T. M., Patzlaff, N. E., Grady, S. R., Heinemann, S. F., & Booker, T. K. (2011). α4β2 nicotinic acetylcholine receptors on dopaminergic neurons mediate nicotine reward and anxiety relief. *The Journal of Neuroscience, 31*, 10891–10902.

Milad, M. R., Orr, S. P., Lasko, N. B., Chang, Y., Rauch, S. L., & Pitman, R. K. (2008). Presence and acquired origin of reduced recall for fear extinction in PTSD: results of a twin study. *Journal of Psychiatric Research, 42*, 515–520.

Moran, V. E. (2012). Cotinine: beyond that expected, more than a biomarker of tobacco consumption. *Frontiers in Pharmacology, 3*, 173.

Patel, R., Spreng, R. N., Shin, L. M., & Girard, T. A. (2012). Neurocircuitry models of posttraumatic stress disorder and beyond: a meta-analysis of functional neuroimaging studies. *Neuroscience and Biobehavioral Reviews, 36*, 2130–2142.

Perkins, K. A., & Grobe, J. E. (1992). Increased desire to smoke during acute stress. *British Journal of Addiction, 87*, 1037–1040.

Peters, J., Kalivas, P. W., & Quirk, G. J. (2009). Extinction circuits for fear and addiction overlap in prefrontal cortex. *Learning and Memory, 16*, 279–288.

Picciotto, M. R., & Corrigall, W. A. (2002). Neuronal systems underlying behaviors related to nicotine addiction: neural circuits and molecular genetics. *The Journal of Neuroscience, 22*, 3338–3341.

Pietrzak, R. H., Goldstein, R. B., Southwick, S. M., & Grant, B. F. (2011). Medical comorbidity of full and partial posttraumatic stress disorder in United States adults: results from wave 2 of the National Epidemiological Survey on Alcohol and Related Conditions. *Psychosomatic Medicine, 73*, 697–707.

Pizzimenti, C. L., & Lattal, K. M. (2015). Epigenetics and memory: causes, consequences and treatments for post-traumatic stress disorder and addiction. *Genes, Brain, and Behavior, 14*, 73–84.

Pomerleau, O. F., & Pomerleau, C. S. (1987). The effects of a psychological stressor on cigarette smoking and on subsequent behavioral and physiological responses. *Psychophysiology, 24*, 278–285.

Porrino, L. J., Smith, H. R., Nader, M. A., & Beveridge, T. J. R. (2007). The effects of cocaine: a shifting target over the course of addiction. *Progress in Neuro-Psychopharmacology and Biological Psychiatry*, *31*, 1593–1600.

Portugal, G. S., Wilkinson, D. S., Turner, J. R., Blendy, J. A., & Gould, T. J. (2012). Strain-dependent effects of acute, chronic, and withdrawal from chronic nicotine on fear conditioning. *Neurobiology of Learning and Memory*, *97*, 482–494.

Quirk, G. J., & Mueller, D. (2008). Neural mechanisms of extinction learning and retrieval. *Neuropsychopharmacology*, *33*, 56–72.

Qureshi, S. U., Pyne, J. M., Magruder, K. M., Schulz, P. E., & Kunik, M. E. (2009). The link between post-traumatic stress disorder and physical comorbidities: a systematic review. *The Psychiatry Quarterly*, *80*, 87–97.

Rauch, S. A., Grunfeld, T. E., Yadin, E., Cahill, S. P., Hembree, E., & Foa, E. B. (2009). Changes in reported physical health symptoms and social function with prolonged exposure therapy for chronic posttraumatic stress disorder. *Depression and Anxiety*, *26*, 732–738.

Rezvani, A. H., Caldwell, D. P., & Levin, E. D. (2005). Nicotinic-serotonergic drug interactions and attentional performance in rats. *Psychopharmacology*, *179*, 521–528.

Schnurr, P. P., Friedman, M. J., Foy, D. W., Shea, M. T., Hseih, F. Y., Lavori, P. W., et al. (2003). Randomized trial of trauma-focused group therapy for posttraumatic stress disorder: results from a department of veterans affairs cooperative study. *Archives of General Psychiatry*, *60*, 481–489.

Schnurr, P. P., Lunney, C. A., Bovin, M. J., & Marx, B. P. (2009). Post-traumatic stress disorder and quality of life: extension of findings to veterans of the wars in Iraq and Afghanistan. *Clinical Psychology Review*, *29*, 727–735.

Shalev, A., Bleich, A., & Ursano, R. J. (1990). Posttraumatic stress disorder: somatic comorbidity and effort tolerance. *Psychosomatics*, *31*, 197–203.

Singh, A., Potter, A., & Newhouse, P. (2004). Nicotinic acetylcholine receptor system and neuropsychiatric disorders. *IDrugs*, *7*, 1096–1103.

Snyder, F. R., Davis, F. C., & Henningfield, J. E. (1989). The tobacco withdrawal syndrome: performance decrements assessed on a computerized test battery. *Drug and Alcohol Dependence*, *23*, 259–266.

Solomon, Z., & Mikulincer, M. (1987). Combat stress reactions, post traumatic stress disorder and somatic complaints among Israeli soldiers. *Journal of Psychosomatic Research*, *31*, 131–137.

Stein, M. B., Kennedy, C. M., & Twamley, E. W. (2002). Neuropsychological function in female victims of intimate partner violence with and without posttraumatic stress disorder. *Biological Psychiatry*, *52*, 1079–1088.

Thorndike, F. P., Wernicke, R., Pearlman, M. Y., & Haaga, D. A. F. (2006). Nicotine dependence, PTSD symptoms, and depression proneness among male and female smokers. *Addictive Behaviors*, *31*, 223–231.

Tian, S., Gao, J., Han, L., Fu, J., Li, C., & Li, Z. (2008). Prior chronic nicotine impairs cued fear extinction but enhances contextual fear conditioning in mice. *Neuroscience*, *153*, 935–943.

Tipps, M. E., Raybuck, J. D., & Lattal, M. (2014). Substance abuse, memory, and post-traumatic stress disorder. *Neurobiology of Learning and Memory*, *112*, 87–100.

US Department of Health and Human Services. (2014). *The health consequences of smoking: 50 years of progress a report of the surgeon general*. Atlanta, GA: US Department of Health and Human Services, Centers for Disease Control and Prevention, National Center for Chronic Disease Prevention and Health Promotion Office on Smoking and Health.

Varani, A. P., Moutinho, L. M., Bettler, B., & Balerio, G. N. (2012). Acute behavioural responses to nicotine and nicotine withdrawal syndrome are modified in GABA(B1) knockout mice. *Neuropharmacology*, *63*, 863–872.

Vasterling, J. J., Brailey, K., Constans, J. I., & Sutker, P. B. (1998). Attention and memory dysfunction in posttraumatic stress disorder. *Neuropsychology*, *12*, 125–133.

Vasterling, J. J., Duke, L. M., Brailey, K., Constans, J. I., Allain, A. N., & Sutker, P. B. (2002). Attention, learning and memory performances and intellectual resources in Vietnam veterans: PTSD and no disorder comparisons. *Neuropsychology, 16,* 5–14.

Vujanovic, A. A., Marshall-Berenz, E., Beckham, J. C., Bernstein, A., & Zvolensky, M. J. (2010). Posttraumatic stress symptoms and cigarette deprivation in the prediction of anxious responding among trauma-exposed smokers: a laboratory test. *Nicotine & Tobacco Research, 12,* 1080–1088.

White, H. K., & Levin, E. D. (1999). Four-week nicotine skin patch treatment effects on cognitive performance in Alzheimer's disease. *Psychopharmacology, 143,* 158–165.

Wilkenson, D. S., & Gould, T. J. (2013). Withdrawal from chronic nicotine and subsequent sensitivity to nicotine challenge on contextual learning. *Behavioral Brain Research, 250,* 58–61.

World Health Organization. (2008). *WHO report on the global tobacco epidemic: The MPOWER package.* Geneva: World Health Organization.

Yehuda, R., Keefe, R. S., Harvey, P. D., Levengood, R. A., Gerber, D. K., Geni, J., et al. (1995). Learning and memory in combat veterans with posttraumatic stress disorder. *The American Journal of Psychiatry, 152,* 137–139.

Zeitlin, R., Patel, S., Solomon, R., Tran, J., Weeber, E. J., & Echeverria, V. (2012). Cotinine enhances the extinction of contextual fear memory and reduces anxiety after fear conditioning. *Behavioural Brain Research, 228,* 284–293.

Zovkic, I. B., & Sweatt, J. D. (2013). Epigenetic mechanisms in learned fear: implications for PTSD. *Neuropsychopharmacology, 38,* 77–93.

Nicotine Withdrawal and Depression: Clinical Studies—A Four-Factor Model for More Accurate Characterization

D.G. Gilbert[1], M.L. Pergadia[2]

[1]Southern Illinois University–Carbondale, Carbondale, IL, United States;
[2]Florida Atlantic University, Boca Raton, FL, United States

INTRODUCTION

Hajek, Taylor, and McRobbie (2010) recently concluded, "In highly dependent smokers that report that smoking helps them cope with stress, smoking cessation is associated with lowering of stress. Whatever immediate effects of smoking may have on perceived stress, overall it may generate or aggravate negative emotional states. The results provide reassurance to smokers worried that stopping smoking may deprive them of a valuable resource." Similarly, outstanding researchers at M. D. Anderson Cancer Center and Brown University recently concluded, "This [their] study adds to a burgeoning body of research demonstrating that significant improvements in psychological functioning can be observed among those who successfully quit smoking even in the most severe psychiatric group [clinical depression]" (Mathew et al., 2013). The present chapter addresses the confidence that we can have in this "quitting smoking makes you feel good" conclusion, versus the view of others, including smokers, that quitting smoking increases both short- and long-term negative affect. It is important to accurately characterize the short- and long-term effects (trajectories) of smoking abstinence on psychological functioning because accurate beliefs about these trajectories have important clinical and theoretical implications.

Negative Affective States and Cognitive Impairments in Nicotine Dependence
http://dx.doi.org/10.1016/B978-0-12-802574-1.00017-X

Depressive vulnerability (history of major depressive disorders, subclinical depressive symptoms, and anhedonia) is associated with greater smoking prevalence, relapse, and nicotine dependence (reviewed by Weinberger, Mazure, Morlett, & Mckee, 2013; Weinberger, Pilver, Desai, Mazure, & McKee, 2012a, 2012b); however, evidence reviewed in this chapter indicates that while findings suggest that increases in withdrawal symptoms are greater in individuals high in depressive vulnerability, the relationships of such depression-related risk to withdrawal symptom severity and trajectories, or what may be described as *mental health measures* preceding or following reduction or cessation of smoking, are not well characterized because of methodological limitations of most relevant studies.

As part of the goal of assessing relationships of depressive traits to withdrawal symptoms, one of the major themes of this chapter is that the evidence on which the *feel better soon and live happily ever after* interpretation of clinical outcome studies is flawed by a tendency of many investigators to underplay the importance of obvious methodological limitations of their studies and the failure to assess and to control for a number of powerful, yet much less well-recognized biasing influences on self-reported abstinence symptoms. As described in this chapter, a review of the literature suggests that these flaws may be especially strong in the case of individuals high in depressive vulnerability and when using measures of depressive symptoms. Overall, the goals of this chapter include (1) the evaluation of findings and methodological issues in the assessment of smoking/nicotine abstinence, including withdrawal symptoms generally, but with a primary focus on symptoms in individuals high in depressive vulnerability; (2) a brief overview of findings by those attempting to characterize the effects of depressive traits on nicotine withdrawal symptom trajectories; and (3) the presentation of a four-factor model (4FM) of methodological limitations that bias most studies in the area, especially ones that assess abstinence trajectories in those high in depressive vulnerability. The 4FM of potential data bias is provided as a template for conceptualizing the results of studies to date and for the development of future more definitive studies of the effects of smoking abstinence.

Consistent with established recommendations (Shiffman, West, & Gilbert, 2004), we define *withdrawal* as a syndrome of behavioral, affective, cognitive, and physiological symptoms, typically transient, emerging upon cessation or reduction of tobacco use, which may cause distress or impairment of behavioral function. *Offset effects* (effects due to removal of a direct nicotine effect) are sustained effects of cessation or reduction of tobacco use that may also cause distress or impairment. Withdrawal and offset effects (jointly referred to as abstinence effects) are important as potential predictors of relapse, as mediators and markers of treatment effects, and as clinical phenomena in their own right (Shiffman et al., 2004).

Nicotine and smoking withdrawal symptom severity and trajectories are not well characterized because of a number of methodological problems and associated biases that are highlighted by the 4FM of abstinence symptom trajectory estimation bias. These problematic biases in self-reported abstinence symptom scores are related to the failure to control for and to carefully assess the impact of these four factors that may bias withdrawal symptom scores, particularly the scores in any retained study sample. These 4FM biases result from (1) nonrandom progressive subject loss due to study dropout and relapse in individuals with depressive vulnerability and more generally in individuals with the most severe withdrawal symptoms and stressful life events; (2) the strong tendency for scores on measures of negative affect and withdrawal symptoms to decrease substantially with repeated testing across time (given a constant environment stress potential); (3) increased prequit anticipatory negative affect and withdrawal symptom scores in the week or so prior to quit attempts; and (4) variation in individual and contextual factors that modulate affect and abstinence symptom scores and influence study completion.

In the following assessment of the 4FM of abstinence effects estimation bias, selective relapse and study dropout are the easiest to conceptualize. However, the three remaining components of the 4FM are more difficult to immediately grasp and therefore are discussed using a series of Figs. 17.1–17.6, most of which were derived from studies explicitly designed to assess baseline stability and drift of abstinence-related measures. In these studies, nicotine withdrawal symptoms were measured using the Shiffman–Jarvik Withdrawal scale (Shiffman & Jarvik, 1976), the Beck Depression Inventory (BDI) (Beck & Steer, 1987), and the Profile of Mood States (McNair, Lorr, & Droppleman, 1971), assessments that are frequently used to characterize abstinence symptoms.

FACTOR 1: DIFFERENTIAL RELAPSE AND DROPOUT

It is important to recognize that withdrawal symptom abstinence curves only characterize the responses of the select group of successful abstainers. In one of the first studies in this area, Cohen and Lichtenstein (1990) reported that 12 participants (8% of the sample) successfully abstained from smoking and reported progressively less stress across 6 months of abstinence relative to baseline and relative to 57 individuals who never quit and to 81 who quit for fewer than 24h. In the above-noted study by Mathew et al. (2013, p. 28), 6% of quitters maintained abstinence and reported less negative affect than nonabstainers, while in a study by Hajek et al. (2010), 41% maintained abstinence and reported less "stress at the moment". The question arises as to what was unique about the minority group of abstainers in each of these studies and in virtually all studies using similar high-relapse methods without random assignment to abstainer versus nonabstainer status. A potential answer is hinted at by the Hajek et al. (2010) measure of negative affect—less stress at the moment. Individuals may maintain abstinence because their environment provided lower levels of stress (eg, McKee, Maciejewski, Falba, & Mazure, 2003; Wewers, 1988). Thus, low levels of environmental stressors may "cause" abstinence, rather than the other way around. It seems unlikely that many individuals in the abstainer groups in these clinical studies recently lost their job, had a relationship breakup, or experienced another random or nonrandom stressful event that increased their anxiety, stress, and temptation to smoke. In addition, genetic and other biological factors may be unique to those who maintain abstinence. These questions can be asked of all clinical studies showing decreased stress and negative affect (or elevated positive affect) in successful abstainers, relative to those who fail to maintain abstinence. The critically important fact is that clinical studies and virtually all other studies have high selective retention in their samples that maintain abstinence relative to failure to maintain abstinence. Stated simply, most clinical outcome studies are correlational in nature, and correlation does not equal causation.

For example, one might consider individuals who take antidepressant medications. Do antidepressants cause depression, or is it the other way around? Fortunately, well-designed randomized clinical trials indicate that, relative to placebos, antidepressants reduce rather than cause depression. However, when attempting to infer causation from smoking abstinence versus nonabstinence, only a few studies have randomly assigned smokers to quit or to continue smoking, and these studies do not support the "quick recovery to feeling better" hypothesis. Furthermore, given the belief among smokers that smoking reduces stress, it is reasonable to hypothesize that those experiencing the greatest degree of stress are more likely to relapse, as well as to drop out of the study (Shiffman et al., 2004). The empirical literature supports the proximal "stress leads to relapse" hypothesis (Shiffman & Paty, 2006). Given that individuals high in depressive vulnerability tend to have more severe withdrawal symptoms (Gilbert et al., 1998, 2002; Weinberger et al., 2012a) and relapse rates (Gilbert, Crauthers, Mooney, & McClernon, 1999; Weinberger et al., 2012a), one would expect them to be selectively excluded from abstainer groups and thus to provide lower estimates of negative affect in the abstainer groups. Additional support of this possibility comes from retrospective studies, in which smokers commonly cite a desire for relief from negative affect as a chief reason for smoking (Brandon & Baker, 1991; Piper et al., 2004), and often attribute relapses to acute negative affect (Brandon, Tiffany, & Baker, 1986; Shiffman, 1982).

The hypothetical effects of selective attrition (relapse and dropout) on Negative Affect/Depressive state scores as a function of degree of subject

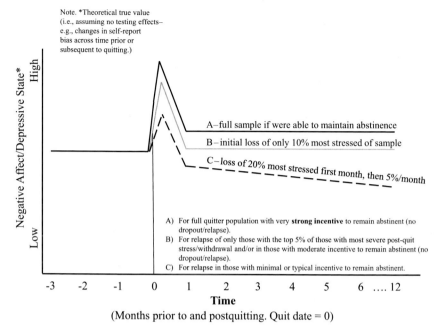

Note. *Theoretical true value
(i.e., assuming no testing effects–
e.g., changes in self-report
bias across time prior or
subsequent to quitting.)

A–full sample if were able to maintain abstinence

B–initial loss of only 10% most stressed of sample

C–loss of 20% most stressed first month, then 5%/month

A) For full quitter population with very **strong incentive** to remain abstinent (no dropout/relapse).
B) For relapse of only those with the top 5% of those with most severe post-quit stress/withdrawal and/or in those with moderate incentive to remain abstinent (no dropout/relapse).
C) For relapse in those with minimal or typical incentive to remain abstinent.

Time

(Months prior to and postquitting. Quit date = 0)

FIGURE 17.1   The hypothetical effects of selective attrition on Negative Affect/Depressive state scores as a function of degree of subject loss present a yet-to-be seen Condition A, where there is no selective relapse, as in the case of no relapse or study dropout. In Condition B, a small percentage (eg, 10%) of the total sample who are the most acutely stressed fail to quit, but there is no subsequent selective relapse (ie, the unlikely situation in which even the most acutely stressed or depressed, or those experiencing the most severe abstinence effects, do not relapse subsequently). Condition C depicts a case in which there is a tendency for those most distress intolerant to relapse as stressors occur during the year after quitting. Note that this figure depicts a hypothetical situation that includes no downward drift or other testing effects and no upward drift due to anticipation of the quit date.

loss are presented in Fig. 17.1. While this figure is a theoretical construction, the lower abstinence score values reflect the mathematical fact that those with the highest negative affect/abstinence scores were eliminated from the abstinent smoker sample. It is based on a compelling literature finding that proximal stress and generalized high levels of distress promote relapse (Shiffman & Paty, 2006; Shiffman et al., 2004). Despite the warning of previous reviews (eg, Shiffman et al., 2004) that clinical and correlational studies have serious errors due to selection bias, the field seems to have recently seen a resurgence of the view that selection factors can be corrected for by logic argumentation or simple post-hoc statistical corrections. In this regard, it may be instructive to recall the hormone replacement therapy (HRT) disaster of late twentieth-century medicine. For several decades, virtually all physicians and patients were convinced of the benefits of the therapy for the heart and health. Subsequently, and without apparent need in the eyes of most, the US National Institutes of Health (NIH) conducted a large randomized clinical trial, the results of which compellingly demonstrated that the very medicine that all thought to benefit was increasing risk of disease in women. Among other things, the randomized clinical trial demonstrated that HRT increased risk of cardiovascular disease and breast cancer rather than preventing them (Rossouw et al., 2002). Nonrandomized, biased samples played a serious role in the generation of the previous earnest but erroneous belief in the health benefits of HRT (Stampfer & Colditz, 1991). Appropriate scientific curiosity dictates that one wonders whether these HRT findings provide a lesson for caution in the interpretation of withdrawal symptom trajectories and the "quitting makes you feel better" hypothesis.

A recent study by Shahab et al. (2015) is relevant to the question of the direction of the relationship of differential dropout and abstinence versus relapse (nonabstinence) in depressive states. The study was designed to identify reciprocal, longitudinal relationships between smoking cessation and depression among older smokers. Within the English Longitudinal Study of Aging, changes in smoking status and depression were assessed across time in recent ex-smokers and smokers ($n = 2375$). Latent growth curve analysis indicated that depression predicted continued smoking longitudinally but not the other way around. Shahab and colleagues concluded that "in older smokers," depressive vulnerability acts as "an important barrier to quitting, although quitting has no long-term impact on depression." These conclusions, based on this sophisticated study using a large sample, highlight the methodological issues involved in attempting to better understand the effect of smoking status on prospective depression-related measures. While baseline and prospective depressive symptoms are predictive of continued smoking, there was much less variance (or change) in smoking behaviors in the prospective prediction of depression (ie, very few of these older smokers were quitting), and it is reasonable to suspect that those who were not able to quit smoking may have had a worsening of depressive symptoms had they quit.

Findings from two other recent studies highlight similar issues. In one population-based study, reduction in smoking was concluded to be associated with reduced risk for prospective problems related to anxiety, mood, drug, and alcohol (Cavazos-Rehg et al., 2014). However, here again, very few smokers quit across the prospective period, obviating the ability to assess the potential impact from those smokers who were not able to quit or cut down on smoking, and who may have experienced relapse-related nicotine withdrawal symptoms upon quit efforts. The second recent study, a systematic review and meta-analysis, concluded that quitting smoking was associated with a reduction in symptoms associated with depression and anxiety (Taylor et al., 2014). This meta-analysis combined different types of studies (eg, cohort and treatment studies), and, interestingly, in subsidiary sensitivity analysis that only included studies with complete data on participants, the effect of smoking cessation on prospective depressive symptoms was no longer significant, highlighting again the importance of selection and/or attrition bias in understanding outcomes and interpretation of results.

STUDIES EXPLICITLY DESIGNED TO CHARACTERIZE ABSTINENCE EFFECTS

The National Institute on Drug Abuse (NIDA) has funded four studies (Gilbert et al., 1998, 2002, 2009) designed explicitly to better characterize the effects of smoking abstinence on smoking withdrawal symptoms and offset effects for 31 or more days using a novel design in which smokers were randomized to quit smoking or to delay quitting smoking during the period of time when the quit groups were being paid large sums of money to maintain biochemically verified abstinence. Besides being random-ized to quit "immediately" or to delay quitting until after the immediate group had gone through their 31, 45, or 67-day paid abstinence period, these studies included multiple baseline assessments twice per week for 5 weeks (10 baseline assessments) in the study that will be our primary focus here, but for only 3 weeks in the first of these studies (six baseline assessments). These multiple baseline assessments were included to dem-onstrate baseline stability, something that the principal investigator (PI) expected to observe given the reported reliability of these measures. How-ever, as nature soon taught the PI, relative rank as assessed by the test–retest correlations used in traditional reliability estimates is not equivalent to the stability of group mean values. One can have perfect correlation reliability ($r = 1.0$), yet have the group means decrease or increase by any value as the relative rankings among individuals or variables remain con-stant. This point is emphasized here in the discussion of the problem of baseline drift in abstinence scores.

Though all four of the above-noted NIDA-funded studies to character-ize abstinence effects resulted in largely similar effects, this chapter focuses on the findings of the second (Gilbert et al., 2002) because it had the lon-gest prequit baseline of the series of studies and also had the largest sam-ple of quitting without pharmacotherapy to promote abstinence. Smoking abstinence responses were characterized in 96 female dependent smok-ers. Participants completed subjective state measures twice per week for 5 weeks and were then randomly assigned to a group required to abstain for 31 days or a control group that continued to smoke. Financial incentives for biochemically verified abstinence resulted in an 81% completion rate in both the quit and smoke groups. Of the 96 participants who completed the baseline phase, 67 were randomly assigned (by a 70:30 odds ratio) to the quit group and 29 were assigned to the smoke group. This 70:30 ratio was used to maximize power to detect individual differences in responses to quitting while maintaining adequate control group power. Of the 67 assigned to the quit group, 54 (81%) completed all aspects of the study and smoked fewer than a total of 10 cigarettes across the 31-day abstinence period and never smoked more than three cigarettes on any 1 day, and 30 remained fully abstinent. Quitters who were not fully abstinent smoked an average of 2.8 cigarettes total during the 31-day quit phase. Reasons for study dropout included relapses (smoking more than a total of 10 cigarettes across the 31-day abstinence period or more than three cigarettes in a single day: 12 individuals in the quit group), scheduling problems (one quit-group individual and one smoke-group individual), and low prequit baseline cotinine values (one smoke-group individual). Completion of all aspects of the study resulted in each participant earning $400 minus any penalties for smoking up to 10 cigarettes. The first five cigarettes cost $10 each; for each additional cigarette beyond five to 10, the cost was $25, for a maximum total of $175 for 10 cigarettes. No payment at all occurred if the participant smoked more than 10 cigarettes total over the 31 days. Nicotine and cotinine concentrations were determined from blood samples collected once a week during the 5-week baseline and then at Days 1, 3, 10, 17, and 31 post quit. Additionally, saliva samples for cotinine assays were obtained approximately every 96h subsequent to quitting and at any additional monitoring session if CO concentration indicated the possibility of smoking (CO 4 parts per million [ppm]). Cotinine and nicotine concentrations were assayed using gas chromatography.

As is seen in subsequent figures, abstinence-related increases in depression, tension, anger, and irritability exhibited little tendency to return to appropriately chosen prequit levels and remained significantly elevated above smoke-group levels. Trait depression and neuroticism predicted larger increased abstinence-associated negative affect (see Gilbert et al., 2002) for specific correlations, but generally, both trait depression as assessed by the MMPI Depression scale and by the NEO-PI depression scale correlated with abstinence-associated increases in POMS Depression and BDI Depression scores and POMS Anxiety in the range of $r = 0.45$.

The first author was fortunate to be the PI on these NIH studies and now turns to how the findings of the first of these studies were a great surprise to him given his expectations based on previous findings with less well-controlled studies.

FACTOR 2: DOWNWARD DRIFT IN SELF-REPORTED NEGATIVE AFFECT

One of the greatest surprises of the first of these controlled studies was the very large downward drift in withdrawal score and negative affect measure scores across the prequit baseline period (Fig. 17.2). Given that

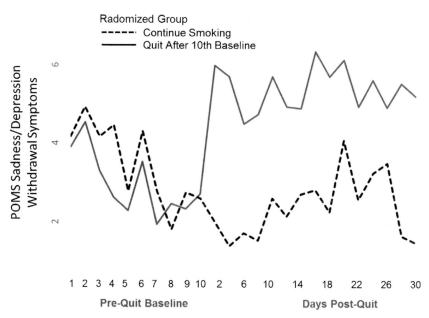

FIGURE 17.2   POMS Sadness/Depression symptom scores during a 5-week (10 assessments) baseline period prior to quitting and at 2-day intervals during the postquit period,
when the quit group was randomized to quit smoking at Day 0. The Continue-to-Smoke
group was randomized from the same sample as the quit group, and biochemical verification
of abstinence (salivary cotinine and nicotine) was assessed throughout the abstinence period
to assure compliance with quit and smoking status of each subject.

the literature reported these dependent measures of negative affect and
withdrawal to have quite high test–retest reliability, it was assumed that
the baseline scores would project pretty much in a straight line until an
assessment or two before the quit date, when the anticipation of quitting
might slightly elevate the scores. The PI was so surprised that he was
convinced that there was an error in his data, yet dozens of hours of
analyses kept revealing the same pattern across virtually all of our
measures of withdrawal symptoms and negative affect—symptoms
progressively decreased (drifted lower) from about 100% of the first baseline
session value to a value about 40–50% lower by the fifth or sixth session
(Study 1=Gilbert et al., 1998; Study 2=Gilbert et al., 2002). Our initial
question was "Are we doing something we were not aware of that was
somehow biasing our findings?"

Our subsequent review of studies using multiple baselines over several weeks or more revealed a substantial literature demonstrating the
same downward drift testing effect that we had observed. This literature

includes assessment of clinical populations and control groups across multiple sessions (Ahava, Iannone, Grebstein, & Schirling, 1998; Arrindell, 2001; Atkenson, Calhoun, Resick, Ellis, 1982; Choquette & Hesselbrock, 1987; Hatzenbuehler, Parpal, & Matthews, 1983; Sharpe & Gilbert, 1998). Atkenson et al. (1982) assessed female rape victims who were matched with nonvictimized controls. In this study, both groups demonstrated the downward drift testing effect over the course of an 18-month follow-up. Interestingly, downward drift is rarely discussed in literature where it is most important (eg, studies of intervention efficacy), possibly because the admission of and controlling for such drift makes interventions and therapies frequently appear to be much less efficacious than they are purported to be. In one of the few nicotine-related studies mentioning drift, McChargue and Collins (1998, p. 207) state that "downward trend during nondeprivation days supported the idea of stabilizing response patterns before deprivation. This trend suggests that other effects may contaminate deprivation effects without an adequate control."

The first author's laboratory is one of very few that has used multiple prequit baseline assessments for more than a week. In our two studies with the longest times of assessment before quitting (beginning 3 or 5 weeks prior to quit date; Gilbert et al., 1998, 2002), there was a decrease of about 50% in the baseline values of scores on the withdrawal and negative affect measures (see Fig. 17.2). We now turn to other features of the results of these highly controlled, randomized studies.

The effects of abstaining from smoking versus continuing to smoke on POMS Sadness/Depression scores are presented in Fig. 17.2. Both quit and smoke groups exhibit a downward drift in depression scores across the first 5–8 baseline assessments, then exhibit a slight increase across the three sessions just prior to the quit date. There is an initial downward drift in Sadness/Depression scores across the first 5–8 prequit assessments, amounting to about a 50% reduction in these scores in both groups. Individuals were not randomized until after completion of the 10-week baseline period. The scores for the quit group and smoking control group do not converge after abstinence. These and subsequent figures are unpublished findings that came from a study described in detail by Gilbert et al. (2002).

In Fig. 17.3, it can be seen that during the distal downward baseline period (first five prequit baseline assessments [A]), a main effect of Time emerged [$F(4/372)=11.01$, $p<0.001$], something consistent with a large literature showing the above-noted downward drift testing effect in measures of negative affect. The high trait depression group exhibited a greater downward drift in their BDI scores than the low trait depression group, as indicated by a significant Group × Time interaction [$F(4/372)=3.37$, $p=0.017$]. Analysis across both high and low NEO-PI Depression groups across the 10 prequit assessments also revealed that downward BDI drift sessions were highly significant [Time, $F(9/729)=7.15$, $p<0.001$].

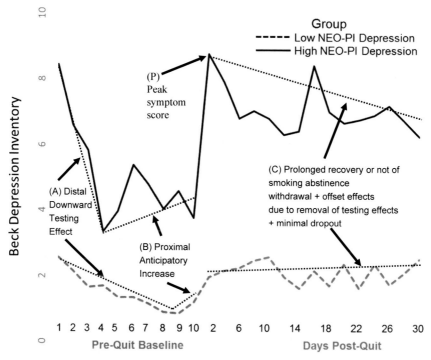

FIGURE 17.3 Beck Depression Inventory (BDI) scores across time in quitters only as a function of low versus high trait Depression scores on the Neuroticism Extraversion Openness-Personality Inventory (NEO-PI). If only 1–3 baseline assessments are used, the downward testing drift would not only impact the prequit baseline score values but also substantially reduce the magnitude of the withdrawal symptom score increases (P – A difference) subsequent to smoking. Higher NEO-PI Depression, NEO-PI Anxiety, and Minnesota Multiphasic Personality Inventory-2 (MMPI) Depression scores were significantly associated with greater increases in BDI scores during the first days of abstinence, whereas only NEO-PI Anxiety and MMPI Depression were significantly associated with increases in BDI during the last few days of the 31-day abstinence period (Gilbert et al., 2002).

As expected, NEO-PI trait depression was associated with much greater levels of absolute BDI scores [Group, $F(1/81) = 15.49$, $p < 0.001$].

Fig. 17.3 also allows the reader to see that whether or not the quit groups return to prequit baseline abstinence symptom levels depends on what part of the prequit baseline is used. There is good reason to believe that the downward drift testing effect also occurs in other studies using only one or a few baseline assessments, something that likely seriously underestimates the severity of abstinence symptoms given that the upward increase in abstinence symptoms would be counteracted by the downward testing effect that is generally maximal over the first 3–6 assessments.

Finally, it is useful to consider studies of nicotine replacement therapy (NRT); relative to placebo therapy, NRT almost universally results in decreases in negative affect and other abstinence symptoms, rather than making people feel worse. These placebo-controlled studies of NRT demonstrate that these beneficial effects of NRT persist well beyond the point at which relapsers begin to show elevated negative affect relative to abstainers (eg, Gilbert et al., 2009). Interestingly, NRT studies tend to demonstrate downward shifts in negative affect/abstinence severity in both the placebo control and NRT groups (eg, Gross & Stitzer, 1989), even though a great majority of publications do not discuss this fact even when depicted in their figures.

FACTOR 3: QUIT-DATE PROXIMAL UPWARD BASELINE DRIFT

The slight upward drift during the 3–5 assessments most proximal to the quit date in Figs. 17.2 and 17.3 and in Figs. 17.4 and 17.5 is frequently observed and frequently commented on in the abstinence literature and may contribute to the almost universal failure to acknowledge or observe prequit baseline downward drift effects in cessation studies. Strong et al. (2009) recently formally assessed and statistically analyzed the progressive increases in negative affect and decreases in positive affect they observed during their three baseline assessments shortly before their study quit date. Their proximal drifts were statistically significant and potentially clinically important, as well as critical to think about in interpreting their findings. They should be praised for their efforts. But, what would have happened if they had acquired six, 10, or more assessments more distal to the quit date? Would these more distal assessments have demonstrated a downward drift testing effect that should have been incorporated into their modeling of the actual effects of abstinence? We think so, on both accounts.

Upward baseline drift, if above the yet-to-be-defined "true" baseline, would have the effect of making it appear that initial withdrawal symptoms are less severe than they actually are, assuming that the highest point or points upward are used as a baseline. Given this fact, individuals with the greatest upward drift would exhibit the greatest attenuation. The Gilbert et al. (2002) data, presented here in Figs. 17.3–17.5, show that individuals high in NEO-PI trait depression exhibited larger upward drifts in withdrawal symptoms proximal to the quit date. Thus, estimates of withdrawal symptom severity in individuals high in depressive traits may be attenuated relative to elevations above their "true" baseline values. This possibility combined with the findings seen in these figures that high-trait individuals exhibited far greater abstinence-associated increases in negative affect and Shiffman–Jarvik Withdrawal scores provides evidence in support of the view that depression-vulnerable individuals are more likely

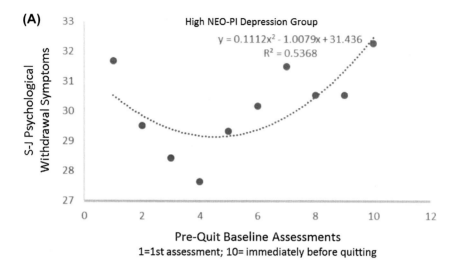

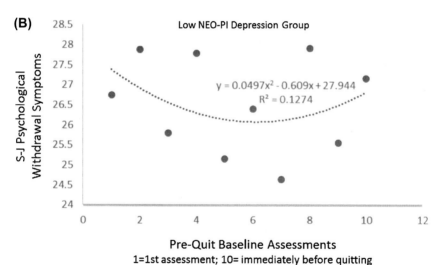

FIGURE 17.4   A and B: Differences in the second-order curvilinear relationship across time for Shiffman–Jarvik Withdrawal Scores in those high in NEO-PI trait depression and those low in this trait.

to relapse because they experience more severe increases in withdrawal symptoms, as well as because their overall symptom scores are so high.

In Fig. 17.4, we mathematically model differences in the curvilinear baseline trajectories for Shiffman–Jarvik Psychological Withdrawal Symptoms for smokers high in NEO-PI trait depression and those low in this trait.

Fig. 17.4 shows that Shiffman–Jarvik Withdrawal scores initially decreased across the first five assessments due to the downward testing

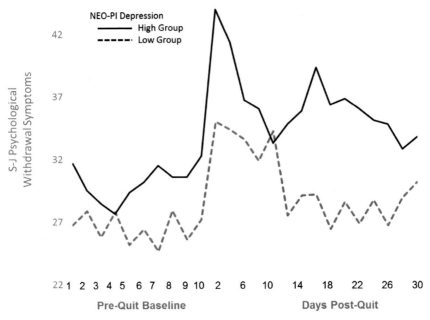

FIGURE 17.5 Shiffman–Jarvik Psychological Withdrawal Symptom scores in those high versus those low (below the median) in NEO-PI trait depression show that scores decreased across the first five assessments in the high trait depression group, but across the first 7 days in the low depression group, followed by the presumably anticipatory increase in scores proximal to quitting that began earlier and were much stronger in those high in trait depression than those low in this trait. Note also that high-depressive-trait individuals reported postquit withdrawal scores that remained substantially greater than prequit levels, while those in the low-depression group approximated baseline levels, though never fully returned to baseline. The degree of withdrawal symptom elevation depends on what is considered the true baseline value for the withdrawal score. The patterns largely reflect those seen with pre- and postquit changes observed with BDI and POMS Depression scores; however, POMS and BDI Depression scores exhibited far larger downward drifts during the distal prequit period (see Figs. 17.2 and 17.3).

effect (distal factor), followed by an increase in abstinence symptoms more proximal to quitting smoking. It is hypothesized that the proximal increase reflects anticipatory anxiety and other negative affect, while the larger earlier downward slope reflects the testing effects observed in many studies not involving anticipatory anxiety or when the distal stressor is preceded by a longer period of time and with multiple testings. There is a linear ($r^2 = 0.80$) downward slope across the first five baseline assessments for Shiffman–Jarvik Psychological Withdrawal Symptoms $(Y) = 12.52 - 2.24x$ (assessment session [ie, ½ week]). That is, during times distal to quitting, for every assessment, there was a downward drift of 2.24 withdrawal score units. In contrast, during the final four baseline sessions (7–10), there was an upward slope where Shiffman–Jarvik Psychological Withdrawal

Symptoms (Y) $= 2.25x + 0.22x$ (assessment session [ie, ½ week]). The important question is: which baseline—proximal, distal, or even more distal than assessed—reflects the typical prequit baseline of smokers?

THE UPS AND DOWNS OF AFFECTIVE DRIFT AND WITHDRAWAL SCORES

Fig. 17.6 depicts the theoretical effects of distal proximal downward testing drift and of upward quit anticipation drift on self-reported negative affect and depressive state scores and is meant to emphasize the question of what is the appropriate baseline for studies of abstinence symptoms. The figure also begs the question of how long prior to quitting should the baseline assessments be made and the potential impact of when the eventual quitter is coming into treatment. The sensitivity of measures of abstinence effects to upward baseline drifts associated with the onset of the quit date prompts the question of what other factors may influence upward or downward baseline drift. Many studies use clinical populations with serious health issues that would be expected to have large and prognosis-dependent effects on measures of abstinence, including positive and

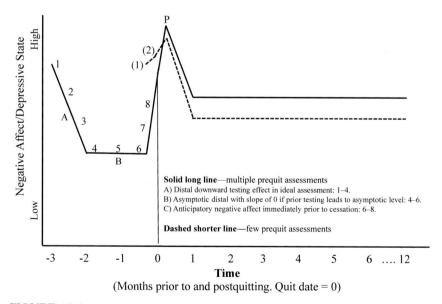

FIGURE 17.6 Depressive states and other forms of negative affect vary at baseline as a function of a wide variety of factors ranging from testing effects (points 1–4) through anticipatory affect induced by impending quit efforts.

negative affect. Similarly, depressive disorders are typically time-limited and vary in intensity. How these affect-inducing stressors impact smoking trajectories in studies to date is a question begging for answers, but they are far beyond what simple clinical evaluations can provide.

FACTOR 4: LONG- AND SHORT-TERM CHRONODYNAMIC LIFE CHANGES AND EVENTS

Abstinence studies rarely assess individual-specific time-varying temporal dynamics of life changes and events. It is reasonable to hypothesize that the chronodynamics of life changes and events impact both prequit baselines and postquit scores on abstinence symptoms and affect indices. For example, biological and medical factors that influence pressures to quit smoking in some individuals may escalate or resolve as a function of time and have large time-varying biological and psychological impacts on depressive and other abstinence-related states. Hospital studies of medically compromised individuals may be especially impacted by such variations and would likely benefit from the characterization of such variables. Meta-analyses in the area would benefit from a consideration of these factors.

Fluctuations across time in mood states, stressors, and health have not to date been analyzed in a detailed or fine-grained manner across the years, months, and moments prior or subsequent to quitting. However, a study by McCarthy, Piasecki, Fiore, and Baker (2006) made good progress in this direction by assessing mood, craving, and hunger assessed four times daily using an electronic diary (ED) for 3 weeks prior to quitting and 3 weeks after quitting. Some smokers reported anticipatory increases in negative affect prior to the quit date, and larger increases in anticipatory negative affect predicted failure to maintain abstinence months later. On average, negative affect abstinence symptoms did not improve across the 3-week postquit assessment period. Mood fluctuations associated with recent episodic ED event reports increased following the quit date. Epidemiological studies have assessed fluctuations in mood states, stressors, and health across time (Weinberger et al., 2012b), but typically sample information annually or less frequently, thereby preventing the identification of more rapidly changing lead–lag relationships among smoking status, affect, symptoms, and specific events. Infrequent sampling also prevents the characterization of rhythmic oscillations in time that occur in association with depressive disorders, mentrual cycle phases, and variations across periods of health and illness. More sophisticated data samples involving sampling at higher frequencies and across longer durations of time will be required of future studies if knowledge concerning these chronodynamic patterns of life changes and events are to be included in the modeling of how slow (low frequency) and rapidly oscillating (high frequency) or critical single events influence prequit baseline values and the interpretation of postquit symptom magnitude and duration.

The statistical and conceptual software for chronodynamic analyses are widely available to researchers and are referred to in terms of spectral analysis, coherence analysis, sequential analysis, and other time series analyses. The benefits of such analyses are widely recognized in other research fields. For example, slow and rapid variations and their covariation with other variations across time are a powerful tool in astronomy to detect variations in light and location, in the field of electroencephalography and functional magnetic resonance imaging scans of brain activity, and in biology and many other fields. A number of studies have used spectral frequency and coherence analyses of variations in depression across time (time series) to help identify cyclical variations in mood (spectral analysis) and mood covariates across varying periods of time (coherence and cross-correlation) (eg, Reid, Towell, & Golding, 2000).

Assessing where the smoker or abstainer is in their chronodynamic life and event cycles will be a challenge for the field in the coming years. Characterization of this information will depend on large and costly experimental studies using procedures such as ecological momentary sampling over long periods of time with high frequency (McCarthy et al., 2006; Shiffman & Paty, 2006). In the meantime, detailed follow-back timelines of life changes, events, and affective states may provide some insight into baseline and postquit chronodynamics.

In summary, factor 4 addresses the notion that individual differences in variability in short and long-term stressors, life circumstances, and biological functioning are important missing pieces of our characterization of baseline and abstinence symptoms. Did the person decide to quit just after learning of a serious medical diagnosis or when especially stress free? In those with seasonal affective disorder, what season is it? More accurate and fine-grained characterization of prequit baseline symptoms and abstinence-related symptoms could provide important new knowledge about abstinence symptom trajectories in depression-prone individuals and others, and thereby may lead to more efficacious interventions.

OTHER VALUABLE DESIGNS

Abstinence and Anhedonia

Cook et al. (2015) used ecological momentary sampling for 5 days before quitting and for 10 days after quitting to assess anhedonia and other withdrawal symptoms in 1175 smokers, and they found that "after controlling for pre-quit negative affect and pre-quit craving, higher pre-quit anhedonia significantly increased the likelihood of smoking at the initial abstinence and 8-week abstinence time points. Likewise, post-quit anhedonia predicted initial abstinence, days to relapse, and 8-week point-prevalence abstinence.... Finally, greater pre-to post-quit change in anhedonia predicated earlier lapse, after controlling for change in craving and negative affect." Fifty-six percent "(844) either relapsed or dropped out of the study by 8 weeks post-quit" (Cook, personal communication, June 5, 2015). Cook further noted, "I think you could be correct that those with the most severe anhedonia may have dropped out of the study."

Longitudinal Epidemiological Studies Using Complex Modeling and Controls

Longitudinal epidemiological studies frequently attempt to control for a large variety of potential confounders, though they cannot adequately control for changes in external stressors and other factors that happen between assessments. Nonetheless, in their recent multivariate growth curve analysis of longitudinal data from 1272 older smokers, Shahab et al. (2015) concluded, "In older smokers, depression appears to act as an important barrier to quitting, although quitting has no long-term impact on depression." This finding may be viewed as being at odds with the "quitting smoking makes you feel better" hypothesis.

SUMMARY, CONCLUSIONS, AND NEW DIRECTIONS

The 4FM was used to assess the degree to which clinical, epidemiological, and research findings on smoking abstinence symptoms may be biased or otherwise confounded. We conclude that these four threats to accurate characterization of withdrawal symptoms are pervasive and that claims that smoking causes stress and negative affect while continued abstinence decreases negative affect are premature, are potentially wrong, and could even prove to be counterproductive in the treatment of smokers attempting to quit. One can imagine that for smokers attempting to quit smoking, who may be experiencing severe withdrawal symptoms, validation and treatment of such symptoms are vitally important. We agree with the conclusions of the review by Shiffman et al. (2004) that new experimental designs will be required to accurately characterize withdrawal symptom trajectories.

Extremely high rates of nonrandom selective dropout, a lack of no-quit control groups, and the failure to account for the repeated-measurements effect make valid interpretations impossible. The result of this selective dropout is that the abstainers are different in terms of environmental stressors, genetic factors, and likely a host of other factors than those who fail to maintain abstinence. There is good reason to believe that this confound in group makeup makes the fully accurate characterization of withdrawal effect impossible. In comparison with relapsers, abstainers have repeatedly been found to experience fewer abstinence symptoms and less stressful environments. Inevitably, the mean values of negative affect are downwardly biased. That is, only the fittest (least stressed and most psychobiologically robust) are included in the reported mean values. The potential degree of such biasing can be recognized by considering the fact that a majority of quitters in clinical and other studies relapsed and were not included in group means. Findings from a small number of well-controlled experimental studies with randomized quit versus smoke designs suggest that full recovery of abstinence symptoms takes longer than 2 months.

In their recent review of the literature, Weinberger et al. (2012a) concluded, "Although attention to the relationship of depression and smoking cessation outcomes has increased over the past 20 years, little information exists to inform a treatment approach for smokers with Current Major Depressive Disorder, Dysthymia, and Minor Depression... and smoking cessation outcomes, thus suggesting major areas for targeted research. It is clearly important to better characterize the time trajectories of affective risks and benefits of maintaining abstinence so that better interventions can be generated." A recent paper by Blalock, Robinson, Wetter, Schreindorfer, and Cinciripini (2008) reported, "Our findings support Piasecki and colleagues' argument that exclusion of lapsers from analyses of post-cessation withdrawal may result in underestimation of withdrawal severity and may preclude greater understanding of relationships between withdrawal severity and smoking behavior following smoking cessation attempts" (Piasecki, Jorenby, Smith, Fiore, & Baker, 2003). This finding may be expected given the reduced differential "relapse" and exclusion from analysis of the most stressed individuals.

The evidence surveyed in this chapter, and the authors' general impression of the larger literature, is that results of the more rigorous and methodologically sophisticated studies differ from those of less rigorous methods and data analyses. For example, the findings from the reciprocal modeling approach used by Shahab et al. (2015) are consistent with the view that smoking status itself may not lead to depression (particularly given the pool of smokers able to quit), but that depression may impact smoking status. Similarly, the NIDA-sponsored studies designed explicitly to characterize the effects of quitting on abstinence effects provide no strong support for the "quitting smoking makes you feel better" hypothesis. However, it should be noted that these studies have not gone beyond 66 days of abstinence.

References

Ahava, G., Iannone, C., Grebstein, L., & Schirling, J. (1998). Is the beck depression inventory reliable over time? An evaluation of multiple test-retest reliability in a nonclinical college student sample. *Journal of Personality Assessment, 70*(2), 222–231.

Arrindell, W. (2001). Changes in waiting-list patients over time: data on some commonly-used measures. Beware!. *Behaviour Research and Therapy, 39*(10), 1227–1247.

Atkeson, B., Calhoun, K. S., Resick, P. A., & Ellis, E. M. (1982). Victims of rape: repeated assessment of depressive symptoms. *Journal of Consulting and Clinical Psychology, 50,* 96–102.

Beck, A., & Steer, R. (1987). *Beck depression inventory manual.* San Antonio, TX: Harcourt Brace Janovich.

Blalock, J. A., Robinson, J. R., Wetter, D. W., Schreindorfer, L. S., & Cinciripini, P. M. (2008). Nicotine withdrawal in smokers with current depressive disorders undergoing intensive smoking cessation treatment. *Psychology of Addictive Behavior, 22*(1), 122–128. http://dx.doi.org/10.1037/0893-164X.22.1.122 ict Behav.

Brandon, T. H., & Baker, T. (1991). The Smoking Consequences Questionnaire: the subjective expected utility of smoking in college students. *Psychological Assessment, 3,* 484–491.

Brandon, T. H., Tiffany, S. T., & Baker, T. B. (1986). The process of smoking relapse. In F. Tims, & C. Leukefeld (Eds.), *Relapse and recovery in drug abuse* (pp. 104–117). Washington, DC: U.S. Government Printing Office. NIDA Research Monograph No. 72.

Cavazos-Rehg, P. A., Breslau, N., Hatsukami, D., Krauss, M. J., Spritznagel, E. L., Grucza, R. A., et al. (2014). Smoking cessation is associated with lower rates of mood/anxiety and alcohol use disorders. *Psychological Medicine, 14*(44), 2523–2535. http://dx.doi.org/10.1017/S0033291713003206.

Choquette, K., & Hesselbrock, M. (1987). Effects of retesting with the Beck and Zung depression scales in alcoholics. *Alcohol and Alcoholism, 22*(3), 277–283.

Cohen, S., & Lichtenstein, E. (1990). Perceived stress, quitting smoking, and smoking relapse. *Health Psychology, 9,* 466–478.

Cook, J. W., Piper, M. E., Leventhal, A. M., Schlam, T. R., Fiore, M. C., & Baker, T. B. (2015). Anhedonia as a component of the tobacco withdrawal syndrome. *Journal of Abnormal Psychology, 124,* 215–225.

Gilbert, D. G., Crauthers, D. M., Mooney, D. K., & McClernon, F. J. (1999). Effects of monetary contingencies on smoking relapse: influence of trait depression, personality, and habitual nicotine intake. *Experimental and Clinical Psychopharmacology, 7*(2), 1–8.

Gilbert, D. G., McClernon, F. J., Rabinovich, N., Plath, L. C., Jensen, R. A., & Meliska, C. J. (1998). Effects of smoking abstinence on mood and craving in men: influences of negative-affect-related personality traits, habitual nicotine intake, and repeated measurements. *Personality and Individual Differences, 25,* 399–423.

Gilbert, D. G., McClernon, F. J., Rabinovich, N. E., Plath, L. C., Masson, C. L., Anderson, A. E., et al. (2002). Mood disturbance fails to resolve across 31 days of cigarette abstinence in women. *Journal of Consulting and Clinical Psychology, 70,* 142–152.

Gilbert, D. G., Zuo, Y., Rabinovich, N. E., Riise, H., Needham, R., & Huggenvik, J. I. (2009). Neurotransmission-related genetic polymorphisms, negative affectivity traits, and gender predict tobacco abstinence symptoms across 44 days with and without nicotine patch. *Journal of Abnormal Psychology, 118,* 322–334.

Gross, J., & Stitzer, M. L. (1989). Nicotine replacement: ten-week effects on tobacco withdrawal symptoms. *Psychopharmacology, 98,* 334–341.

Hajek, P., Taylor, T., & McRobbie, H. (2010). The effect of stopping smoking on perceived stress levels. *Addiction, 105,* 1466–1471.

Hatzenbuehler, L., Parpal, M., & Matthews, L. (1983). Classifying college students as depressed or nondepressed using the Beck Depression Inventory: an empirical analysis. *Journal of Consulting and Clinical Psychology, 51*(3), 360–366.

Mathew, A. R., Robinson, J. D., Norton, P. J., Cinciripini, P. M., Brown, R. A., & Blalock, J. A. (2013). Affective trajectories before and after a quit attempt among smokers with current depressive disorders. *Nicotine and Tobacco Research, 15*, 1807–1815. http://dx.doi.org/10.1093/ntr/ntt036.

McCarthy, D. E., Piasecki, T. M., Fiore, M. C., & Baker, T. B. (2006). Life before and after quitting smoking: an electronic diary study. *Journal of Abnormal Psychology, 115*, 454–466.

McChargue, D. E., & Collins, F. L. (1998). Differentiating withdrawal patterns between smokers and smokeless tobacco users. *Experimental and Clinical Psychopharmacology, 6*, 205–208.

McKee, S. A., Maciejewski, P. K., Falba, T., & Mazure, C. M. (2003). Sex differences in the effects of stressful life events on changes in smoking status. *Addiction, 98*, 847–855.

McNair, L. M., Lorr, M., & Droppelman, L. F. (1971). *Manual for the profile of mood states*. San Diego, CA: Education and Industrial Testing Service.

Piasecki, T. M., Jorenby, D. E., Smith, S. S., Fiore, M. C., & Baker, T. B. (2003). Smoking withdrawal dynamics: I. Abstinence distress in lapsers and abstainers. *Journal of Abnormal Psychology, 112*(1), 3–13.

Piper, M., Piasecki, T., Federman, E., Bolt, D., Smith, S., Fiore, M., et al. (2004). A multiple motives approach to tobacco dependence: the Wisconsin Inventory of Smoking Dependence Motives (WISDM-68). *Journal of Consulting and Clinical Psychology, 72*(2), 139–154.

Reid, S., Towell, A. D., & Golding, J. F. (2000). Seasonality, social zeitgebers and mood variability in entrainment of mood: implications for seasonal affective disorder. *Journal of Affective Disorders, 59*(1), 47–54.

Rossouw, J. E., Anderson, G. L., Prentice, R. L., LaCroix, A. Z., Kooperberg, C., Stefanick, M. L., et al. (2002). Risks and benefits of estrogen plus progestin in healthy postmenopausal women: principal results from the Women's Health Initiative randomized controlled trial. *JAMA, 288*(3), 321–333.

Shahab, L., Gilchrist, G., Hagger-Johnson, G., Shankar, A., West, E., & West, R. (2015). Reciprocal associations between smoking cessation and depression in older smokers: findings from the English Longitudinal Study of Ageing. *The British Journal of Psychiatry: The Journal of Mental Science*. http://dx.doi.org/10.1192/bjp.bp.114.153494 published online May 21, 2015.

Sharpe, J. P., & Gilbert, D. G. (1998). Effects of repeated administration of the Beck Depression Inventory and other measures of negative mood states. *Personality and Individual Differences, 24*, 457–463.

Shiffman, S. (1982). Relapse following smoking cessation: a situational analysis. *Journal of Consulting and Clinical Psychology, 50*, 71–86.

Shiffman, S. M., & Jarvik, M. E. (1976). Smoking withdrawal symptoms in two weeks of abstinence. *Psychopharmacology, 50*, 35–39.

Shiffman, S., & Paty, J. (2006). Smoking patterns and dependence: contrasting chippers and heavy smokers. *Journal of Abnormal Psychology, 115*, 509–523. http://dx.doi.org/10.1037/0021-843X.115.3.509.

Shiffman, S., West, R. J., & Gilbert, D. G. (2004). Recommendation for the assessment of tobacco craving and withdrawal in smoking cessation trials. Work Group on the Assessment of Craving and Withdrawal in Clinical Trials. *Nicotine and Tobacco Research, 6*, 599–614.

Stampfer, M. J., & Colditz, G. A. (1991). Estrogen replacement therapy and coronary heart disease: a quantitative assessment of the epidemiologic evidence. *Preventive Medicine, 20*(1), 47–63.

Strong, D. R., Kahler, C. W., Leventhal, A. M., Abrantes, A. M., Lloyd-Richardson, E., Niaura, R., et al. (2009). Impact of bupropion and cognitive-behavioral treatment for depression on positive affect, negative affect, and urges to smoke during cessation treatment. *Nicotine and Tobacco Research, 11*, 1142–1153. http://dx.doi.org/10.1093/ntr/ntp111.

Taylor, G., McNeill, A., Girling, A., Farley, A., Lindson-Hawley, N., & Aveyard, P. (2014). Change in mental health after smoking cessation: systematic review and meta-analysis. *BMJ, 13*(348). http://dx.doi.org/10.1136/bmj.g1151 g1151.

Weinberger, A., Mazure, C., Morlett, A., & Mckee, S. (2013). Two decades of smoking cessation treatment research on smokers with depression: 1990–2010. *Nicotine and Tobacco Research, 15*(6), 1014–1031. http://dx.doi.org/10.1093/ntr/nts213.

Weinberger, A. H., Pilver, C. E., Desai, R. A., Mazure, C. M., & McKee, S. A. (2012a). The relationship of dysthymia, minor depression, and gender to changes in smoking for current and former smokers: longitudinal evaluation of the U.S. population. *Drug and Alcohol Dependence.* http://dx.doi.org/10.1016/j. drugalcdep.2012.06.028.

Weinberger, A. H., Pilver, C. E., Desai, R. A., Mazure, C. M., & McKee, S. A. (2012b). The relationship of major depressive disorder and gender to changes in smoking for current and former smokers: longitudinal evaluation in the US population. *Addiction, 107*(10), 1847–1856. http://dx.doi.org/10.1111/j.1360-0443.2012.03889.x.

Wewers, M. E. (1988). The role of postcessation factors in tobacco abstinence: stressful events and coping responses. *Addictive Behaviors, 13*, 297–302.

18

Neuroimaging Insights Into the Multifaceted Nature of the Nicotine Withdrawal Syndrome

M.T. Sutherland[1], J.A. Yanes[1], E.A. Stein[2]

[1]Florida International University, Miami, FL, United States;
[2]National Institute on Drug Abuse/NIH, Baltimore, MD, United States

INTRODUCTION

Five decades of antismoking public health initiatives have decreased the prevalence of adult cigarette smokers in the United States by nearly 60%,[1] yet cessation rates for those who currently smoke are notoriously low. Although 69% of smokers endorse a desire to quit and 52% try to do so within a given year, only ~6% achieve sustained cessation (CDC, 2011). This disparity between the desire to stop smoking and actual quit rates highlights the need for novel approaches to expedite the evolution of cessation interventions. The nicotine withdrawal syndrome (NWS) is a major barrier to quitting and includes hallmark features such as mood disturbances, cognitive impairment, and reward deficits (Cook et al., 2015; Hughes, 2007; Lerman et al., 2007). Nicotine delivery reverses abstinence-induced dysregulation of affective (Kassel, Stroud, & Paronis, 2003), cognitive (Heishman, Taylor, & Henningfield, 1994), and reward processes (Kenny & Markou, 2006), suggesting that early relapse occurs, in part, to relieve these symptoms, thereby perpetuating smoking via negative reinforcement (Baker, Piper, McCarthy, Majeskie, & Fiore, 2004). Although individual differences in specific symptomatology and time course complicate characterization of the NWS, most attempts to quit fail within the

---

[1]From 1965 to 2013, the percentage of US adults endorsing daily smoking decreased from 42.4% to 17.8%.

Negative Affective States and Cognitive Impairments in Nicotine Dependence
http://dx.doi.org/10.1016/B978-0-12-802574-1.00018-1

first week (Hughes, 1992), implicating early abstinence as a critical intervention period.

One principal reason for the currently low quit rates is the still-limited understanding of the fundamental neurobiological mechanisms underlying various facets of the NWS. Dissecting the NWS into its constituent symptoms and characterizing their respective neural substrates represent one principled approach to facilitate identification of interventional targets, apply strategies to fractionate smokers by core phenotypes, and ultimately implement personalized treatment (Lerman et al., 2007). The emergence of noninvasive neuroimaging techniques has opened a new vista to enhance understanding of the human brain mechanisms contributing to abstinence-induced emotional, cognitive, and reward alterations. While it has been traditionally assumed that dysregulation of these psychological processes is attributable to aberrant activity *within* circumscribed brain regions, an emergent view regarding such dysregulation as also a function of aberrant interactions *between* distributed regions (Koob & Volkow, 2010; Sutherland, McHugh, Pariyadath, & Stein, 2012). Whereas functional magnetic resonance imaging (fMRI) task paradigms have been essential for delineating the consequences of nicotine withdrawal *within* regions (eg, Lawrence, Ross, & Stein, 2002; Xu et al., 2005), an alternative, task-independent measure – resting-state fMRI (rs-fMRI) and the application of intrinsic functional connectivity (iFC) analyses – is proving useful for interrogating aberrant interactions *between* regions (eg, Hong et al., 2009; Sutherland et al., 2013a). Thus, a more complete and coherent framework to appreciate the multifaceted nature of the NWS is likely to emerge by considering both activity within (via task-based fMRI) and interactions between brain regions (via task-independent rs-fMRI).

Toward such a goal, this chapter highlights emerging evidence linking specific regional, circuit, and network-level functional brain alterations with three facets of the NWS: affective disturbances, cognitive impairment, and reward dysregulation. We first review evidence indicating that negative affect among abstinent smokers is linked with the amygdala and its interconnected circuitry, particularly the insula. Next, we consider findings suggesting that cognitive impairment during abstinence is linked with *decreased* activity in a network of regions associated with task-relevant information processing (ie, the executive control network) and *increased* activity in a network of regions associated with task-irrelevant information processing (ie, the default-mode network). Third, we highlight results linking dysregulated processing of nondrug-related reward with aberrant activity in the striatum. We conclude by listing some considerations for future neuroimaging research aimed at helping more people stop smoking.

AFFECTIVE DISTURBANCES

Abstinence-induced negative affect (eg, anxiety and irritability) is a major impediment to quitting (Baker et al., 2004; Hughes, 2007; Kassel et al., 2003), promotes relapse (Piper et al., 2011), and can be relieved by cigarette smoking or pharmacologic cessation aids (Patterson et al., 2009; Perkins, Karelitz, Conklin, Sayette, & Giedgowd, 2010). The role of the amygdala in affect-related processes is well established (LeDoux, 2003), and amygdala activity varies as a function of an individual's state or trait anxiety levels (Carlson, Greenberg, Rubin, & Mujica-Parodi, 2011; Stein, Simmons, Feinstein, & Paulus, 2007). The neural substrates mediating negative affect during drug abstinence are centered on the amygdala and its interconnected circuitry (Koob & Le Moal, 2005; Koob & Volkow, 2010). As such, aberrations in amygdala activity and/or its functional connectivity with other brain regions represent plausible targets for the alleviation of abstinence-induced negative affect and smoking cessation interventions.

Emerging evidence suggests that hyperactivity *within* the amygdala is critically linked with smoking abstinence (Mihov & Hurlemann, 2012). For example, in overnight deprived smokers, greater amygdala activity co-varies with increased self-reported withdrawal symptoms (Sutherland et al., 2013b) and tobacco craving (Wang et al., 2007). Specifically, using perfusion MRI, Wang et al. (2007) assessed regional cerebral blood flow (rCBF) and self-reported craving in smokers under abstinent (>12 h) and satiated conditions. Those authors noted that increased rCBF in the amygdala, among other regions (eg, insula), positively correlated with *abstinence-induced* urges to smoke. Similarly, increased amygdala responsivity to smoking-related images has also been linked with *cue-induced* urges to smoke (Chase, Eickhoff, Laird, & Hogarth, 2011; Smolka et al., 2006) and greater relapse susceptibility (Janes et al., 2010). These findings indicate that individual differences in abstinence- or cue-induced amygdala hyperactivity are associated with clinically relevant measures, including withdrawal symptoms, craving severity, and smoking relapse itself.

On the other hand, cigarette smoking or administration of pharmacologic cessation aids reduces amygdala activity among abstinent smokers (Franklin et al., 2011; Loughead et al., 2010, 2013; Rose et al., 2003; Sutherland et al., 2013b; Zubieta et al., 2005). For example, Zubieta et al. (2005) observed that smoking a nicotine-containing cigarette, compared with a denicotinized cigarette, decreased rCBF in the bilateral amygdala of overnight deprived smokers. Similarly, administration of varenicline, a nicotinic acetylcholine receptor (nAChR) partial agonist, decreased right amygdala rCBF at rest (Franklin et al., 2011) and bilateral amygdala activity during fMRI tasks probing working memory (Loughead et al., 2010) or emotional processing (Loughead et al., 2013; Sutherland et al., 2013b). Specifically, Sutherland et al. (2013b) examined the impact of varenicline and nicotine on behavioral performance and amygdala activity among overnight deprived smokers performing an emotional face matching task. When considering smokers as a single homogeneous group, varenicline and nicotine modulated reaction times (RTs) and heart rate, yet appeared to have no significant impact on amygdala activity. However, in an exploratory analysis that parsed participants into subgroups that either did or did not show robust RT improvements following drug administration, varenicline and nicotine modulated amygdala reactivity in only a subset of smokers. In the smoker subset showing RT improvements, varenicline and nicotine also decreased abstinence-induced amygdala hyperactivity (Fig. 18.1A). In contrast, drug administration did not modulate amygdala function in the smoker subset failing to show RT improvements, as that cohort displayed a more moderate level of amygdala reactivity during abstinence (ie, in the absence of drugs). Such outcomes suggest individual differences in abstinence- and drug-induced effects on amygdala activity. Collectively, these neuroimaging findings indicate that downregulation of activity *within* the amygdala may partly underlie the beneficial clinical effects of cessation interventions, particularly in those individuals experiencing greater negative affect (Piper et al., 2011) and/or those indicating smoking for anxiety reduction or relaxation (Rose et al., 2007).

Moving toward a circuit-level conceptualization, converging evidence also implicates functional interactions *between* the amygdala and insula as a neural substrate of negative affect in general and during nicotine withdrawal in particular. First, the amygdala and insula are anatomically (Baur, Hanggi, Langer, & Jancke, 2013) and functionally (Roy et al., 2009) connected, and co-occurring hyperactivity of these structures is often noted in task-based fMRI studies assessing pathological (Etkin & Wager, 2007) or experimentally induced anxiety (Carlson et al., 2011). Second, task-independent rs-fMRI studies have observed stronger amygdala–insula iFC in adolescent and adult anxiety disorders (Hamm et al., 2014; Sripada et al., 2012) where such hyperconnectivity positively correlates with anxiety severity (Roy et al., 2013). Third, using both rs-fMRI and diffusion tensor imaging, Baur et al. (2013) provided evidence relating individual differences in nonpathological state and trait anxiety with amygdala–insula functional and structural connectivity. Specifically, among healthy participants, increased amygdala–insula *functional connectivity* positively correlated with *state* anxiety levels, whereas increased *structural connectivity* (ie, tract-based axial diffusivity) within an amygdala–insula white matter pathway positively correlated with *trait* anxiety levels. With respect to nicotine, the insula is critically involved in the maintenance of addiction (Naqvi, Rudrauf, Damasio, & Bechara, 2007), and amygdala–insula interactions are hypothesized to play a role at multiple stages of the addiction cycle (Naqvi & Bechara, 2010; Sutherland et al., 2012). The insula is thought to monitor abstinence-induced bodily sensations and, in turn,

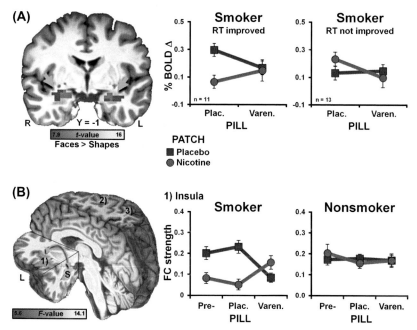

FIGURE 18.1 Amygdala hyperactivity and amygdala–insula hyperconnectivity may contribute to abstinence-induced negative affect in some smokers. (A) Amygdala reactivity (assessed by comparing responses to emotional faces versus geometric shapes) was differentially modulated by transdermal nicotine (PATCH) and orally administered varenicline (PILL) across smoker subgroups. Pharmacologically induced decreases in amygdala reactivity were only observed in the smoker subgroup showing elevated amygdala reactivity during abstinence (Smoker, RT improved) *(Figure adapted from Sutherland, M.T., Carroll, A.J., Salmeron, B.J., Ross, T.J., Hong, L.E., & Stein, E.A. (2013b). Individual differences in amygdala reactivity following nicotinic receptor stimulation in abstinent smokers. NeuroImage, 66, 585–593.).* (B) Amygdala–insula functional coupling during abstinence was reduced by nicotine and varenicline. Sutherland et al. (2013a) identified brain regions whose iFC strength with a left amygdala seed (S, green) was altered by pharmacologic cessation aids. The graphs depict drug-induced changes in iFC between the amygdala and insula (1). Drug-induced changes were observed only among smokers, suggesting that aberrations in amygdala–insula iFC are linked with the state of nicotine withdrawal. Similar drug-induced changes in iFC were observed in precentral (2) and superior parietal (3) regions *(Figure adapted from Sutherland, M.T., Carroll, A.J., Salmeron, B.J., Ross, T.J., Hong, L.E., & Stein E.A. (2013a). Down-regulation of amygdala and insula functional circuits by varenicline and nicotine in abstinent cigarette smokers. Biological Psychiatry, 74, 538–546.).* **Pre-**: before beginning study pill administration; **Plac.**: during placebo pill administration; **Varen.**: during active varenicline pill administration.

modify affective and motivational processes through interactions with other brain regions, including the amygdala and ventromedial prefrontal cortex (vmPFC). Providing experimental support for this perspective, Sutherland et al. (2013a) observed that hyperconnectivity in an amygdala–insula functional circuit was downregulated by nicotine and varenicline among abstinent smokers (Fig. 18.1B). Such decreased amygdala–insula functional coupling may also contribute, in part, to the amelioration of withdrawal-related negative affect.

The studies above highlight the utility of examining activity *within* the amygdala and interactions *between* the amygdala and other regions to provide insight into the neurobiological underpinnings of abstinence-induced negative affect. Taken together, emerging results suggest that amygdala hyperactivity and amygdala–insula hyperconnectivity may underlie aspects of the NWS. As such, the normalization of amygdala activity and/or its functional interactions with other regions may represent neurobiological intervention targets, particularly for those smokers experiencing greater degrees of affective disturbances during the early stages of quitting.

COGNITIVE IMPAIRMENTS

Withdrawal-related cognitive impairments (eg, in working memory and sustained attention) are increasingly recognized as barriers to quitting (Ashare, Falcone, & Lerman, 2014; Lerman et al., 2007), are predictive of relapse (Patterson et al., 2010), and can be ameliorated by nicotine or other pharmacologic cessation aids (Heishman et al., 1994; Patterson et al., 2009). Neuroimaging efforts have converged on the view that efficient goal-directed cognition is facilitated by activation of some brain regions and yet deactivation of others (Anticevic et al., 2012; Dosenbach et al., 2006; Hu, Chen, Gu, & Yang, 2013). Those brain regions showing task-induced *activation* are grouped into two ensembles, the so-called executive control network (ECN) and the salience network (SN; Seeley et al., 2007). In contrast, those regions consistently showing task-induced *deactivation* are collectively referred to as the default-mode network (DMN; Raichle et al., 2001). Whereas the ECN, composed of lateral prefrontal and parietal regions, is generally associated with externally oriented information processing and attention, the DMN, anchored by the posterior cingulate cortex (PCC), medial PFC, and parahippocampal gyri, is generally associated with internally oriented mental processes (eg, mind-wandering). The SN, consisting of the bilateral insulae and anterior cingulate cortex (ACC), is thought to facilitate processing of the currently most homeostatically relevant stimuli arising from internal or external sources by toggling the relative activity between the competitively interacting ECN and DMN (Fox et al., 2005; Uddin, 2015). Accordingly, failures to adequately deactivate DMN regions or activate ECN regions (Eichele et al., 2008; Hu et al., 2013) as well as maladaptive interactions between nodes of these networks (Kelly, Uddin, Biswal, Castellanos, & Milham, 2008) represent putative mechanisms contributing to suboptimal goal-directed cognition in healthy individuals and across neuropsychiatric disorders (Anticevic et al., 2012; Menon, 2011). As such, alterations in within-network activity (ie, ECN activation and DMN deactivation) and/or between-network interactions (eg, SN–DMN and ECN–DMN) represent emergent targets to relieve abstinence-induced cognitive impairments (Hahn et al., 2007; Lerman et al., 2014; Sutherland, Liang, Yang, & Stein, 2015b; Sutherland et al., 2012).

Task-based fMRI evidence suggests that decreased activation of regions *within* the ECN as well as reduced deactivation of regions *within* the DMN are linked to abstinence-induced cognitive impairments. Such performance deficits and associated alterations in regional activations and deactivations have been characterized by assessing smokers under abstinent (24–72 h) versus satiated conditions with a working memory (n-back) task (Ashare et al., 2013; Falcone et al., 2013; Loughead et al., 2009, 2015). These studies have consistently observed abstinence-induced *decreases* in working memory-related *activations* within the bilateral dorsolateral PFC (dlPFC) and medial frontal–cingulate gyrus (MF/CG) (core ECN and SN nodes), particularly during the most difficult task conditions (ie, 2- and 3-back). In addition, these studies have also observed *reduced* working memory-related *suppression* of PCC and vmPFC function (core DMN nodes). Indicative of individual differences and clinical relevance, these abstinence-induced alterations in activation and deactivation patterns vary as a function of age (Falcone et al., 2013) or genetics (Ashare et al., 2013; Loughead et al., 2009), are linked with task performance (Falcone et al., 2013; Loughead et al., 2010), and, critically, can predict future smoking relapse (Loughead et al., 2015). Whereas decreased ECN activations may be indicative of a failure to recruit sufficient task-relevant cognitive resources (Ashare et al., 2014), decreased DMN deactivations suggest the persistent engagement of task-irrelevant information processing (Anticevic et al., 2012). Collectively, these findings suggest that decreased activity in ECN regions and/or reduced suppression of DMN regions contribute, in part, to cognitive impairments that perpetuate smoking and/or precipitate relapse among some individuals.

In contrast to abstinence-induced effects, nAChR agonist administration increases activity within some ECN regions and suppresses activity within some DMN regions. Specifically, Loughead et al. (2010) observed that varenicline administration relative to placebo increased working memory-related activations in the bilateral dlPFC and MF/CG while also enhancing deactivations in the PCC, vmPFC, and parahippocampus among 3-day abstinent smokers. Nicotine-induced increases of ECN activation and/or enhancements of DMN suppression similarly have been observed during smoking abstinence when considering alternative cognitive domains such as visuospatial attention (Hahn et al., 2007), sustained attention (Beaver et al., 2011; Lawrence et al., 2002), selective and divided attention, and stimulus detection (Hahn et al., 2009). For example, nicotine replacement to minimally deprived smokers (~3 h) enhanced deactivation of core DMN nodes (eg, PCC and medial PFC) during a spatial attention task, such that greater deactivations correlated with better performance (Hahn et al., 2007). Nicotine-induced increased activity within the lateral parietal and prefrontal cortices, thalamus, and dorsal ACC also accompanies behavioral improvements among deprived smokers performing sustained-attention tasks (Beaver et al., 2011; Lawrence et al., 2002). These findings link nicotine-induced modulation of brain activation and deactivation patterns with task performance.

As such, multiple recent narrative reviews have advocated that *one* mechanism by which nAChR agonists exert pro-cognitive effects is by decreasing activity within some task-irrelevant regions (eg, DMN nodes) while increasing activity within some task-related regions (eg, ECN nodes) (Bentley, Driver, & Dolan, 2011; Jasinska, Zorick, Brody, & Stein, 2014; Newhouse, Potter, Dumas, & Thiel, 2011; Sutherland et al., 2012, 2015b). Providing quantitative support for this network-level perspective, Sutherland et al. (2015a) conducted a meta-analysis of pharmacologic fMRI studies assessing the impact of nAChR agonists on human brain function across diverse task paradigms. That meta-analysis identified convergent nAChR drug-induced activity *decreases* in multiple regions, including the PCC, vmPFC, and right parahippocampus (DMN nodes), among other regions (Fig. 18.2A). In contrast, convergent drug-induced activity *increases* were observed in lateral frontoparietal cortices and the MF–CG (ECN nodes), as well as in the thalamus and cuneus. Collectively, these findings suggest that nAChR agonist-induced decreases in DMN activity and increases in ECN activity may contribute to negative reinforcement mechanisms perpetuating smoking as well as the efficacy of cessation interventions, particularly among those individuals experiencing greater withdrawal-related cognitive impairments (Patterson et al., 2010).

Moving beyond the impact of abstinence *within* regions, aberrations in the functional interactions *between* core nodes of the DMN, ECN, and SN may also contribute to facets of the NWS. For example, Sutherland et al. (2012, 2015b) synthesized a network-level heuristic framework proposing that the insula (a core SN node) tracks withdrawal-induced physiological sensations during abstinence and, in turn, orients attention toward this homeostatically salient internal state by biasing activity toward the DMN and away from the ECN. Whereas the SN in general and insula in particular register physiological signals associated with homeostatic disequilibrium (Craig, 2010), enhanced SN–DMN interactions are theorized to modify affective, cognitive, and motivational processes prompting the organism to respond to and alleviate such a state (Naqvi & Bechara, 2010; Sutherland et al., 2012). As such, one hypothesis is that early abstinence is associated with elevated functional coupling between the insula (SN) and DMN, which may contribute to withdrawal symptoms, tobacco craving, and/

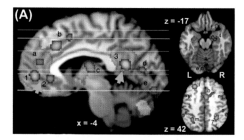
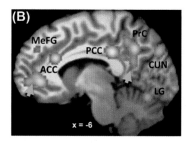
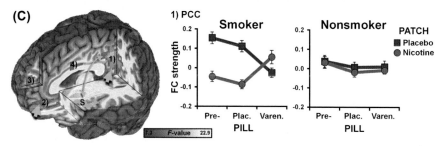

FIGURE 18.2 Alterations in within-network activity and/or between-network interactions may contribute to cognitive impairment in some smokers. (A) Meta-analysis results showing regions of convergent decreases (blue) and increases (red) in activity following nAChR agonist administration. Across pharmacologic fMRI studies, nAChR agonist administration decreased activity in DMN regions (ie, vmPFC, PCC, and parahippocampus) and increased activity in regions overlapping the ECN (ie, lateral prefrontal and parietal regions). Templates of the DMN (purple transparency) and ECN (yellow transparency) are overlaid for visualization of overlap with these large-scale networks. *(Figure adapted from Sutherland, M.T., Ray, K.L., Riedel, M.C., Yanes, J.A., Stein, E.A., & Laird, A.R. (2015a). Neurobiological impact of nicotinic acetylcholine receptor agonists: an activation likelihood estimation meta-analysis of pharmacologic neuroimaging studies. Biological Psychiatry, 78, 711-720).* (B) Meta-analysis results showing regions of convergent activity increases in response to smoking-related images. In contrast to nAChR-agonist-induced *decreases* (shown in A, blue), smoking cues *increase* activity, notably in the vmPFC and PCC *(Figure adapted from Engelmann, J.M., Versace, F., Robinson, J.D., Minnix, J.A., Lam, C.Y., Cui, Y., et al. (2012). Neural substrates of smoking cue reactivity: a meta-analysis of fMRI studies. NeuroImage, 60, 252–262.).* (C) Insula–DMN functional coupling during smoking abstinence was reduced by nicotine and varenicline. Sutherland et al. (2013a) identified brain regions whose iFC strength with a functionally defined left insula seed (S, green) was altered by pharmacologic cessation aids. The graphs depict drug-induced changes in iFC between the insula and PCC (1). Similar drug-induced changes in iFC were observed in the vmPFC (2), dorsomedial PFC (3), and midcingulate (4) *(Figure adapted from Sutherland, M.T., Carroll, A.J., Salmeron, B.J., Ross, T.J., Hong, L.E., & Stein E.A. (2013a). Down-regulation of amygdala and insula functional circuits by varenicline and nicotine in abstinent cigarette smokers. Biological Psychiatry, 74, 538–546.).*

or cognitive impairments. Indirectly supporting this hypothesis, elevated activity within the insula and core DMN nodes (eg, PCC and vmPFC) has been observed during smoking abstinence and following drug cue presentation (Fig. 18.2B) (Engelmann et al., 2012; Wang et al., 2007). Providing more direct support, Sutherland et al. (2013a) conducted a pharmacologic rs-fMRI study examining the impact of nicotine and varenicline on the insula's iFC with other brain regions among overnight deprived smokers. They observed that iFC between the insula and core DMN nodes (ie, PCC, vmPFC, and parahippocampus) was downregulated by nicotine and varenicline (Fig. 18.2C). Furthermore, elevated functional coupling between the insula and regions showing nAChR drug-induced iFC changes (ie, PCC, medial PFC, and parahippocampus) was also positively correlated with greater self-reported withdrawal symptoms and slower RT in a subsequent face-matching task. Further relating similar between-network interactions with clinically relevant measures, abstinence-induced increases in SN–DMN and decreases in SN–ECN coupling have been linked with elevated tobacco craving, suboptimal task performance, and reduced deactivation of the vmPFC and PCC during a subsequent working memory task (Lerman et al., 2014). Lastly, Weiland, Sabbineni, Calhoun, Welsh, and Hutchison (2015) observed reduced iFC strength within the DMN and ECN of smokers compared with nonsmokers, which may also relate to cognitive impairments. These initial rs-fMRI findings suggest that alterations in the functional interactions between the SN, DMN, and ECN may underlie aspects of the NWS, given that such interactions are modulated by pharmacologic cessation aids, associated with self-reported withdrawal symptoms, and predictive of alterations in the brain and behavior (Lerman et al., 2014; Sutherland et al., 2013a).

Taken together, the studies discussed in this section highlight the utility of examining alterations of within-network activity and between-network interactions to provide insight into the neural substrates mediating abstinence-induced cognitive impairments. Specifically, a failure to suppress task-irrelevant DMN activity, an inability to recruit sufficient task-related ECN activity, increased insula–DMN, and/or decreased SN–ECN functional interactions currently represent plausible network-level mechanisms contributing to suboptimal goal-directed cognition. As such, a desirable characteristic of efficacious smoking cessation interventions may be the normalization of activity within and/or between these large-scale networks, particularly among those smokers experiencing more pronounced cognitive disturbances during the initial stages of quitting.

REWARD DYSREGULATION

Abstinence-induced anhedonia is an increasingly recognized, clinically significant facet of the NWS (Dawkins, Powell, West, Powell, & Pickering, 2006; Leventhal, Ramsey, Brown, LaChance, & Kahler, 2008) that is relieved by nicotine administration (Cook et al., 2015; Dawkins et al., 2006) and predictive of relapse (Cook et al., 2015). The role of the mesocorticolimbic dopaminergic (DAergic) circuitry in processing reinforcing stimuli, including those associated with drugs of abuse, is well established (Delgado, 2007; Haber & Knutson 2010; Wise, 2009). Dysregulated reward processing associated with an extended drug use history is mediated by neuroadaptations (and/or preexisting vulnerabilities) in the striatum that may manifest as both hypersensitivity to drug-related reward and concomitant hyposensitivity to nondrug-related reward (Berridge & Robinson 1998; Der-Avakian & Markou 2012; Koob & Le Moal 2005). Consistent with hypersensitivity to drug-related reward, increased activity in the striatum, medial PFC, and ACC is commonly observed following drug cue presentation to individuals addicted to various substances (Chase et al., 2011; Engelmann et al., 2012). Conversely, diminished striatal activity during the processing of nondrug-related reward (eg, money) has been observed, although not consistently, among drug addicts (Balodis & Potenza, 2015). As such, functional aberrations in the striatum or, more generally, the DAergic circuitry represent plausible neurobiological targets to reduce reward deficits in some smokers.

Accumulating evidence suggests a link between smoking and hypoactivity *within* the striatum to nondrug-related rewards, which may be further exacerbated by smoking deprivation. For example, *nondeprived* smokers compared with nonsmokers or occasional smokers show reduced activity in the caudate, putamen, and ventral striatum when processing aspects of monetary reward such as gain magnitude and temporal proximity of reward (Buhler et al., 2010; Kobiella et al., 2014; Luo, Ainslie, Giragosian, & Monterosso, 2011; Martin-Soelch, Missimer, Leenders, & Schultz, 2003). Specifically, using a delay discounting task, Luo et al. (2011) observed hypoactivity within the ventral and dorsal striatum among nondeprived smokers, particularly during anticipation of delayed rewards. Similar "trait-like" deficits in striatal functioning also have been noted in the context of a nondrug reward-learning (juice) paradigm (Rose et al., 2012). Such functional alterations, perhaps independent of "state-like" effects (ie, withdrawal), are corroborated by evidence of structural alterations in smokers' DAergic circuitry. In contrast to reductions in prefrontal (eg, vmPFC) cortical thickness and volume (Fritz et al., 2014; Kuhn, Schubert, & Gallinat, 2010), larger dorsal striatal (putamen) volumes have been observed among smokers (Franklin et al., 2014) where volumetric increases positively correlate with greater lifetime cigarette use (Das, Cherbuin, Anstey, Sachdev, & Easteal, 2012) and smoking urges (Janes, Park, Farmer, & Chakravarty, 2015).

Striatal hypoactivity also has been observed, although not consistently (Addicott et al., 2012), when assessing *minimally deprived and abstinent* smokers in monetary reward-processing tasks (Fedota et al., 2015; Peters et al., 2011; Rose et al., 2013; Sweitzer et al., 2014; Wilson et al., 2014). Providing compelling evidence that abstinence modulates reward processing, Sweitzer et al. (2014) conducted an fMRI study among smokers assessing neural responses to both monetary and smoking rewards under abstinent (24h) and satiated conditions. In a double dissociation fashion, they observed that anticipatory-related striatal (ie, bilateral caudate) and medial PFC activity during abstinence (versus satiety) was *attenuated* for *monetary* rewards, and yet *elevated* for *smoking* rewards. Critically, individual differences in such abstinence-induced striatal hypoactivity to monetary reward is predictive of poorer outcomes regarding withdrawal symptoms, craving severity (Sweitzer et al., 2014), and ability to refrain from smoking (Wilson et al., 2014). Speaking to the complex interactions of neurobiological, pharmacological, and psychological processes, striatal activity is also modulated by expectations about smoking opportunity (Wilson, Sayette, Delgado, & Fiez, 2008) or beliefs about having been administered nicotine (Gu et al., 2015). Given that the magnitude of striatal (and vmPFC) activity likely indexes the relative value of stimuli (Bartra, McGuire, & Kable, 2013), these initial findings suggest that greater hypoactivity within the DAergic circuitry may contribute to more pronounced reward dysregulation during abstinence.

On the other hand, nAChR agonists enhance reward processing in the DAergic circuitry when considering animal models (Kenny & Markou 2006; Spiller et al., 2009) or deprived smokers (Fedota et al., 2015; Rose et al., 2013; Sweitzer et al., 2014). In rats, both nicotine and varenicline administration reduce intracranial self-stimulation thresholds, suggesting that nAChR agonists acutely render the DAergic circuitry hypersensitive to nondrug-related rewards (Kenny & Markou 2006; Spiller et al., 2009). In humans, nicotine increases caudate activity to monetary reward-predicting cues among overnight-abstinent smokers (Sweitzer et al., 2014) and to reward magnitude-predicting cues among minimally deprived smokers (vs. nonsmokers) (Rose et al., 2013). Recently, Fedota et al. (2015) conducted a pharmacologic fMRI study that probed the impact of nicotine and varenicline on the neural correlates of anticipatory reward processing among overnight abstinent smokers (>12h) and nonsmokers. They observed hypoactivation among abstinent smokers (vs. nonsmokers) in multiple striatal regions (ie, the nucleus accumbens, caudate, and putamen) and the ACC in response to monetary reward-predicting cues. Critically, nicotine administration to smokers augmented reward-related hypoactivity in the putamen (Fig. 18.3) and ACC, thereby "normalizing" activity levels to those observed among nonsmokers under placebo conditions. Suggesting that such nicotine-induced effects are not constrained to individuals with an extended smoking history, nicotine administration also increased reward-related activity in the putamen and ACC of nonsmokers. These neuroimaging findings are consistent with nicotine-induced enhancement of neural activity in response to nondrug-related

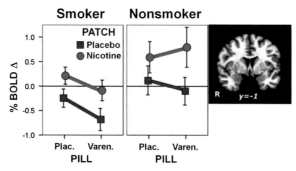

FIGURE 18.3 Abstinence-induced striatal hypoactivity to nondrug-related reward is reduced by nicotine administration. Fedota et al. (2015) observed that nicotine administration (blue) relative to placebo (red) increased responses to reward-predicting cues in the putamen among both smokers and nonsmokers. Critically, administration of nicotine to abstinent smokers appeared to "normalize" putamen activity to the level observed among nonsmokers assessed under placebo patch conditions. *Figure adapted from Fedota, J.R., Sutherland, M.T., Salmeron, B.J., Ross, T.J., Hong, L.E., & Stein, E.A. (2015). Reward anticipation is differentially modulated by varenicline and nicotine in smokers.* Neuropsychopharmacology, 40, 2038-46.

rewards and also suggest that abstinence-related reductions in such activity may contribute to the continuation and/or resumption of cigarette smoking among some individuals.

The studies discussed here highlight the utility of examining activity within the DAergic circuitry in general and the striatum in particular to provide insight into smoking-related reward dysregulation. Taken together, these results suggest that striatal hypoactivity in response to properties of nondrug-related rewards is linked with an extended smoking history, which may be exacerbated by nicotine withdrawal and ameliorated to some degree by nAChR agonists. As such, normalization of DAergic hypoactivity to nondrug-related rewards may represent a neurobiological intervention target for those experiencing anhedonia when trying to quit.

SUMMARY AND FUTURE CONSIDERATIONS

We considered three aspects of the NWS and the putative regional, circuit, and network-level brain alterations associated with each. Specifically, we highlighted neuroimaging evidence linking: (1) negative affect with amygdala hyperactivity and amygdala–insula hyperconnectivity; (2) cognitive impairment with alterations of within-network activity (ie, DMN deactivations and ECN activations) and between-network connectivity (eg, insula–DMN iFC); and (3) reward dysregulation with hypoactivity in the striatum and DAergic circuitry to nondrug-related rewards.

Emphasizing clinical relevance, more profound brain alterations associated with these three aspects of the NWS typically indicate poorer outcomes on smoking-related behaviors, including relapse. Enhanced insight into the multifaceted nature of the NWS and the contributing neurobiology may expedite identification of brain targets for improved interventions, strategies to parse smokers by core phenotypes, and the ability to tailor treatment for a given individual.

Despite progress toward these ultimate goals, several considerations remain for future research aimed at helping more people stop smoking. One consideration will be to further characterize individual differences regarding the impact of abstinence on specific withdrawal symptoms and neurobiological substrates. Such research emphasizing the perspective that individuals continue to smoke for different reasons, or combinations of reasons, may facilitate the evolution of multiple interventions each with a precise neurobiological target. Such an armamentarium of options could allow for personalized treatment employing the best single strategy or combination of strategies most likely to prove efficacious. Another consideration will be to characterize the potential overlap between the neurobiology associated with cigarette smoking and other psychiatric conditions. Given that smokers are typically overrepresented among individuals diagnosed with a psychiatric disorder, it is plausible that some individuals smoke to reduce clinical symptoms such as anxiety (eg, anxiety disorders), cognitive impairments (eg, attention deficit hyperactivity disorder and schizophrenia), and/or reward-processing deficits (eg, depression). Improved understanding of nAChR agonist-induced effects on these psychological and neurobiological processes will be relevant not only to smoking cessation applications, but also to treatment strategies for other psychiatric conditions. Finally, another consideration will be to delineate the degree to which alterations in brain function and structure are antecedents or consequences (or both) of smoking (eg, Peters et al., 2011). Identification of neuroimaging-based antecedents of smoking could be employed to target prevention efforts toward those individuals most in need. The neuroimaging findings discussed in this chapter suggest the intriguing possibility that continued research further characterizing alterations in dissociable neurocircuitry could one day be leveraged to identify optimal individualized cessation interventions, account for smoking comorbidity among psychiatric conditions, and yield brain-based predictors of future drug use.

Acknowledgments

The authors are supported by a grant from the National Institute on Drug Abuse (NIDA, MTS: K01-DA037819) and the NIDA Intramural Research Program (EAS). The content is solely the responsibility of the authors and does not necessarily represent the official views of the National Institutes of Health.

References

Addicott, M. A., Baranger, D. A., Kozink, R. V., Smoski, M. J., Dichter, G. S., & McClernon, F. J. (2012). Smoking withdrawal is associated with increases in brain activation during decision making and reward anticipation: a preliminary study. *Psychopharmacology (Berlin)*, *219*, 563–573.

Anticevic, A., Cole, M. W., Murray, J. D., Corlett, P. R., Wang, X. J., & Krystal, J. H. (2012). The role of default network deactivation in cognition and disease. *Trends in Cognitive Sciences*, *16*, 584–592.

Ashare, R. L., Falcone, M., & Lerman, C. (2014). Cognitive function during nicotine withdrawal: implications for nicotine dependence treatment. *Neuropharmacology, 76*(Pt B), 581–591.

Ashare, R. L., Valdez, J. N., Ruparel, K., Albelda, B., Hopson, R. D., Keefe, J. R., et al. (2013). Association of abstinence-induced alterations in working memory function and COMT genotype in smokers. *Psychopharmacology (Berlin)*, *230*, 653–662.

Baker, T. B., Piper, M. E., McCarthy, D. E., Majeskie, M. R., & Fiore, M. C. (2004). Addiction motivation reformulated: an affective processing model of negative reinforcement. *Psychological Reviews, 111*, 33–51.

Balodis, I. M., & Potenza, M. N. (2015). Anticipatory reward processing in addicted populations: a focus on the monetary incentive delay task. *Biological Psychiatry, 77*, 434–444.

Bartra, O., McGuire, J. T., & Kable, J. W. (2013). The valuation system: a coordinate-based meta-analysis of BOLD fMRI experiments examining neural correlates of subjective value. *NeuroImage, 76*, 412–427.

Baur, V., Hanggi, J., Langer, N., & Jancke, L. (2013). Resting-state functional and structural connectivity within an insula-amygdala route specifically index state and trait anxiety. *Biological Psychiatry, 73*, 85–92.

Beaver, J. D., Long, C. J., Cole, D. M., Durcan, M. J., Bannon, L. C., Mishra, R. G., et al. (2011). The Effects of nicotine replacement on cognitive brain activity during smoking withdrawal studied with simultaneous fMRI/EEG. *Neuropsychopharm, 36*, 1792–1800.

Bentley, P., Driver, J., & Dolan, R. J. (2011). Cholinergic modulation of cognition: insights from human pharmacological functional neuroimaging. *Progress in Neurobiology, 94*, 360–388.

Berridge, K. C., & Robinson, T. E. (1998). What is the role of dopamine in reward: hedonic impact, reward learning, or incentive salience? *Brain Research Brain Research Reviews, 28*, 309–369.

Buhler, M., Vollstadt-Klein, S., Kobiella, A., Budde, H., Reed, L. J., Braus, D. F., et al. (2010). Nicotine dependence is characterized by disordered reward processing in a network driving motivation. *Biological Psychiatry, 67*, 745–752.

Carlson, J. M., Greenberg, T., Rubin, D., & Mujica-Parodi, L. R. (2011). Feeling anxious: anticipatory amygdalo-insular response predicts the feeling of anxious anticipation. *Social Cognitive and Affective Neuroscience, 6*, 74–81.

CDC. (2011). Quitting smoking among adults: United States, 2001-2010. *Morbidity and Mortality Weekly Report, 60*, 1513–1519.

Chase, H. W., Eickhoff, S. B., Laird, A. R., & Hogarth, L. (2011). The neural basis of drug stimulus processing and craving: an activation likelihood estimation meta-analysis. *Biological Psychiatry, 70*, 785–793.

Cook, J. W., Piper, M. E., Leventhal, A. M., Schlam, T. R., Fiore, M. C., & Baker, T. B. (2015). Anhedonia as a component of the tobacco withdrawal syndrome. *Journal of Abnormal Psychology, 124*, 215–225.

Craig, A. D. (2010). The sentient self. *Brain Structure & Function, 214*, 563–577.

Das, D., Cherbuin, N., Anstey, K. J., Sachdev, P. S., & Easteal, S. (2012). Lifetime cigarette smoking is associated with striatal volume measures. *Addiction Biology, 17*, 817–825.

Dawkins, L., Powell, J. H., West, R., Powell, J., & Pickering, A. (2006). A double-blind placebo controlled experimental study of nicotine: I–effects on incentive motivation. *Psychopharmacology (Berlin), 189*, 355–367.

Delgado, M. R. (2007). Reward-related responses in the human striatum. *Annals of the New York Academy of Sciences, 1104*, 70–88.

Der-Avakian, A., & Markou, A. (2012). The neurobiology of anhedonia and other reward-related deficits. *Trends in Neurosciences, 35*, 68 77.

Dosenbach, N. U. F., Visscher, K. M., Palmer, E. D., Miezin, F. M., Wenger, K. K., Kang, H. S. C.S.C., et al. (2006). A core system for the implementation of task sets. *Neuron, 50*, 799–812.

Eichele, T., Debener, S., Calhoun, V. D., Specht, K., Engel, A. K., Hugdahl, K., et al. (2008). Prediction of human errors by maladaptive changes in event-related brain networks. *PNAS, 105*, 6173–6178.

Engelmann, J. M., Versace, F., Robinson, J. D., Minnix, J. A., Lam, C. Y., Cui, Y., et al. (2012). Neural substrates of smoking cue reactivity: a meta-analysis of fMRI studies. *NeuroImage, 60*, 252–262.

Etkin, A., & Wager, T. D. (2007). Functional neuroimaging of anxiety: a meta-analysis of emotional processing in PTSD, social anxiety disorder, and specific phobia. *The American Journal of Psychiatry, 164*, 1476–1488.

Falcone, M., Wileyto, E. P., Ruparel, K., Gerraty, R. T., Laprate, L., Detre, J. A., et al. (2013). Age-related differences in working memory deficits during nicotine withdrawal. *Addiction Biology, 19*, 907–917.

Fedota, J. R., Sutherland, M. T., Salmeron, B. J., Ross, T. J., Hong, L. E., & Stein, E. A. (2015). Reward anticipation is differentially modulated by varenicline and nicotine in smokers. *Neuropsychopharmacology, 40*, 2038–2046.

Fox, M. D., Snyder, A. Z., Vincent, J. L., Corbetta, M., Van Essen, D. C., & Raichle, M. E. (2005). The human brain is intrinsically organized into dynamic, anticorrelated functional networks. *PNAS, 102*, 9673–9678.

Franklin, T., Wang, Z., Suh, J. J., Hazan, R., Cruz, J., Li, Y., et al. (2011). Effects of varenicline on smoking cue-triggered neural and craving responses. *Archives of General Psychiatry, 68*, 516–526.

Franklin, T. R., Wetherill, R. R., Jagannathan, K., Johnson, B., Mumma, J., Hager, N., et al. (2014). The effects of chronic cigarette smoking on gray matter volume: influence of sex. *PLoS One, 9*, e104102.

Fritz, H. C., Wittfeld, K., Schmidt, C. O., Domin, M., Grabe, H. J., Hegenscheid, K., et al. (2014). Current smoking and reduced gray matter volume-a voxel-based morphometry study. *Neuropsychopharmacology, 39*, 2594–2600.

Gu, X., Lohrenz, T., Salas, R., Baldwin, P. R., Soltani, A., Kirk, U., et al. (2015). Belief about nicotine selectively modulates value and reward prediction error signals in smokers. *Proceedings of National Academy of Sciences of the United States of America, 112*, 2539–2544.

Haber, S. N., & Knutson, B. (2010). The reward circuit: linking primate anatomy and human imaging. *Neuropsychopharmacology, 35*, 4–26.

Hahn, B., Ross, T. J., Wolkenberg, F. A., Shakleya, D. M., Huestis, M. A., & Stein, E. A. (2009). Performance effects of nicotine during selective attention, divided attention, and simple stimulus detection: an fMRI study. *Cerebral Cortex, 19*, 1990–2000.

Hahn, B., Ross, T. J., Yang, Y., Kim, I., Huestis, M. A., & Stein, E. A. (2007). Nicotine enhances visuospatial attention by deactivating areas of the resting brain default network. *The Journal of Neuroscience, 27*, 3477–3489.

Hamm, L. L., Jacobs, R. H., Johnson, M. W., Fitzgerald, D. A., Fitzgerald, K. D., Langenecker, S. A., et al. (2014). Aberrant amygdala functional connectivity at rest in pediatric anxiety disorders. *Biology of Mood & Anxiety Disorders, 4*, 15.

Heishman, S. J., Taylor, R. C., & Henningfield, J. E. (1994). Nicotine and smoking: a review of effects on human performance. *Experimental and Clinical Psychopharmacology, 2*, 345–395.

Hong, L. E., Gu, H., Yang, Y., Ross, T. J., Salmeron, B. J., Buchholz, B., et al. (2009). Association of nicotine addiction and Nicotine's actions with separate cingulate cortex functional circuits. *Archives in General Psychiatry, 66*, 431–441.

Hu, Y., Chen, X., Gu, H., & Yang, Y. (2013). Resting-state glutamate and GABA concentrations predict task-induced deactivation in the default mode network. *The Journal of Neuroscience, 33*, 18566–18573.

Hughes, J. R. (1992). Tobacco withdrawal in self-quitters. *Journal of Consulting and Clinical Psychology, 60*, 689–697.

Hughes, J. R. (2007). Effects of abstinence from tobacco: valid symptoms and time course. *Nicotine & Tobacco Research, 9*, 315–327.

Janes, A. C., Park, M. T., Farmer, S., & Chakravarty, M. M. (2015). Striatal morphology is associated with tobacco cigarette craving. *Neuropsychopharmacology, 40*, 406–411.

Janes, A. C., Pizzagalli, D. A., Richardt, S., Frederick, B. D., Chuzi, S., Pachas, G., et al. (2010). Brain reactivity to smoking cues prior to smoking cessation predicts ability to maintain tobacco abstinence. *Biological Psychiatry, 67*, 722–729.

Jasinska, A. J., Zorick, T., Brody, A. L., & Stein, E. A. (2014). Dual role of nicotine in addiction and cognition: a review of neuroimaging studies in humans. *Neuropharmacology, 84*, 111–122.

Kassel, J. D., Stroud, L. R., & Paronis, C. A. (2003). Smoking, stress, and negative affect: correlation, causation, and context across stages of smoking. *Psychological Bulletin, 129*, 270–304.

Kelly, A. M. C., Uddin, L. Q., Biswal, B. B., Castellanos, F. X., & Milham, M. P. (2008). Competition between functional brain networks mediates behavioral variability. *NeuroImage, 39*, 527–537.

Kenny, P. J., & Markou, A. (2006). Nicotine self-administration acutely activates brain reward systems and induces a long-lasting increase in reward sensitivity. *Neuropsychopharmacology, 31*, 1203–1211.

Kobiella, A., Ripke, S., Kroemer, N. B., Vollmert, C., Vollstadt-Klein, S., Ulshofer, D. E., et al. (2014). Acute and chronic nicotine effects on behaviour and brain activation during intertemporal decision making. *Addiction Biology, 19*, 918–930.

Koob, G. F., & Le Moal, M. (2005). Plasticity of reward neurocircuitry and the 'dark side' of drug addiction. *Nature Neuroscience, 8*, 1442–1444.

Koob, G. F., & Volkow, N. D. (2010). Neurocircuitry of addiction. *Neuropsychopharmacology, 35*, 217–238.

Kuhn, S., Schubert, F., & Gallinat, J. (2010). Reduced thickness of medial orbitofrontal cortex in smokers. *Biological Psychiatry, 68*, 1061–1065.

Lawrence, N. S., Ross, T. J., & Stein, E. A. (2002). Cognitive mechanisms of nicotine on visual attention. *Neuron, 36*, 539–548.

LeDoux, J. (2003). The emotional brain, fear, and the amygdala. *Cellular and Molecular Neurobiology, 23*, 727–738.

Lerman, C., Gu, H., Loughead, J., Ruparel, K., Yang, Y., & Stein, E. A. (2014). Large-scale brain network coupling predicts acute nicotine abstinence effects on craving and cognitive function. *JAMA Psychiatry, 71*, 523–530.

Lerman, C., LeSage, M. G., Perkins, K. A., O'Malley, S. S., Siegel, S. J., Benowitz, N. L., et al. (2007). Translational research in medication development for nicotine dependence. *Nature Reviews Drug Discovery, 6*, 746–762.

Leventhal, A. M., Ramsey, S. E., Brown, R. A., LaChance, H. R., & Kahler, C. W. (2008). Dimensions of depressive symptoms and smoking cessation. *Nicotine & Tobacco Research, 10*, 507–517.

Loughead, J., Ray, R., Wileyto, E. P., Ruparel, K., O'Donnell, G. P., Senecal, N., et al. (2013). Brain activity and emotional processing in smokers treated with varenicline. *Addiction Biology, 18*, 732–738.

Loughead, J., Ray, R., Wileyto, E. P., Ruparel, K., Sanborn, P., Siegel, S., et al. (2010). Effects of the alpha 4 beta 2 partial agonist varenicline on brain activity and working memory in abstinent smokers. *Biological Psychiatry, 67*, 715–721.

Loughead, J., Wileyto, E. P., Ruparel, K., Falcone, M., Hopson, R., Gur, R., et al. (2015). Working memory-related neural activity predicts future smoking relapse. *Neuropsychopharmacology, 40,* 1311–1320.

Loughead, J., Wileyto, E. P., Valdez, J. N., Sanborn, P., Tang, K., Strasser, A. A., et al. (2009). Effect of abstinence challenge on brain function and cognition in smokers differs by COMT genotype. *Molecular Psychiatry, 14,* 820–826.

Luo, S., Ainslie, G., Giragosian, L., & Monterosso, J. R. (2011). Striatal hyposensitivity to delayed rewards among cigarette smokers. *Drug and Alcohol Dependence, 116,* 18–23.

Martin-Soelch, C., Missimer, J., Leenders, K. L., & Schultz, W. (2003). Neural activity related to the processing of increasing monetary reward in smokers and nonsmokers. *The European Journal of Neuroscience, 18,* 680–688.

Menon, V. (2011). Large-scale brain networks and psychopathology: a unifying triple network model. *Trends in Cognitive Sciences, 15,* 483–506.

Mihov, M., & Hurlemann, R. (2012). Altered amygdala function in nicotine addiction: insights from human neuroimaging studies. *Neuropsychologia, 50,* 1719–1729.

Naqvi, N. H., & Bechara, A. (2010). The insula and drug addiction: an interoceptive view of pleasure, urges, and decision-making. *Brain Structure & Function, 214,* 435–450.

Naqvi, N. H., Rudrauf, D., Damasio, H., & Bechara, A. (2007). Damage to the insula disrupts addiction to cigarette smoking. *Science, 315,* 531–534.

Newhouse, P. A., Potter, A. S., Dumas, J. A., & Thiel, C. M. (2011). Functional brain imaging of nicotinic effects on higher cognitive processes. *Biochemical Pharmacology, 82,* 943–951.

Patterson, F., Jepson, C., Loughead, J., Perkins, K., Strasser, A. A., Siegel, S., et al. (2010). Working memory deficits predict short-term smoking resumption following brief abstinence. *Drug and Alcohol Dependence, 106,* 61–64.

Patterson, F., Jepson, C., Strasser, A. A., Loughead, J., Perkins, K. A., Gur, R. C., et al. (2009). Varenicline improves mood and cognition during smoking abstinence. *Biological Psychiatry, 65,* 144–149.

Perkins, K. A., Karelitz, J. L., Conklin, C. A., Sayette, M. A., & Giedgowd, G. E. (2010). Acute negative affect relief from smoking depends on the affect situation and measure but not on nicotine. *Biological Psychiatry, 67,* 707–714.

Peters, J., Bromberg, U., Schneider, S., Brassen, S., Menz, M., Banaschewski, T., et al. (2011). Lower ventral striatal activation during reward anticipation in adolescent smokers. *The American Journal of Psychiatry, 168,* 540–549.

Piper, M. E., Schlam, T. R., Cook, J. W., Sheffer, M. A., Smith, S. S., Loh, W. Y., et al. (2011). Tobacco withdrawal components and their relations with cessation success. *Psychopharmacology (Berlin), 216,* 569–578.

Raichle, M. E., MacLeod, A. M., Snyder, A. Z., Powers, W. J., Gusnard, D. A., & Shulman, G. L. (2001). A default mode of brain function. *PNAS, 98,* 676–682.

Rose, J. E., Behm, F. M., Salley, A. N., Bates, J. E., Coleman, R. E., Hawk, T. C., et al. (2007). Regional brain activity correlates of nicotine dependence. *Neuropsychopharmacology, 32,* 2441–2452.

Rose, J. E., Behm, F. M., Westman, E. C., Mathew, R. J., London, E. D., Hawk, T. C., et al. (2003). PET studies of the influences of nicotine on neural systems in cigarette smokers. *American Journal of Psychiatry, 160,* 323–333.

Rose, E. J., Ross, T. J., Salmeron, B. J., Lee, M., Shakleya, D. M., Huestis, M., et al. (2012). Chronic exposure to nicotine is associated with reduced reward-related activity in the striatum but not the midbrain. *Biological Psychiatry, 71,* 206–213.

Rose, E. J., Ross, T. J., Salmeron, B. J., Lee, M., Shakleya, D. M., Huestis, M. A., et al. (2013). Acute nicotine differentially impacts anticipatory valence- and magnitude-related striatal activity. *Biological Psychiatry, 73,* 280–288.

Roy, A. K., Fudge, J. L., Kelly, C., Perry, J. S., Daniele, T., Carlisi, C., et al. (2013). Intrinsic functional connectivity of amygdala-based networks in adolescent generalized anxiety disorder. *Journal of the American Academy of Child and Adolescent Psychiatry, 52,* 290–299, e2.

Roy, A. K., Shehzad, Z., Margulies, D. S., Kelly, A. M. C., Uddin, L. Q., Gotimer, K., et al. (2009). Functional connectivity of the human amygdala using resting state fMRI. *Neuro-Image, 45*, 614–626.

Seeley, W. W., Menon, V., Schatzberg, A. F., Keller, J., Glover, G. H., Kenna, H., et al. (2007). Dissociable intrinsic connectivity networks for salience processing and executive control. *The Journal of Neuroscience, 27*, 2349–2356.

Smolka, M. N., Buhler, M., Klein, S., Zimmermann, U., Mann, K., Heinz, A., et al. (2006). Severity of nicotine dependence modulates cue-induced brain activity in regions involved in motor preparation and imagery. *Psychopharmacology (Berlin), 184*, 577–588.

Spiller, K., Xi, Z. X., Li, X., Ashby, C. R., Jr., Callahan, P. M., Tehim, A., et al. (2009). Varenicline attenuates nicotine-enhanced brain-stimulation reward by activation of alpha4beta2 nicotinic receptors in rats. *Neuropharmacology, 57*, 60–66.

Sripada, R. K., King, A. P., Garfinkel, S. N., Wang, X., Sripada, C. S., Welsh, R. C., et al. (2012). Altered resting-state amygdala functional connectivity in men with posttraumatic stress disorder. Journal of psychiatry & neuroscience. *Journal of Psychiatry & Neuroscience, 37*, 241–249.

Stein, M. B., Simmons, A. N., Feinstein, J. S., & Paulus, M. P. (2007). Increased amygdala and insula activation during emotion processing in anxiety-prone subjects. *The American Journal of Psychiatry, 164*, 318–327.

Sutherland, M. T., Carroll, A. J., Salmeron, B. J., Ross, T. J., Hong, L. E., & Stein, E. A. (2013a). Down-regulation of amygdala and insula functional circuits by varenicline and nicotine in abstinent cigarette smokers. *Biological Psychiatry, 74*, 538–546.

Sutherland, M. T., Carroll, A. J., Salmeron, B. J., Ross, T. J., Hong, L. E., & Stein, E. A. (2013b). Individual differences in amygdala reactivity following nicotinic receptor stimulation in abstinent smokers. *NeuroImage, 66*, 585–593.

Sutherland, M. T., Ray, K. L., Riedel, M. C., Yanes, J. A., Stein, E. A., & Laird, A. R. (2015a). Neurobiological impact of nicotinic acetylcholine receptor agonists: an activation likelihood estimation meta-analysis of pharmacologic neuroimaging studies. *Biological Psychiatry, 78*, 711–720.

Sutherland, M. T., Liang, X., Yang, Y., & Stein, E. A. (2015b). Beyond functional localization: advancing the understanding of addiction-related processes by examining brain connectivity. In S. Wilson (Ed.), *The Wiley-Blackwell handbook on the neuroscience of addiction*. Hoboken, NJ: Wiley-Blackwell. ISBN13: 9781118472248.

Sutherland, M. T., McHugh, M. J., Pariyadath, V., & Stein, E. A. (2012). Resting state functional connectivity in addiction: lessons learned and a road ahead. *NeuroImage, 62*, 2281–2295.

Sweitzer, M. M., Geier, C. F., Joel, D. L., McGurrin, P., Denlinger, R. L., Forbes, E. E., et al. (2014). Dissociated effects of anticipating smoking versus monetary reward in the caudate as a function of smoking abstinence. *Biological Psychiatry, 76*, 681–688.

Uddin, L. Q. (2015). Salience processing and insular cortical function and dysfunction. *Nature Reviews Neuroscience, 16*, 55–61.

Wang, Z., Faith, M., Patterson, F., Tang, K., Kerrin, K., Wileyto, E. P., et al. (2007). Neural substrates of abstinence-induced cigarette cravings in chronic smokers. *The Journal of Neuroscience, 27*, 14035–14040.

Weiland, B. J., Sabbineni, A., Calhoun, V. D., Welsh, R. C., & Hutchison, K. E. (2015). Reduced executive and default network functional connectivity in cigarette smokers. *Human Brain Mapping, 36*, 872–882.

Wilson, S. J., Delgado, M. R., McKee, S. A., Grigson, P. S., MacLean, R. R., Nichols, T. T., et al. (2014). Weak ventral striatal responses to monetary outcomes predict an unwillingness to resist cigarette smoking. *Cognitive Affective & Behavioral Neuroscience, 14*, 1196–1207.

Wilson, S. J., Sayette, M. A., Delgado, M. R., & Fiez, J. A. (2008). Effect of smoking opportunity on responses to monetary gain and loss in the caudate nucleus. *Journal of Abnormal Psychology, 117*, 428–434.

Wise, R. A. (2009). Roles for nigrostriatal–not just mesocorticolimbic–dopamine in reward and addiction. *Trends in Neurosciences, 32,* 517–524.

Xu, J., Mendrek, A., Cohen, M. S., Monterosso, J., Rodriguez, P., Simon, S. L., et al. (2005). Brain activity in cigarette smokers performing a working memory task: effect of smoking abstinence. *Biological Psychiatry, 58,* 143–150.

Zubieta, J. K., Heitzeg, M. M., Xu, Y. J., Koeppe, R. A., Ni, L. S., Guthrie, S., et al. (2005). Regional cerebral blood flow responses to smoking in tobacco smokers after overnight abstinence. *American Journal of Psychiatry, 162,* 567–577.

Index

Printed in the United States
By Bookmasters